MEDICINE IN AN AGE OF COMMERCE AND EMPIRE

Medicine in an Age of Commerce and Empire

Britain and its Tropical Colonies, 1660–1830

MARK HARRISON

OXFORD
UNIVERSITY PRESS

OXFORD
UNIVERSITY PRESS

Great Clarendon Street, Oxford OX2 6DP

Oxford University Press is a department of the University of Oxford.
It furthers the University's objective of excellence in research, scholarship,
and education by publishing worldwide in

Oxford New York

Auckland Cape Town Dar es Salaam Hong Kong Karachi
Kuala Lumpur Madrid Melbourne Mexico City Nairobi
New Delhi Shanghai Taipei Toronto

With offices in

Argentina Austria Brazil Chile Czech Republic France Greece
Guatemala Hungary Italy Japan Poland Portugal Singapore
South Korea Switzerland Thailand Turkey Ukraine Vietnam

Oxford is a registered trade mark of Oxford University Press
in the UK and in certain other countries

Published in the United States
by Oxford University Press Inc., New York

First published 2010

British Library Cataloguing in Publication Data
Data available

Library of Congress Cataloging in Publication Data
Data available

Typeset by SPI Publisher Services, Pondicherry, India
Printed in Great Britain
on acid-free paper by
MPG Books Group, Bodmin and King's Lynn

ISBN 978–0–19–957773–6

1 3 5 7 9 10 8 6 4 2

Acknowledgements

I began this book as a Wellcome Trust Senior Research Fellow at the University of Oxford in 2000 and it was envisaged as part of a five-year research project which encompassed various aspects of medicine in Britain's tropical colonies. After less than a year, I was fortunate enough to become Director of the Wellcome Unit for the History of Medicine at the University of Oxford and with the kind permission of the Wellcome Trust was able to turn my fellowship grant into a project grant. This enabled me to employ a Research Assistant who subsequently became my co-worker on the project: Dr Pratik Chakrabarti. The amount of source material relating to our subject was so vast, and the themes so numerous, that we soon decided to split the project in two. Pratik concentrated more on the immediate locality of medical practice in the East and West Indies, while I focused on the intellectual history of medicine and the dissemination of ideas and practices around the British Empire. This book represents the fruits of that labour, and first and foremost I wish to thank the Wellcome Trust for making it possible and Pratik for sharing ideas and information. Although this book has been written wholly by me, it should be seen as the outcome of our stimulating discussions over the best part of a decade.

Since beginning this project, I have received assistance from many people and have benefited greatly from the feedback and suggestions of numerous scholars. Particular thanks go to Professor Christopher Lawrence who reviewed the entire manuscript for Oxford University Press and made many useful suggestions. I also owe a special debt of gratitude to Loreen Salleh who read the entire manuscript and helped improve both its readability and accuracy. I have also been fortunate enough to discuss many of my ideas with students taking my advanced paper class in 'Disease, Medicine and Colonialism before 1900' and my further subject in 'Medicine, Empire and Improvement'. My former research students have been a source of inspiration, too, and I should particularly like to thank Dr Erica Charters, Dr Sanchari Dutta, Dr Ryan Johnson, Dr Kate Kelly, Dr Amna Khalid, Dr Saurabh Mishra, Dr Ishita Pande, and Dr Samiksha Sehrawat who all helped in various ways. Carol Brady and Belinda Michaelides at the Wellcome Unit have been great colleagues and have helped me enormously in many ways. I also owe a great debt to Dr Sloan Mahone who took over as Acting Director during my absence on research leave and to Dr Sabine Clarke for taking on some of my teaching in my absence.

In addition, I should like to thank the following people for making valuable suggestions and sharing ideas over the years, many of which found their way into this book in some form: Professor Warwick Anderson, Professor David Arnold, Dr Guy Attewell, Dr Sanjoy Bhattacharya, Professor Laurence Brockliss,

Dr Karen Brown, Professor W. F. Bynum, Professor Hal Cook, Professor Pietro Corsi, Professor Suranjan Das, Professor Geoffrey Hudson, Dr Margaret Jones, Dr Deep Kanta Lahiri Choudhury, Professor Deepak Kumar, Professor Harry Marks, Dr Projit Bihari Mukharji, Dr Biswamoy Pati, Professor Douglas Peers, Dr Margaret Pelling, Professor John Pickstone, the late Professor Roy Porter, Dr Anna Marie Roos Benton, Professor Nicolaas Rupke, Mr Norris Saakwa-Mante, Professor Paul Slack, Dr Kavita Sivaramakrishnan, Dr Simon Smith, Professor Sanjay Subrahmanyam, Dr Helen Sweet, Dr Louella Vaughan, Professor John Harley Warner, Dr David Washbrook, and Professor Michael Worboys.

I also wish to thank the Wellcome Library for granting me permission to publish images from their iconographic collection; Routledge publishers for permission to publish parts of two chapters that I wrote in edited works: Biswamoy Pati and Mark Harrison (eds.), *The Social History of Health and Medicine in Colonial India* (2009) and Hormoz Ebrahimnejad (ed.), *The Development of Modern Medicine in Non-Western Countries* (2009).

Most of all I would like to thank Loreen and my family for their love and forbearance.

Contents

List of illustrations ix
List of abbreviations x

Introduction 1

PART I MEDICINE AS NATURAL HISTORY

1. Climate, fever, and medicine before 1700 29
2. 'Accidents of the air': Sydenham and Boerhaave in the tropics 47
3. The medicine of warm climates 64
4. Pathology, physiology, and race 89

PART II TROPICAL THERAPEUTICS

1. Inflamed bodies 121
2. Exotics and antiseptics 130
3. Empire of experiment 146
4. A therapeutic revolution 172

PART III ILLS OF EMPIRE

1. Invalids and entrepreneurs 211
2. The voyager returns 227
3. Albion's coast is sick 237
4. The prospect of invasion 254

Conclusion 287
Bibliography 293
Index 339

List of illustrations

I.1	James Lind, MD, Wellcome Images, V003579	73
I.2	Benjamin Moseley, MD, Wellcome Images, V0004144	82
II.1	Sir James McGrigor, Wellcome Images, M0019464	170
II.2	Robert Jackson, Wellcome Images, V0026607	182
III.1	James Johnson, MD, Wellcome Images, M0013753	232
III.2	Thomas Trotter, MD, Wellcome Images, M0017886	239
III.3	The Torrid Zone, Wellcome Images, L0010581	259

All of the above images are reproduced with the kind permission of the Wellcome Library, London.

List of abbreviations

APAC	Asia, Pacific and African Collections
BCA	Birmingham City Archives
BL	British Library
BRO	Bristol Record Office
DRO	Derbyshire Record Office
GCRO	Gloucestershire County Record Office
MPP	Madras Public Proceedings
MSA	Maharashtra State Archives
NMM	National Maritime Museum
RAMC	Royal Army Medical Corps (Muniment Collection)
RCPE	Royal College of Physicians and Surgeons of Edinburgh
SCA	Sheffield City Archives
SCUG	Special Collections, University of Glasgow Library
U of N	University of Newcastle
WBSA	West Bengal State Archives
WL	Wellcome Library

Introduction

ORIENTATION

In 1817, Dr Charles Maclean celebrated 'the great independence of mind' which prevailed among medical practitioners in the East and West Indies and the 'increased freedom of investigation' and 'discriminating practice' which resulted from it.[1] As a former Army and East India Company surgeon, it is hardly surprising that Maclean should have elevated their medical achievements, but he went further than that. In his view, practitioners working in the colonies had been in the vanguard of reform, having contributed much to the 'immense changes' which had transformed British medicine in the early years of the century.[2] The colonies afforded medical practitioners opportunities unparalleled in Great Britain, while exposing them to an enormous variety of disease environments and medical traditions. In these exotic locations – in the hospitals of the Army, Navy, and the East India Company – an empirical and experimental approach to medicine rapidly developed, providing a counterpoint to what Maclean saw as hide-bound tradition and ignorance at home. His views were partisan and idiosyncratic but by no means unique. By the 1820s, practitioners with experience in the colonies were widely regarded as authorities in several areas of British medicine. And yet, the legacy of British colonial expansion to medicine remains obscure. Most historians of medicine see the winds of change blowing from revolutionary Paris. It is said that the techniques developed in Parisian hospitals from the mid-1790s marked a sharp break from the 'neo-classical' notions of disease and medicine which, in modified form, continued to dominate elite medical practice. In these hospitals for the poor, patients were subject to examination as never before and new instruments, such as the stethoscope, were developed for this purpose. Patients who died in the hospitals were also routinely dissected, allowing post-mortem signs of disease to be correlated with symptoms observed among the living. The traditional idea that disease was an imbalance of the humours was thus displaced as its progress was traced through organs and tissues.[3]

[1] Maclean, *Results of an Investigation*, vol. 1, xiii.

[2] Maclean, *Evils of Quarantine Laws*, vii.

[3] Bynum, *Science and the Practice of Medicine*. Classic detailed studies include: Ackerknecht, *Medicine at the Paris Hospital*; Foucault, *The Birth of the Clinic*. See also Pickstone, 'Ways of

According to the conventional narrative, young men from Europe and North America flocked to France after the peace of 1815 to learn these new techniques and avail themselves of opportunities for dissection and post-mortem examination.[4] Through them, and reformist journals in their own countries, medical practitioners learned of the pathological investigations of Xavier Bichat and the diagnostic techniques of physicians such as R. T. Laennec. These and other important changes associated with hospital-based practice – meticulous record-keeping, 'clinical trials', and so forth – became the hallmarks of medical modernity in the early part of the nineteenth century.[5] In Britain, their principal exponents tended to be surgeon-apothecaries who established journals and institutions to rival those of the London-based medical elite – the Royal College of Physicians – which they portrayed as effete and backward-looking.[6]

In reality, the situation was not so clear-cut. Recent scholarship has shown that some established practitioners, including fellows of the Royal College, had also embraced 'science' and were seeking to modernize their profession in similar ways to surgeons and apothecaries.[7] A strong case has also been made for a cumulative process of change rather than a sudden rupture in medical theory and practice in the 1790s.[8] According to some historians, the 'clinico-pathological' approach which became the hallmark of Paris medicine had its origins in the infirmaries of Edinburgh and Vienna and the anatomy schools of London.[9] Morbid anatomy and therapeutic experimentation was also undertaken in charitable infirmaries well before the 1790s,[10] while in philosophical circles it was fashionable for the deceased to leave their bodies for dissection.[11]

One ought not to exaggerate the extent to which medicine was consumed by the fever of reform in the decades prior to the French Revolution, but a significant and growing number of medical practitioners were seeking an empirical basis for medicine: one that would replace what they regarded as sterile

Knowing: Towards a Historical Sociology of Science, Technology and Medicine'; idem, *Ways of Knowing: A New History of Science, Technology and Medicine.* For the characteristics of 'Paris medicine', see La Berge and Hannaway, 'Paris Medicine'.

[4] Maulitz, 'Channel Crossing'; Bonner, *Becoming a Physician*; Warner, *Against the Spirit of System.*

[5] For the classical definition of 'hospital medicine', see Jewson, 'The Disappearance of the Sick Man from Medical Cosmology'.

[6] Warner, 'The Idea of Science in English Medical Education'.

[7] Vaughan, '"Improvements in the Art of Healing"'.

[8] For Scotland, see: Risse, *Hospital Life in Enlightenment Scotland*; Lawrence, 'Medicine as Culture'; Rosner, *Medical Education in the Age of Improvement.* For England, see Lawrence, *Charitable Knowledge*; Vaughan, '"Improvements in the Art of Healing"'. For France, see Brockliss, 'Before the Clinic'; Gelfand, *Professionalizing Modern Medicine.*

[9] Keel, *L'Avenement de la Médicine Clinique Moderne en Europe*; idem, 'Was Anatomical and Tissue Pathology a Product of the Paris Clinical School or Not?'

[10] Fissell, *Patients, Power, and the Poor,* 140–4; 162–70, 199–200; Lawrence, *Charitable Knowledge.*

[11] Bateson, '"Open a Few Corpses"'.

speculation and system-building. The rise of consumer society may have played a part in these changes by opening up new opportunities for medical practice and the sale of medical goods.[12] Incessant warfare was an equally important stimulus to innovation; the relatively disciplined environment of military and naval hospitals, and their increasing separation from civil society, provided considerable scope for clinical observation, dissection, and therapeutic trials.[13] But what little we know about these institutions is based on documents and publications relating to hospitals in the British Isles. We possess very few accounts of military and naval medicine in other parts of the British Empire or, indeed, of the few civilian establishments that then existed beyond Britain's shores.[14]

This book provides the first detailed account of how commercial and imperial expansion affected British medicine at a time of momentous change. It argues that imperial wars, territorial annexation, and colonial trade made a deep impact upon British medicine, providing a major stimulus to the emergence of what was known as 'rational' or 'scientific' medicine. Although it largely endorses Charles Maclean's claims about the innovative nature of medicine in the East and West Indies, the book stresses the importance of seeing these developments as part of a general drive for medical, social, and political reform. But, however we choose to frame it, the medical world of the 'long eighteenth century' was one in which the tropical colonies loomed large, on account of either the work undertaken there or the prominent role which practitioners with colonial experience came to play in professional institutions and debates. On reflection, it is difficult to see how it could have been otherwise. Many practitioners cut their teeth in the Army, the Navy, and the East India Company, and the knowledge and values which they imbibed early in their careers had a lasting effect. Through their increasingly numerous publications, they began to communicate their ideas to medical practitioners who had never ventured beyond Britain and to alter the theory and practice of medicine at home. Their first-hand knowledge was vital to a nation that depended increasingly on its commercial links with distant parts of the globe and which was engaged in regular and expansive conflicts with its imperial rivals. Thousands of soldiers, sailors, and merchants perished annually, creating a massive drain on the imperial exchequer. Thousands more returned from the colonies as invalids suffering from fevers, hepatitis, and chronic dysentery,

[12] See Jenner and Wallis (eds.), *Medicine and the Market*; Porter, 'Health Care in Enlightenment England'; Bynum and Porter (eds.), *Medical Fringe and Medical Orthodoxy*; Jewson, 'Medical Knowledge and the Patronage System'.

[13] See Tröhler, 'Quantification in British Medicine and Surgery'; Bynum, 'Cullen and the Study of Fevers in Britain'; Charters, 'Disease, War and the Imperial State'; Alsop, 'Warfare and the Creation of British Imperial Medicine'; Kelly, '"Not Surgeons Alone, but Medical Officers"'. For France, see Brockliss and Jones, *The Medical World of Early Modern France*, 689–717; Vess, *Medical Revolution in France*, 23–39.

[14] One of the few exceptions is Sheridan, *Doctors and Slaves*.

and with them came the prospect of diseases from abroad; of the appearance of deadly new maladies on Britain's shores.

Colonial exploration and settlement stimulated the development of British medicine in numerous ways. Direct access to the bazaars of Asia and the opportunity to prospect for remedies unknown in Europe opened up new therapeutic possibilities. Interaction on various levels with Indian and African medical practitioners provided insights into how such remedies might be employed and, in some cases, suggested alternative uses for drugs already familiar in the West. Encounters with climates very different from those of Europe also encouraged medical practitioners to investigate the relationship between environment and disease, developing the neo-Hippocratic approach adumbrated by the English physician Thomas Sydenham at the end of the seventeenth century. In the military and naval hospitals of India and the Caribbean, and in some other settlements, British practitioners had the opportunity to match meteorological observations with those made at the bedside and, increasingly, with the results of pathological investigations conducted post-mortem. In Britain, the supply of bodies for dissection was still severely restricted, but there were no such constraints in the colonies, where cadavers were plentiful. Practitioners working in colonial hospitals were thus able to compare post-mortem findings with the symptoms of disease in living patients, giving rise to a system of medicine not unlike that which later developed in revolutionary Paris.

As the medical establishments of India and the West Indies grew in size, which they did rapidly during the eighteenth century, they became more confident in articulating their distinctiveness. Most tropical practitioners prided themselves on their independence and cared little for traditional sources of professional authority. By the end of the eighteenth century, there was a recognizable genre of medical literature which catered specifically for those venturing to warm climates.[15] It placed great emphasis upon observation and urged its readers to reject much of what they had learned in Britain. It did not steer clear of, and even courted, controversy. Colonial medicine was pre-eminently a medicine of place: an epitome of knowledge distilled from a variety of learned traditions, folklore, and scientific investigation.[16] But those who had served in the colonies regarded their experience as relevant to the problems faced by medical practitioners in Britain, too, and they firmly believed that their skills and knowledge were transferable. Indeed, they were usually in regular contact with like-minded colleagues at home and saw their work as an extension of a broader project of professional reform which drew inspiration from numerous sources.

[15] Arnold (ed.), *Warm Climates and Western Medicine*; idem, 'India's Place in the Tropical World'.

[16] Livingstone, *Putting Science in its Place*.

Through their contacts in Britain, and just as often on their own account, practitioners who gained experience in the colonies began subtly but profoundly to alter the nature of British medicine. Pathological observations made in military and naval hospitals began to inform new theories of disease causation and courses of treatment. Former colonial practitioners also found employment in fever hospitals and other medical institutions recently established in Britain. There, they applied insights derived from their experience overseas, and in many cases continued to use the treatments they had employed in colonial hospitals, albeit in modified form. By the end of the eighteenth century, experience in colonial outposts could offer distinct advantages. Those who had the benefit of working overseas were regarded as authorities on ailments such as fevers, dysentery, and hepatitis; some even ascended to the pinnacle of their profession. Theirs was not the usual route – via Oxbridge and the Royal College of Physicians – but service in the Army, Navy, or East India Company gave them access to powerful patrons. By this means, as well as through intellectual distinction, they sometimes became royal physicians and dispensers of patronage in their own right.

While most of the surgeons and physicians discussed in this book were employed in military or naval establishments, a minority practised privately. In India, there were a handful of physicians with patrons in the higher echelons of the Company and the Indian royal courts. In the West Indies, a larger number worked as doctors in sugar plantations, where they occupied an often difficult position between masters and slaves. While some exhibited sympathy for the plight of slaves and had relationships with them, they were part of a new disciplinary regime that aimed to protect their employers' human capital and improve its productivity.[17] In some cases, these slave doctors were at odds with military and naval surgeons stationed in the Caribbean, some of whom became prominent abolitionists. But in many respects, this diverse body of practitioners shared a similar outlook. Most stressed the importance of experience and believed that different forms of treatment were necessary for diseases in the tropics, whether they appeared among Europeans, Africans, or Indians. Traditional therapeutic regimes seemed powerless to halt the course of diseases which all too often ended fatally.

The medical establishments of the Company, the Army, and the Navy tended to attract individuals of an independent cast of mind. It is true that many were lured by the prospect of a relatively stable income or simply by a yearning for adventure. But a significant minority relished the opportunity of working overseas in order to further their medical and philosophical interests and to boost their career prospects at home. Many of these were men from the so-called 'Celtic Fringe' or were religious Dissenters blocked from entry into the universities of

[17] Thomas, 'Doctoring Ideology'; Sheridan, *Doctors and Slaves.*

Oxford and Cambridge.[18] Most had received some instruction in the sciences and in medicine at Scottish universities – principally Edinburgh – and/or the London hospitals and anatomy schools. These institutions afforded the most advanced medical instruction then available in Europe and, to some extent, shaped approaches to the theory and practice of medicine overseas. The fact that most colonial practitioners had not attended the ancient English universities also barred them from entering the inner sanctum of professional power: the Royal College of Physicians of London.[19] Although some became licentiates of the College and practised medicine in the metropolis after returning from the colonies, very few became fellows with full voting rights. As such, they tended to operate in different circles and looked for advancement by other means. Some were also engaged in bitter disputes with the College over its exclusiveness, as well as the medical traditions and practices that its fellows defended.

The theme of dissent – religious, political, and professional – runs strongly throughout this book. There were intellectual affinities between the outlook of many practitioners working overseas and their religious views, which were often combined with a radical outlook on political matters. They tended to see the reform of medicine and society as inseparable. Many were linked to circles of Dissenting natural philosophers and medical practitioners in Britain, and with the members of these societies they shared an experimental attitude towards knowledge and a desire that it be applied to useful works. For the most part, they saw the British Empire as a force for good, replacing superstition and despotism with an enlightened, if autocratic, regime. And when it looked as if that regime might itself become tyrannical, they were among the first to criticize it. Some former colonial practitioners played an active role in British politics, too, railing against reactionary government and campaigning for better conditions for the poor and the oppressed.

In the colonies, British practitioners with Dissenting convictions found others of like mind. In India, there were close links between members of the Company's medical establishment and Pietist and Moravian missionaries from northern Europe. They shared similar outlooks on a range of professional and religious

[18] The term 'Dissenter' is normally taken to mean a member of a Protestant church or sect which had refused to accept the 1660–2 re-imposition of episcopacy and the Prayer Book of the Church of England, e.g. Baptists, Presbyterians, Unitarians, and Quakers. Unable to find advancement through the Church or the legal profession, Dissenters were especially drawn to medicine and the natural sciences, as well as commerce. These were all activities which seemed to be progressive in social and even in political terms, as well as providing a means of personal advancement. See Raistrick, *Quakers in Science and Industry*; Thackray, 'Natural Knowledge in Cultural Context'.

[19] At present we have a detailed study of the Army only, and that from the late eighteenth century; however, a mass of impressionistic evidence suggests that what was true of the Army was true of the Navy also, and that the recruitment trends at the end of the century were similar to those earlier on. See Ackroyd et al., *Advancing with the Army*; Brockliss et al., *Nelson's Surgeon*. The significance of Scottish and Irish recruitment is also evident in the case of the medical services of the East India Company; see Crawford, *Roll of the Indian Medical Service*.

matters, their work often being shaped by a rejection of what they saw as corrupt, modern lifestyles. This sometimes manifested itself in a desire to use their medical knowledge for human betterment and sometimes in Romantic celebrations of Indian nature and culture.[20] As in the West Indies, Dissenters highlighted some of the contradictions of colonialism and attempted, albeit unsuccessfully, to resolve them. The connection established between like-minded practitioners in India also opened up important intellectual networks, enabling a free flow of information and ideas about medicine and natural philosophy between British medical establishments in India and centres of learning in northern Europe. Similar connections existed between some of the British practitioners in the West Indies and fellow radicals in North America. A network of reform-minded medical men thus stretched from the Indian to the Atlantic Ocean, contributing to each other's journals, citing each other's publications, and corresponding with one another on a range of professional and political subjects.

The relationship between Dissent and medical innovation was never simple or unidirectional, but there was a close affinity between certain medical theories and practices – pneumatic medicine, for example – and the Dissenting worldview. Methodological simplicity, empiricism, and a desire to sweep away medicine's old regime were often espoused together with other reformist sentiments.[21] However, practitioners with Dissenting views shared these aspirations with some more established figures, including a number of prominent Anglicans and Tories. It is well known that some latitudinarians exhibited a strong interest in Newtonian mechanical philosophy, for example, and that they pursued natural-historical interests not unlike those of rational Dissenters.[22] Such individuals were occasionally to be found working in the colonies, but those who remained in Britain also took a keen interest in the work of colonial practitioners and solicited their views on a range of philosophical and professional matters. Here, the Royal Society of London played an important role at the end of the seventeenth and in the first half of the eighteenth century, encouraging practitioners based overseas to contribute to its *Transactions*. By the early nineteenth century, however, the political complexion – if not the religious background – of many colonial practitioners had changed.[23] In the context of the Napoleonic Wars, radical expressions of political dissent were rare, and most military and

[20] A theme that has fruitfully been explored in Grove, *Green Imperialism* and Sivasundaram, *Nature and the Godly Empire*.

[21] See Wood (ed.), *Science and Dissent in England*.

[22] e.g. Jacob, *The Newtonians and the English Revolution*; Jacob, 'The Anglican Origins of Modern Science'; idem, 'Scientific Culture in the Early English Enlightenment'; Rusnock, 'Hippocrates, Bacon, and Medical Meteorology at the Royal Society'.

[23] During the French Wars between one-quarter and one-third of medical practitioners in the British Army did not belong to the established Church. See Ackroyd et al., *Advancing with the Army*, 93.

naval practitioners tended to be conservative in outlook, though supportive of professional reform and a range of progressive causes. Those, like the tempestuous doctor Charles Maclean, who refused to temper their earlier radicalism, tended to be regarded as liabilities by their former colleagues, who sought a more gradual path to reform.

Although it would be foolish to generalize about the diverse body of practitioners that worked in the colonies, all were shaped to some degree by the context of their medical practice. The vast majority were accustomed to thinking about disease and medicine in terms of groups and this led them to favour universal remedies as opposed to individualized treatments.[24] It also induced them to think of diseases as distinct entities with characteristic signs, symptoms, and trajectories: a tendency encouraged by the growing trend towards record-keeping in military and naval hospitals. Like William Cullen, the Edinburgh professor who had taught many surgeons entering the armed forces and the East India Company, most were extremely interested in the classification of disease. Although they often rejected or modified the scheme favoured by their teacher, they shared Cullen's natural-historical approach to the subject and treated the diseases they encountered much as a botanist would treat plants, classifying them into genera and species, and considering them in relation to other natural phenomena.

Military and naval hospitals in Britain afforded similar opportunities, especially during the Napoleonic Wars, when they played an important role in the investigation of diseases such as ophthalmia.[25] But opportunities for clinical and post-mortem investigation were not as extensive as in colonial institutions. The nature of medical practice in the colonies also differed considerably on account of climatic and epidemiological differences, hence the emergence of a distinct branch of medicine: the medicine of 'warm' or 'hot' climates. The works which constituted this genre overlapped with those on military and naval medicine but were different in several respects. Those on the medicine of warm climates included contributions from non-military practitioners and had unique points of reference. Medical practice in the tropics was also shaped by commercial imperatives in addition to military and naval ones. As well as the medical practitioners who worked on plantations, hundreds were employed by the East India Company on board its cargo vessels and in its trading posts. Trade was the reason why medical establishments initially developed in the East Indies and it formed part of the day-to-day business of medicine until the early nineteenth century. Company surgeons obtained many of their drugs and a great deal of medical knowledge from local bazaars; prospecting for new medicines was also done with a view to their profitability as commodities for export to Europe.[26]

[24] Lawrence, *Medicine and the Making of Modern Britain*, 23.
[25] Pickstone, 'Dearth, Dirt and Fever Epidemics', 141; Kelly, '"Not Surgeons Alone"'.
[26] See Brockway, *Science and Colonial Expansion*; Schiebinger, *Plants and Empire.*

More generally, practitioners with extensive experience overseas tended to favour freedom of trade and were outspoken in their demands for reform or abolition of the quarantine laws, which they claimed were outdated and medically unnecessary. Such views harmonized with the interests of trading corporations such as the East India and Levant Companies and were often expressed by those inconvenienced by quarantine in their voyages between different outposts of empire. Opposition to quarantine was also consistent with radical political views. By the end of the eighteenth century, quarantine was widely portrayed as a vestige of corrupt and unenlightened regimes and its abolition was urged as part of a general programme of reform.

The argument advanced here lends support to those who have stressed the formative influence of colonial trade upon empirically grounded philosophical and medical ideas.[27] But its bearing upon the wider body of literature on colonial medicine is less obvious. As most of these works have focused on the nineteenth and twentieth centuries, their concepts and categories can appear anachronistic when applied to a period in which colonial rule was either emergent (as in India) or based upon a system of slavery which was dismantled in the 1830s. Moreover, the chief concern in most works on medicine in the colonies has been with interventions in the lives of imperial subjects.[28] The aspirations of colonial medicine in the long eighteenth century were more modest: until the early 1800s, the majority of practitioners in the tropical colonies worked in military or naval establishments and concentrated primarily on the health of Europeans. British practitioners did occasionally treat Indian soldiers and sometimes Indian nobility but, apart from that, their work among non-Europeans was largely confined to slave ships and plantations.

But while the main purpose of this book is rather different from most studies of medicine and empire, it sheds light on some of the themes explored in later periods. For example, the racial ideas that underpinned European imperialism at its apogee can only be fully understood in the light of their formation a century before.[29] Historians of the later nineteenth and twentieth centuries have also remarked on the innovative work undertaken by doctors in the colonies and its impact on medicine in Europe and North America.[30] It will be argued here that colonial innovation was important in earlier periods, too, and that it had a formative influence upon the development of what came to be known as 'Western' medicine. Modern medicine, or what was understood as such during the early nineteenth century, was as much a product of the colonies as of the infirmaries of revolutionary Paris; or, for that matter, of the hospitals and anatomy schools of Britain. We ought to think of these institutions not as unique

[27] Cook, *Matters of Exchange*; Harris, 'Long-Distance Corporations'.
[28] Arnold, *Colonizing the Body*.
[29] Ernst and Harris (eds.), *Race, Science and Medicine*; Harrison, *Climates and Constitutions*; Anderson, *The Cultivation of Whiteness*.
[30] Haynes, *Imperial Medicine*; Anderson, *Colonial Pathologies*; Kellar, *Colonial Madness*.

points of origin but as different centres of medical modernity standing in a dynamic relationship to one another. It may strike some readers as perverse to claim that the origins of modern Western medicine lay beyond the West, but in this respect there is no reason why medicine should be different from other realms of human activity. Quite apart from colonial artefacts and commodities, it is now generally recognized that many elements of Western culture were shaped in fundamental ways by colonial expansion.[31] Colonial subjects and characters were commonplace in nineteenth-century literature and art,[32] while national identity – in the case of Britain at least – was forged in the crucible of colonial warfare and the moral questions posed by slavery.[33] These and many similar observations follow naturally from an approach to the history of modernity which stresses the interdependence and interconnectedness of developments across the globe.[34]

But the exact nature of the relationship between the colonies and the imperial centre remains a source of disagreement. Although historians of medicine have had relatively little to say about this subject, in the kindred field of the history of science there has been endless debate about the nature of science in the colonial 'periphery' and its relationship to imperial centres. The period up to 1820 is conventionally regarded as an early 'phase' of colonial science, characterized by strong direction from the centre and a narrowly utilitarian focus on resource exploitation.[35] The role of 'scientists' in the colonies (the term is anachronistic for the period before 1830) is said to be one of 'data-gathering',[36] the important work of interpretation being done in scientific institutions back in Europe; in 'centres of calculation' as some scholars have termed them.[37] But historians are increasingly finding that these models fail to capture the complexities of scientific exchange between different parts of the Empire. The same is true of medicine. Elite institutions such as the Royal Society of London and the University of Edinburgh loom large in what follows, as do the East India Company's Court of Directors, the Admiralty, and the Army Medical Board. But they are only part of the story. The tenor of medical work in the tropical colonies during the period covered in this volume was to reject or radically revise metropolitan orthodoxy. Furthermore, some of the innovations which occurred in the colonies had an important impact upon the development of medicine in Britain itself: not just in the sense of furnishing the British profession with new drugs or empirical

[31] Stoler and Cooper, 'Tensions of Empire'.

[32] Said, *Culture and Imperialism*; MacKenzie, *Orientalism.*

[33] Wilson (ed.), *A New Imperial History*; Hall, *Civilizing Subjects*; Thompson, *Imperial Britain.* On the challenge posed by this new direction in imperial historiography to the history of science, see Stuchtey, 'Introduction' of Stuchtey (ed.), *Science Across the European Empires.*

[34] Pre-eminently, Bayly, *The Birth of the Modern World.*

[35] MacLeod, 'On Visiting the "Moving Metropolis"'.

[36] Kumar, *Science and the Raj*, 65.

[37] Latour's concept has been employed to good effect in Spary, *Utopia's Garden.*

information but also in showing practitioners how such drugs might be used. Even more fundamental were the contributions made by practitioners working in the colonies to pathology, to the clinical description of diseases, and to matters concerning the cause of disease and its prevention.

The means by which this information circulated were far more varied than traditional concepts of colonial science, with their emphasis upon hierarchical relationships, allow.[38] Ties with eminent metropolitan patrons of science such as Sir Joseph Banks are certainly evident, but other networks were equally important. One of these centred on the University of Edinburgh and, to a lesser extent, other Scottish universities. But the relationship of colonial practitioners to their colleagues and professors in Scotland was far from subservient. While most retained great respect for their teachers, they often differed from them on important points of detail, if not always in terms of their basic approach to medicine. Furthermore, not all colonial practitioners had ties with Edinburgh and even for many of those who did, their associations with other institutions or groups were equally, if not more, important. British medical practitioners in the colonies were linked to a variety of lively provincial societies and 'marginal' individuals who shared their reformist views. The connections between these different 'peripheries' were largely unmediated by formal authority. They were transnational, too, extending to other European countries, to the eastern seaboard of America, and even to the colonies of other powers. If we extend our view to encompass all or even most of these networks, terms such as 'centre' and 'periphery' become problematic, what was considered central being very much in the eye of the beholder.[39]

An important starting point in conceptualizing the relationship between medical practitioners in Britain and the colonies is to recognize that ideas and skills could be transferred on different terms. Sometimes relationships were characterized by free exchange of knowledge between individuals who believed that they inhabited an intellectual community. In such cases, the oft-used term 'Republic of Letters' is certainly appropriate,[40] but in other cases the relationships were more formal – as in the case of military and naval chains of command – or entailed commercial transactions. Sometimes knowledge was accepted on trust, based on shared notions of honour and civility, but in other cases it was tested and evaluated before being accepted.[41] The same can be said of 'exchanges' between European practitioners and those from other medical traditions.[42] Medical

[38] For an overview of the extensive literature on this subject, see MacLeod, 'Introduction', in MacLeod (ed.), *Nature and Empire*; Harrison, 'Science and the British Empire'.

[39] Pioneering work in this area includes Wade Chambers and Gillespie, 'Locality in the History of Science'; Endersby, 'A Garden Enclosed'; Sivasundaram, 'Trading Knowledge'; idem, '"A Christian Benares"'.

[40] See Daston, 'The Ideal and Reality of the Republic of Letters'; Goldgar, *Impolite Learning*; Brockliss, *Calvet's Web*.

[41] Bayly, *Empire and Information*; Shapin, *A Social History of Truth*.

[42] Valle, '"The Pleasure of Receiving your Favour"'; Frost, 'The Antipodean Exchange'; Crosby, *The Columbian Exchange*.

commodities and ideas were sometimes purchased from bazaars, sometimes freely obtained, and occasionally plundered or even forcibly extracted. A variety of mechanisms – which grew more formal over time – existed for evaluating information and for bringing non-European treatments into Western pharmacopoeia. Provided that these different forms of knowledge exchange are recognized and that asymmetrical relationships are acknowledged, then the concept of a 'network' of information is serviceable, as is the notion of a 'circulation' of ideas.[43]

In the period covered by this book, the Caribbean and the Indian Ocean were in a continual state of flux, but this volatility gave rise to a fertile and innovative intellectual environment. This era of commercial and imperial expansion, of warfare on a global scale, played a hugely important but largely forgotten part in the transformation of British medicine. Providing as much contextual information as possible, this book moves between general accounts of medical ideas and practices and some more detailed case studies, the aim being to illustrate the dense and often overlapping networks that existed between practitioners in the colonies and elsewhere, as well as the ways in which commercial, professional, political, and religious considerations intertwined to affect their work. The layout of the book is thematic, examining in turn natural-historical investigations of disease, therapeutics, and finally the ways in which empire became associated with a host of new medical problems in Britain, giving colonial practitioners greater influence within their profession and in society more generally. While the book concentrates on the two largest overseas congregations of British medical practitioners – in India and the West Indies – frequent reference is made to other locations such as the Mediterranean, North America, and the coastal settlements of Africa. It was within this expansive geographical framework that a distinctive medicine of 'warm' or 'hot' climates began to emerge.

MEDICINE AND IMPERIAL ECONOMY

Western medical practitioners began to write about the East and West Indies from around the middle of the sixteenth century. The earliest texts were Portuguese, but by the seventeenth century, medical practitioners from other European countries were writing on the diseases and medicines of exotic lands and on the best means of preserving the health of European travellers and settlers. Their observations were augmented by numerous references to disease and to medical practices in travel literature and in the administrative records of trading companies such as the Dutch and English East India Companies. By the end of the seventeenth century, practitioners who had never ventured beyond Europe were also beginning to use medicines imported from the Asian and American colonies,

[43] Raj, *Relocating Modern Science*; Drayton, 'Maritime Networks'; Lester, 'Imperial Circuits and Networks'.

the bark of the cinchona tree being the best-known example.[44] But from that time through to the beginning of the nineteenth century, medical interest in tropical countries began to increase. The reason was economic and military rivalry between European nations which were, or were in the process of becoming, colonial powers.

Conflicts that had their genesis in Europe were played out on a large geographical stage, and disputes over colonial trade brought nations such as England and Holland to war on several occasions during the seventeenth century.[45] By the beginning of the eighteenth century, England, and after the Act of Union in 1707, Great Britain, found itself at war regularly with the Catholic powers of France and Spain, in conflicts that took its armed forces to the East and West Indies, the Mediterranean, and North America. The most important of these conflicts were the War of the Spanish Succession (1702–13), the War of Austrian Succession (1740–8), the Seven Years War (1756–63), the War of American Independence (1775–83), the French Revolutionary Wars (1793–1802), and the Napoleonic Wars (1803–15). As a result of these conflicts, Britain was able to consolidate and expand its position as a colonial power in the West Indies while acquiring new territories elsewhere, such as Gibraltar.[46] The eclipse of French power in India by the middle of the eighteenth century also enabled the British – through the East India Company – to become the dominant European power in India, gaining effective control of much of the subcontinent by the early nineteenth century.[47]

As more Britons settled in the plantation colonies of the West Indies, opportunities arose for the practice of medicine overseas, and by the end of the seventeenth century, a number of physicians, surgeons, and apothecaries had established private practices there, mostly on the economically important islands of Jamaica and Barbados. By the 1720s, if not before, European practitioners were also to be found working on the plantations, where they often combined private practice among Europeans with the treatment of slaves. The high death rate among African slaves on the islands – as well as on the passage across the Atlantic – served as an inducement to provide basic medical care.[48] Traders and plantation owners had a strong economic incentive to prevent disease from occurring and to treat it to the best of their ability. Efforts were made to inoculate

[44] Schiebinger and Swan (eds.), *Colonial Botany.*

[45] Black, *The British Seaborne Empire*, chap. 3; Jones, *The Anglo-Dutch Wars.*

[46] Buckley, *The British Army in the West Indies*; Crewe, *Yellow Jack and the Worm*; Ward, *British West Indian Slavery.*

[47] Bayly, *Indian Society and the Making of the British Empire*; Marshall, *Bengal: The British Bridgehead*; idem (ed.), *The Eighteenth Century in Indian History*; Fisher (ed.), *The Politics of the British Annexation of India*; Alavi (ed.), *The Eighteenth Century in India.*

[48] On mortality and morbidity of African slaves in the Caribbean, see Kiple, *The Caribbean Slave*; idem (ed.), *The African Exchange*; idem, 'Deficiency Diseases in the Caribbean'; Klein and Engermann, 'A Note on Mortality in the French Slave Trade'; Sheridan, *Doctors and Slaves*; Curtin, *The Atlantic Slave Trade.*

slaves against smallpox, to improve hygiene, and to reduce overcrowding; rudimentary hospitals were also established on some plantations.[49] However, slaves continued to receive medical treatment from those among them who possessed knowledge of African medical traditions. British practitioners took note of their remedies and incorporated some of them into their own therapeutic regimes. Their work among slaves also enabled them to observe certain diseases – such as yaws and elephantiasis – which were entirely new to them, and which seemed to affect Africans almost exclusively. Since most medical practitioners remained in the islands for some years, they also had the opportunity to make prolonged observations of local diseases and the conditions in which they developed; some of which they communicated in print or by word of mouth to other practitioners in the Caribbean, North America, and Britain.

Most of the private practitioners who wrote about the diseases of the Caribbean had some formal medical training – usually at one of the Scottish universities – and some possessed medical degrees.[50] In his *History of Jamaica*, Robert Renny, who had studied but never practised medicine, declared: 'In no colony in the world, are medical practitioners to be found, better educated, more attentive, than those of Jamaica.'[51] But there were also many persons practising medicine without any discernible qualification. In 1806, the Army surgeon George Pinckard wrote: 'there are Gentlemen in the medical profession in Barbadoes, who are, equally, an honor to their profession, and an ornament to society. . . . But it is an unhappy truth that there are others who are only pre-eminent in ignorance. . . . They are more illiterate than you can believe, and the very *negro doctors* of the estates too justly vie with them in medical knowledge.'[52] Having fewer opportunities to consult trained practitioners, many of those living on smaller Caribbean islands such as Martinique and Grenada resorted to self-medication, using an array of remedies and tonics recommended by other residents.[53] Letters to and from the West Indies – and other tropical locations – provide valuable insights into such practices and the circulation of medical ideas beyond the profession itself.

But by far the most important centres of medical activity in the East and West Indies were the medical establishments of the armed forces. In the West Indies, these comprised the surgeons (and a few physicians) employed by the Army and the Royal Navy. Some remained in the Caribbean for a number of years, acquiring

[49] Klein and Engermann, 'A Note on Mortality', 271; Vaughan, 'Slavery, Smallpox and Revolution'; Stewart, 'The Edge of Utility'; Sheridan, *Doctors and Slaves*; idem, 'The Guinea Surgeons'.

[50] Kinship networks were important in the settlement of Scottish practitioners on the different Caribbean islands. See Hamilton, *Scotland, the Caribbean and the Atlantic World*, 113–16.

[51] Renny, *An History of Jamaica*, 200.

[52] Pinckard, *Notes on the West Indies*, 1, 388–9. On allegations of malpractice more generally, see Hamilton, *Scotland, the Caribbean and the Atlantic World*, 117–19.

[53] e.g. L. MacLean to William Fitzherbert, 7 November 1770, Fitzherbert of Tissington Papers, D 239 M/F 8269, Derbyshire Record Office [hereafter, DRO].

a detailed knowledge of the diseases of the region, but the majority were members of expeditionary forces which normally spent no more than a few years there – if they were lucky enough to survive. Some 70 to 80 per cent of the British and American force besieged in Cartegena in 1741 perished from disease, as did 40 per cent of the force sent to take Havana in 1762. Mortality was generally lower during the American War of Independence, but still the average mortality rate in the Caribbean was 25 per cent, almost none of it at enemy hands. But perhaps the most spectacular losses were incurred during the war against France in the 1790s. Around 12,500 British troops on the island of St Domingue died during the period 1793 to 1798.[54] These expeditionary forces were particularly vulnerable, as they tended to camp in exposed locations and lacked the immunity to yellow fever which most defending troops had acquired after several years of service.[55]

In addition to the high death rate that accompanied expeditions to the Caribbean, the armed forces were constantly denuded of effective personnel by non-lethal sicknesses. Those who had been admitted to hospital or sent back to Britain as invalids were a great burden financially and militarily. It is rare to find morbidity records for several stations simultaneously but such exist for the year 1767 and give a vivid impression of the drain on manpower in a typical year; that is, one in which there were no large engagements or major epidemics. These returns show that the peacetime sickness rate of British regiments in the West Indies (10.2 per cent of total strength) was more than double those of any other garrison in the Western Hemisphere. Troops stationed on Gibraltar were the next most sickly with a rate of 5 per cent, followed by foot-guards in Britain (4 per cent), troops in Minorca (3.9 per cent) and in North America (3.8 per cent).[56]

British servicemen in India were not as numerous as they were in the Caribbean because the East India Company possessed its own armies – and a marine service – which were composed chiefly of Indians. However, losses among British troops in the region were high at the most unhealthy times of year – the hot and rainy seasons – and were particularly heavy on active service.[57] Even in peacetime, the death toll of Britons in the Indies was high and the burden of sickness often crushing. But in other tropical settlements – most notoriously along the West African Coast – mortality was far higher. No precise figures are available for the eighteenth century, but in the early nineteenth century, West Africa – which had become notorious as the 'White Man's Grave' – invariably topped the mortality league for Britons stationed overseas. The average death rate for British

[54] Geggus, 'Yellow Fever in the 1790s'; idem, *Slavery, War, and Revolution*; Leach, *Roots of Conflict*, 55–61; Kiple, 'Race, War and Tropical Medicine'.

[55] McNeill, 'The Ecological Basis of Warfare in the Caribbean'.

[56] Returns of His Majesty's Forces, October 1767, D.45, X.15, Gloucestershire County Record Office [hereafter, GCRO].

[57] Harrison, *Climates*, chap. 2.

troops in West Africa ranged from 483 to 668 per 1,000 men, whereas for the West Indies it was in the region of 85–138 per 1,000. Mortality in India was considerably lower, ranging from 30 to 75 per 1,000 troops, although still considerably higher than the average of 15 per 1,000 for soldiers stationed in Britain.[58]

To some extent, these losses were borne fatalistically as the inevitable cost of war and commerce in hot climates. Military expeditions may even have been regarded as a way of ridding society of its most useless and disruptive elements.[59] By the mid-eighteenth century, however, there was mounting concern about the losses sustained on tropical expeditions. A series of interconnected developments in technology and tactics made it far more costly to train men for battle.[60] The increasing scale and frequency of warfare during the eighteenth century also meant that skilled manpower was at a premium. The British Army alone grew from 15,851 officers and men in 1715 to 26,314 in the 1730s, and by the end of the War of Austrian Succession had reached 75,516. Even after the conclusion of hostilities, the peacetime establishment was considerably higher than before the war – some 29,132 officers and men – and during the Seven Years War, the number rose to 111,533. These figures do not include the Irish establishment, which, in 1761, provided a further 24,000 officers and men.[61] The expansion of the armed forces placed a heavy burden on the national exchequer and on tax-payers,[62] and provided a powerful stimulus to the conservation of manpower.[63]

Medicine played an increasingly important part in this process, since it was far less expensive to treat a sick or wounded serviceman than to train a replacement. The need for a permanent medical service in the Army and Navy had long been recognized but, at the beginning of the eighteenth century, the numbers of medical practitioners employed in either service – or that of the East India Company – was relatively small. Their professional standing was also low and, lacking the powers of a commissioned officer, they found it difficult to have much influence upon the organization of medical care.[64] However, medical practitioners in the armed forces were acutely aware of the mounting cost of warfare and began to stress the utility of medicine to the state. In his *Œconomical and Medical Observations* (1764), the military surgeon Richard Brocklesby wrote of the 'distresses and death of so many useful members of the Body Politick', when urging medical and hygienic reforms on the Army during the Seven Years

[58] Sheridan, *Doctors and Slaves*, 12. See also Curtin, 'The White Man's Grave'; idem, *The Image of Africa*, chaps 3 and 14; idem, *Death By Migration.*

[59] Bewell, *Romanticism and Colonial Disease*, chap. 2.

[60] See Roberts, *The Military Revolution*; Black, *A Military Revolution?*; idem, *European Warfare 1660–1815*; Parker, *The Military Revolution.*

[61] Guy, *Oeconomy and Discipline*, 9.

[62] Brewer, *The Sinews of Power*, 89–90.

[63] Guy, *Oeconomy and Discipline.*

[64] Gruber von Arni, *Hospital Care*, chap. 7; Cantlie, *A History of the Army Medical Department*, vol. 1.

War.[65] The very title of this work suggests the centrality of economical considerations to military medical reform. Brocklesby's contemporary, Donald Monro, a scion of the famous Edinburgh medical dynasty, set out the argument in greater detail: 'In a commercial Country like our own, where Numbers of Hands are constantly wanted for the carrying on our Manufactories, we have a strong political Argument to add to that drawn from the Dictates of Humanity, why the Life of every individual should be most carefully attended to.' 'The Preservation of the Lives of Soldiers', he concluded, 'is then with us a Matter of the highest Importance, in order to make as low as possible the Number of Recruits who must be perpetually drawn off for Service to War.'[66]

In other words, losses in wartime were not only costly in military terms but had far-reaching consequences for the nation's economy. Significantly, these remarks were made in a report apparently commissioned by George III,[67] showing that the Crown considered the loss of manpower through disease to be a matter of some importance. The economic advantages of improved medical provisions were also stressed by medical practitioners in the Navy. In his *Essay on Diseases incidental to Europeans in Hot Climates* (1768), James Lind wrote that 'The recent examples of the great mortality in hot climates, ought to draw the attention of all the commercial nations of Europe, towards the important object of preserving the health of their countrymen.' 'Unhealthy settlements', he warned, 'require a constant supply of people, and of course drain their mother country of an incredible number, and some of its most useful inhabitants.'[68]

The language of economic and public utility was evident in nearly all the military and naval medical works of the eighteenth century but was most clearly articulated in the writings of Gilbert Blane, a crucially important figure in naval medical reform. Blane enjoyed a close relationship with the Admiralty and was astute in the way in which he framed his arguments for improvements in hygiene, victualling, and medical care. He was always careful to link humanitarian arguments to economical ones: '[E]ven considering men merely as a commodity,' he wrote, 'it could be made evident in an œconomical and political view, independent of moral considerations, that the lives and health of men might be preserved at much less expense and trouble than what are necessary to repair the ravages of disease.'[69] Again, he stressed that 'money would avail nothing to the public defence without a sufficient number of able and healthy men, who are the real resources of a state, and the true sinews of war.'[70] Blane used this phrase on several occasions, presumably believing that it crystallized economic and humanitarian

65 Brocklesby, *Œconomical and Medical Observations*, 27–8.
66 Monro, *An Account of the Diseases which were most frequent in the British Military Hospitals in Germany*, ix.
67 Ibid., iv.
68 Lind, *An Essay on Diseases incidental to Europeans in Hot Climates*, 1808 edn., 8.
69 Blane, *Observations on the Diseases incident to Seamen*, 1st edn., 207.
70 Blane, *Observations*, 3rd edn., 180.

arguments for reform.[71] Other naval surgeons quickly embraced Blane's notion of the sailor as a national commodity. In 1790, Frederick Thomson argued that the health of seamen ought to be preserved even if they are considered 'merely as a commodity',[72] and in 1798 a similar point was made by Elliot Arthy.[73] As Arthy and others pointed out, the loss of life was a particular problem in foreign stations such as the Caribbean; a 'subject of so much national importance', as one writer described it.[74]

The growing awareness that men had an economic value – and the articulation of this in systems of military accounting – provided a powerful stimulus to the improvement of medical provisions in foreign stations and other measures to conserve manpower.[75] The term 'œconomy', which appears so frequently in medical and military literature during the eighteenth century, is also suggestive of new forms of management and discipline that were emerging at this time.[76] For most of the century, the term 'œconomy' referred to good management and discipline rather than simply to the conservation of public money. Such principles underlay measures to improve sanitation, ventilation, and diet in naval vessels,[77] cutting the annual sickness rate among sailors from 37.8 per cent at the height of the War of Independence to 15.2 per cent in 1796, and to only 6.4 per cent in 1806.[78] The military advantages of hygiene were also articulated in the Army; notably, in military manuals such as General Bland's *Treatise on Military Discipline*, which impressed the importance of cleanliness upon regimental officers, reminding them of exemplars such as Vegetius from the Classical world.[79] Some commanders did manage to keep their men relatively free from disease, but hygienic discipline was often neglected or difficult to maintain on active service.[80]

Manpower economy – in all senses of the term – was also the driving force behind the foundation of hospitals for servicemen at home and overseas. By the 1750s, the Navy was sending most of its casualties to makeshift hospitals rather than treating them in private lodging houses as was formerly the case. But these temporary hospitals tended to be poorly run, and it was to put an end to waste and indiscipline that two permanent establishments were constructed at Haslar, near Gosport, and at Stonehouse, near Plymouth. The former began to take

[71] Blane, 'On the Medical Service of the Fleet in the West Indies in the Year 1782', 70.
[72] Thompson, *An Essay on the Scurvy*, iii.
[73] Arthy, *The Seaman's Medical Advocate*, i.
[74] Review of William Fowle's Practical Treatise on the Different Fevers of the West Indies (1800) in *Medical and Physical Journal*, 4 (1800), 354.
[75] Foucault, 'The Politics of Health in the Eighteenth Century'.
[76] Foucault, *Discipline and Punish*.
[77] Lawrence, 'Disciplining Disease'.
[78] Blane, 'On the Comparative Health of the British Navy, from the Year 1779 to the Year 1814, with Proposals for its further Improvement', 40.
[79] Bland, *A Treatise of Military Discipline*, 226.
[80] Harrison, 'Medicine and the Management of Modern Warfare'.

patients in 1754 and was completed in 1761; the latter was partially in use in 1760 and fully open by 1762.[81] Both these hospitals received many patients from the tropical colonies, especially the West Indies, and Haslar in particular became an important site for the production of medical knowledge regarding the diseases of warm climates.

The new naval hospitals had a good reputation and soon became models for military and civilian establishments throughout Europe. At Haslar, for example, 9,862 out of 14,418 patients admitted between 1753 and 1757 were discharged as cured – an impressive 68 per cent,[82] whereas the death rate at this time for those admitted to hospital was generally around 40 per cent.[83] But in the colonies there was nothing to compare with the likes of Haslar. Ambitious plans for a military hospital in the short-lived colony of Tangiers were never realized before the territory was given up in 1684.[84] Hospitals established for other imperial garrisons – such as those in the West Indies – were generally makeshift and insubstantial, often overcrowded and providing scant shelter from the elements. But some hospitals were in more or less continual use throughout the second half of the eighteenth century. Among these were the naval hospitals of Jamaica, Antigua, Barbados, and Gibraltar. The hospital at New Greenwich, Jamaica, was the first of these institutions, being the brainchild of the Commander-in-Chief, Admiral Vernon. It was completed in 1745 but its location, close to marshes and lagoons, led to many deaths from fever amongst patients and staff, and a new institution was constructed in 1756 a few miles away, at Port Royal.[85] In addition to these permanent hospitals, the armed forces continued to make use of private sick quarters (not all of which were poorly run) and general hospitals, which were usually created for the duration of a campaign.[86] This arrangement was widely regarded as unsatisfactory, however, and there were attempts to establish a larger and better naval hospital at Port Royal at the end of the century, following numerous complaints about the standard of care provided for sick and wounded seamen.[87]

Notwithstanding their limitations, the naval hospitals played an important role in warfare in the West Indies, from the point of view of both economy and morale. The same was true of the Army. As Dr Benjamin Moseley pointed out, 'As the restoring [of] soldiers speedily to health is of the first consequence, in climates where a short illness renders them useless . . . and where diseases are

[81] Rodger, *The Wooden World*, 109–12.

[82] Ibid., 196.

[83] Duffy, *The Military Experience in the Age of Reason*, 172.

[84] Gruber von Arni, *Hospital Care*, chap. 1.

[85] Moseley, *A Treatise on Tropical Diseases*, 1st edn., 186; Surgeon's Report, enclosed in F/7, CL, NMM; The Hospital at Jamaica 1739–48, 23, MS 1933, Box 149, Special Collections, National Library of Jamaica.

[86] On the contracting system, see Crimmin, 'The Sick and Hurt Board and the Health of Seamen'.

[87] Office of the Sick and Wounded Seamen to Sir Evan Nepean, DM/F/30, CL, NMM.

inevitable, convenient and proper hospitals are of the utmost importance.' 'The cost of a good hospital', he insisted, 'is nothing in the scale of expence [sic]. It is a solecism in oeconomy to have a bad one. A bad hospital may deprive the state, in a few months, of as many men, whose value would amount, in political calculation, to a sum sufficient to build a good one.' However, he lamented that the hospitals available during the American War in Jamaica fell far short of what was required: 'I lost more value in men at Castile Fort, and at Up Park, in three months, from the miseries of the hospital alone, than would have been adequate to the expence [sic] of erecting a proper one, for all the troops in the island.'[88]

The poor condition of general hospitals was confirmed by many other writers, most notably the Army surgeon Robert Jackson. Writing of his experiences in North America and the Caribbean during the American War of Independence, Jackson complained that the wrong people were usually chosen to command general hospitals (these were still combatant rather than medical officers), and that their aptitude was seldom the most important consideration. Moreover, he insisted, 'general hospitals are ruinous to military discipline . . . they produce sloth and indolence, the worst disease to which a soldier is liable, and . . . they extinguish very speedily the ardour for the service in the field.' 'It is only . . . by habits of exercise, even by toils and fatigue, that men at last attain the properties of good soldiers . . . while it is only by constant practice of such discipline that they are preserved in a state fit for the performance of their duties.' For this reason, Jackson favoured keeping as many of the sick and wounded as possible with the regiment. Only if they remained with the Army, he argued, could discipline be maintained.[89]

It is likely that general hospitals in America and the West Indies during the War of Independence left much to be desired, but their failings may have been exaggerated by Jackson, who saw these institutions as bastions of inexperienced physicians foisted upon the Army by an ineffectual and out-of-touch Medical Board. With this possibility in mind, it is interesting to note that the French appear to have regarded the British general hospitals as a model to be emulated.[90] During the wars against the French in the 1790s, the condition of hospitals was still less than satisfactory in many cases. Some of the larger ones certainly afforded scope for important medical work, but the state of hygiene and discipline was often grim. Writing of his experiences in the West Indies, the surgeon Hector M'Lean lamented that:

> It is particularly difficult to see the early stage of the Remittent [fever] among soldiers. They never complain in the beginning, and have such an aversion to go into an hospital, that they conceal their situation till the disease has confirmed itself in their constitutions.

[88] Moseley, *Treatise*, 155–6.

[89] Jackson, *Treatise on the Fevers of Jamaica*, 419–20.

[90] Memorandum on the reform of the French military hospital service by Dr Vincent Olivier Gouraud, c. 1789, WMS 1721/8, WL.

It is not surprising that soldiers dislike general hospitals; they see very few return, who once enter their gates.[91]

After the wars, the condition of hospitals in the West Indies seems to have declined, if anything, especially in the smaller stations. The hospital sited on The Ridge in Antigua, for instance, was a wooden building capable of holding no more than forty sick men at the most. The Army's Inspector-General of Hospitals, William Fergusson, reported disapprovingly that 'it in no respects deserves the character or possesses any of the conveniences of a hospital, it is merely a barrack very improperly situated on the highest point . . . of a bleak hill top.' The hospital at Monks Hill on the same island was even worse. Its roof was said to be in a ruinous state and the whole hospital bore 'more resemblance to a plantation sick house of an inferior description for negroes than an hospital for British soldiers'. The situation was little better on most islands, but there were occasional surprises, such as the military hospital at St Joseph's, Trinidad, which, though made of wood, was said to have ample and well-ventilated accommodation for the sick.[92]

In the East Indies, most of the hospitals used by the Army and Navy were facilities constructed by the East India Company for their 'factors' (traders and civil servants), its Marine service, and the European soldiers serving in the 'presidency' armies of Bengal, Madras, and Bombay. The most important hospitals under the auspices of the Company were those opened at Madras in 1664, in Bombay in 1670, and in Calcutta in 1708.[93] All three establishments sometimes cared for Crown troops and naval personnel in addition to those employed by the Company, although most naval patients were accommodated in separate sick quarters in Calcutta and Bombay.[94] The hospitals were located within the fortified 'factories' or trading posts established by the Company and were thus reasonably well protected, but most appear to have been inadequate from a medical point of view. In 1750, for example, Andrew Munro, the surgeon of the hospital in Madras, complained to the governor that it was massively overcrowded and that accommodation for staff was being used by the sick. He urged that a house or some other building be hired to provide extra accommodation.[95] Seven years later, his successors Robert Turing and James Wilson reported that many repairs and additions were needed to make the hospital fit for purpose.[96] Problems were also experienced in coordinating medical care between the hospital in Madras and some smaller institutions scattered throughout the region, creating 'great irregularity and confusion' as well as 'extraordinary

[91] M'Lean, *An Enquiry*, 128–9.
[92] William Fergusson, Reports on Hospital Establishments in the West Indies, RAMC 210, WL.
[93] Crawford, *Roll of the Indian Medical Service*, vol. 2, 391–2, 400, 418–22.
[94] Gradish, *The Manning of the British Navy*, 187.
[95] Andrew Munro, Consultation with Governor (Richard Price) in Council, 1 July 1750, Madras Public Proceedings [hereafter, MPP], P/240/8, APAC, BL.
[96] MPP, Nos. 455 and 462, 1757, P/240/15, APAC, BL.

expense'.[97] In Madras, additional accommodation for the hospital was eventually found in a rented house but, in 1768, it was severely damaged by a typhoon and needed to be completely rebuilt.[98] Three years later, it was still not properly constructed, leaving the sick to suffer 'deplorable' conditions during the monsoon rains.[99] However, the hospital at Madras was eventually made more secure and better able to accommodate the large numbers of sick which it regularly received during the rainy season. In 1772, the Chief Engineer of Madras, Patrick Ross, produced a report for a new, purpose-built hospital with proper drains, benches to allow convalescents to sit out on a verandah, an apothecaries' shop, and so forth. The new institution was also to have a separate, detached apartment for 'Contagious Distempers', together with small rooms for 'lunatics' and for Indian medical staff.[100]

The hospital at Madras was in most respects typical of those in the East India Company's settlements. Over time, hospitals in the major towns were transformed from small, cramped quarters within the old forts into larger institutions located in more or less purpose-built accommodation. By the middle of the eighteenth century, these hospitals typically employed two surgeons, two or three surgeons' mates, and a host of Indian hospital assistants, dressers, and medicine-compounders.[101] But outside the larger fortified settlements, the condition of hospitals was far more variable. In 1782, John Ruding reported to the Governor of Fort St George in Madras that the state of the hospital in Chingleput was 'very much out of repair, so much so, that I don't know whither [sic] it would be less expence [sic] to pull it down, and with the old materials build a new one'.[102] Other small hospitals established for the Company's army in Madras presidency, such as that at Masulipatam, appeared to be in a reasonable condition but normally accommodated no more than half a dozen patients.[103]

It was only in the presidency towns of Madras, Calcutta, and Bombay that hospitals were capable of providing the kind of environment that was conducive to medical innovation. There, there were sufficient numbers of patients housed for long enough to permit protracted clinical observation. The fact that these larger hospitals employed Indians who had some experience of practising varieties of traditional medicine may have eased exchange of information and the incorporation of new remedies into British practice. The proximity of hospitals to native bazaars in the presidency towns also encouraged the use of local remedies, as did the fact that supplies of medicines from Britain seldom arrived

[97] MPP, No. 197, April 1760, P/240/18, APAC, BL.

[98] MPP, No. 215, 29 March 1768, P/240/26; Nos. 827 and 829, 1 November 1768, P/240/27, APAC, BL.

[99] MPP, No. 1007, 20 December 1770, P/240/30, APAC, BL.

[100] MPP, No. 597, 25 July 1772; No. 864, 20 October 1772, APAC, BL.

[101] MPP, No. 177, 26 February 1762, P/240/20; Nos. 91–2, 30 January 1764, APAC, BL.

[102] Ruding to Lord George Macartney, President and Governor of Fort St George, 16 January 1782, Macartney Papers, WMS 5746/1, WL.

[103] James Hodges to Macartney, 17 April 1783, WMS 5746/1, WL.

intact, if at all.[104] Necessity was thus the mother of invention when it came to the treatment of disease but the relatively disciplined environment of military hospitals enabled new therapies to be subjected to trial and their results systematically recorded. Hospitals also kept accurate records of the numbers admitted and discharged, as well as the nature of the illness. Few of these have survived to the present day, but those that have indicate that record-keeping was done thoroughly. They also provide a snap-shot of the diseases typically encountered in the Company's hospitals and the likelihood of survival. The returns for the Calcutta hospital in 1767, for example, show that the most common causes of admission in that year (and in the other years for which records are available) were 'fever' and 'flux' (dysentery) in that order, with just over 10 per cent of fever cases dying in hospital and nearly 14 per cent of flux cases. The majority of patients (56 per cent) spent longer than two weeks in hospital, thus providing ample opportunity for observation of their symptoms.[105] The high death rate also provided hospital surgeons with a steady stream of cadavers for dissection.

Practitioners working in colonial hospitals readily shared their observations with one another in a desperate attempt to combat the deadly diseases of the tropics. More often than not, they did so by word of mouth, sometimes travelling great distances to visit each other's institutions. However, the nature of the medical community differed considerably from place to place. In India, which had a large medical establishment, the bulk of which consisted of Company surgeons on long service (some 624 by 1824),[106] there was more continuity and it was probably easier to learn what was happening in other presidency towns than it was for information to be shared between the scattered and often isolated hospitals of the West Indies. Nevertheless, by the end of the eighteenth century, there was a good deal of contact between practitioners working across the tropics and in other warm climates. Their isolation was overcome through correspondence networks and various print media, which linked practitioners throughout the English-speaking world and beyond. From the 1820s, medical and physical societies and medical colleges also began to emerge in the East and West Indies, some of which produced their own journals.[107] These societies and their organs

[104] Pratik Chakrabarti, '"Neither of meate nor drinke"'.

[105] See Hospital Admissions, Fort William, Calcutta, 1767; and for 1752 (July–December only) and 1763, L/MIL/10/130, APAC, BL. For a fuller discussion, see Harrison, 'Disease and Medicine in the Armies of British India, 1750–1830'.

[106] Arnold, *Science, Technology and Medicine in Colonial India*, 58.

[107] e.g. *Jamaica Physical Journal*. The first edition of the journal appeared in 1834 and had 76 subscribers, mostly inhabitants of the island. Its founding followed the establishment of a College of Physicians and Surgeons on the Island, enabled by the passage of the Jamaica Medical Act of 1832. See issue 1 (1834), 1–2, 42. In India, the first exclusively medical journal was the *Transactions of the Medical and Physical Society of Calcutta*. The Society met for the first time in 1823 and its transactions appeared two years later. A Medical College – the first in India – was established in the same city in 1835. See Harrison, 'Was There an Oriental Renaissance in Medicine?'; idem, 'Medicine and Orientalism'.

fostered a distinctive set of medical ideas and practices. But the burgeoning print culture of the late eighteenth and early nineteenth centuries also enabled medical practitioners to share their work with a much wider audience in Britain, North America, and Continental Europe. In this way, they were able to exert a profound effect upon Western medicine at a crucial, formative stage in its history.

PART I

MEDICINE AS NATURAL HISTORY

Introduction to Part I

The hospitals established in the Indies were among the most important sites of innovation in British medicine. Despite their many limitations, they fostered a proudly independent medical culture that was antagonistic to the bastions of medical tradition. This part of the book shows how practitioners working in these hospitals rejected the genteel, text-based medicine of the physician elite for an avowedly empirical form of medicine supported by the twin pillars of bedside observation and post-mortem dissection. Although the same trends were evident in Britain, in the colonies the pace of change was quicker and the impact on medical theory and practice more profound. Taking advantage of unparalleled opportunities for dissection and the correlation of morbid signs with symptoms in living patients, practitioners in the colonies constructed detailed natural histories of disease. Their methods were complemented by the systematic investigation of external phenomena which appeared to have a bearing on the causes and prognosis of the same maladies. Knowledge acquired in the wards and at the dissecting table was augmented by that obtained from barometers, thermometers, and other such instruments. These developments had close parallels in Britain, too, but meteorology figured less prominently at home than it did in the tropics, where the awesome power of nature made an enormous impression.

By the mid-seventeenth century, climate was central to the theory and practice of medicine in India and the West Indies, serving as the framework for what would become a new genre of medical literature. But despite the growing distinctiveness of tropical medical practice, colonial surgeons and physicians began to make important contributions to medicine in Britain. There, too, the nature, causation, and treatment of fevers had become matters of urgency. The massive scale and scope of warfare during the eighteenth century, and the increasing tendency to attach an economic value to the lives of soldiers and sailors, meant that the prevention and treatment of disease received greater attention. At the same time, the devastation caused by yellow fever in North America and the Mediterranean suggested that Britain, too, could be at risk from tropical maladies.

The nature of fevers probably excited more controversy than any other subject in British medicine during this period. Practitioners diverged sharply, not only on matters of theory and practice, but over how, if at all, their disputes could be resolved. The relative merits of many different forms of enquiry and evidence were vociferously debated: natural history versus anatomy; observation and experiment versus reason and tradition; individual case histories versus statistical tables. The bitterness and rancour generated by these disputes is understandable if we bear in mind that they were often enmeshed with political and religious upheavals and inseparable from questions of professional authority.[1] Perhaps the most important of these was the challenge mounted by surgeons, apothecaries, and other practitioners to the monopoly and influence of the Royal College of Physicians in London. Medical practitioners in the colonies were among the most vociferous critics of the College and of the medical institutions which were dominated by its fellows.

Part I of this book examines these issues in relation to theories of disease causation or aetiology. Aetiology was of fundamental importance to medicine and many related areas of natural philosophy: it went to the heart of Man's relationship to his environment. But the collapse of the Aristotelian-Galenic paradigm during the seventeenth century left medicine bereft of certainties. Numerous competing claims were being made about the workings of the human body and its governing principles: chemists, mechanists, and more traditionally minded physicians vied with one another, each seeking to unlock the secrets of Nature.[2] Colonial expansion added another dimension to these debates, posing new challenges and creating new opportunities for the observation of disease. Freed from the usual constraints of medicine at home, practitioners in the colonies embarked on a quest for knowledge which transformed the theory and practice of medicine in Britain, its Empire, and beyond.

[1] e.g. Cunningham, 'Sydenham versus Newton'; Cook, *The Decline of the Old Medical Regime*; Martensen, 'Hippocrates and the Politics of Medical Knowledge'.

[2] Maclean, *Logic, Signs and Nature in the Renaissance*; French, *Medicine before Science*.

1

Climate, fever, and medicine before 1700

Until the early seventeenth century, few writers on fever departed significantly from ancient Greek, Roman, or Arabic texts, leaving the authority of Galen and Avicenna more or less intact. All regarded the essence of fever as excessive bodily heat, although there was plenty of disagreement over its nature and causes. Practitioners differed, for example, over whether this heat was natural, arising within the body, or extraneous, or a mixture of the two.[1] These age-old debates lost much of their significance following the publication of William Harvey's *De Motu Cordis* (1628), in which he famously advanced his theory of the circulation of the blood. From then on, heat came to be regarded more as an effect than a cause of fever.[2] This was one of several important changes that transformed thinking about fever during the seventeenth century and which had a bearing upon medical theory and practice in the tropics. Most of these had their origins in Europe, in challenges to the Aristotelian-Galenic system mounted by enthusiasts for chemical medicine,[3] or experimental natural philosophy.[4] But medical practitioners in the tropics also participated in the reclassification and redefinition of fevers which was taking place in Europe. Their contribution lay chiefly in the natural-historical investigation of disease: in the exploration of maladies in relation to their environment and in post-mortem dissection.

In respect of the former, though not the latter, practitioners in India and the Caribbean followed in the footsteps of the English physician Thomas Sydenham (1624–89). Together with the philosopher Francis Bacon, Sydenham was to become one of the iconic figures of English medical reform during the eighteenth and early nineteenth centuries, and certainly one of the most celebrated by British practitioners working in the tropics. Sydenham's support for Parliament and the Commonwealth seems to have prevented his advancement at the court of

[1] Brain, *Galen on Bloodletting*, 10–12.

[2] Lonie, 'Fever Pathology in the Sixteenth Century'.

[3] Debus, *The English Paracelsians*, 180–2; King, *The Road to Medical Enlightenment*, 37–62; Wear, *Knowledge and Practice in English Medicine*, 368–72, 428–33; Rattansi, 'The Helmontian-Galenist Controversy'; Webster, 'English Medical Reformers'; Cook, 'The Society of Chemical Physicians'; Cleruzio, 'From van Helmont to Boyle'.

[4] e.g. Thomas Willis (1621–75), *Diatribe duae Medico-Philosophicae*. See Frank, *Harvey and the Oxford Physiologists*; Webster, *The Great Instauration*, 153–74; Bates, 'Thomas Willis and the Fevers Literature of the Seventeenth Century'.

Charles II and, despite holding the necessary qualifications, he never became a fellow of the Royal College of Physicians, holding the rank of licentiate.[5] However, one should not necessarily assume that this reflected Sydenham's standing as a doctor. He may have been content with being a licentiate of the college, for it permitted him to escape the governing duties of a fellow; his standing among fellows of the College may also have been greater than some historians have claimed.[6] While Sydenham was possibly more conservative, medically, than some historians like to believe, for subsequent generations he came to represent the reforming impulse in medicine. In particular, his work on disease represented an empirical tendency in physic which stemmed from the Hippocratic revival of the Renaissance and the inductive philosophy of Bacon. Like Hippocrates, Sydenham was famed for his careful observation of diseases as they appeared in patients and of the meteorological conditions which produced them. His approach was based on Books I and III of the *Epidemics* and bore a strong resemblance to Book I in particular, with close attention to such factors as wind direction, temperature, and rainfall.[7] Although Sydenham eschewed speculation about the essential causes of epidemics, it seemed evident to him that peculiar states of the atmosphere, which he termed 'constitutions' of the air or 'epidemic furniture', produced characteristic types of disease. Thus, one year might be marked by continued fever and another by plague. According to Sydenham, these diseases occurred when certain 'particles of air' – noxious to human and animal life – entered into the body through respiration, mixing with the blood, and imbuing the whole organism with what he called a 'morbifick contagion'.[8] By the latter, he did not mean that diseases became contagious in the sense understood today but that they spread within the body as its humours putrefied. In Sydenham's view, the disease state consisted in the body's attempt to free itself of morbific matter.[9] 'What . . . is the Plague', he wrote, 'but a complication of Symptoms, by which Nature uses to cast out the malignant Particles . . . or other eruptions that were drawn in by the Air.'[10]

This renewed sensitivity to meteorological conditions was a major development in theories of fever. According to Sydenham, the varieties of disease were infinite, depending on the unique disposition of each epidemic constitution. Yet, he believed that it was possible to order diseases as different types, in much the same way as botanists classified plants. The classification of disease had to be painstaking, cautious, and provisional, and observations repeated as often as possible in the manner recommended by Bacon.[11] This empirical approach to

5 Cook, 'Sydenham, Thomas (*bap.* 1624, *d.* 1689)', *DNB.*
6 I owe this important insight to Mr Simon Howes.
7 'Epidemics', Books I & III, in Lloyd (ed.), *Hippocratic Writings.*
8 *The Whole Works of that Excellent Practical Physician, Dr Thomas Sydenham*, 1.
9 Wear, *Knowledge and Practice*, 457–60.
10 Sydenham, *Works*, 2.
11 French, *Medicine before Science*, 191–2; Sydenham, *Works*, 36, 59.

the study of disease probably owed much to Sydenham's association with natural philosophers such as Robert Boyle, his friend and neighbour, and the physician-philosopher John Locke. Like them, he insisted that the only sound basis for knowledge was observation.[12] There has been a tendency to overstate Sydenham's debt to Boyle, although it is clearly evident in his view of the air as impregnated with minute particles; a view expressed clearly in Boyle's *General History of the Air* (1692). But of particular significance in these respects is Sydenham's reading of the Hippocratic texts. Like other seventeenth-century writers, he selected those features of the Hippocratic corpus which were most compatible with his own approach to medicine. 'His' Hippocrates was the author of the *Epidemics* and *Airs, Waters and Places*; an empirical physician who learned from a careful study of nature.[13] In portraying Hippocrates as an inductive physician, Sydenham stood in a long line of practitioners who stressed experiential, practical medicine in opposition to the canonical authority of Classical texts. In England, this shift away from Galenic orthodoxy was bound up with the challenge mounted to the Royal College of Physicians, led by practitioners without university qualifications such as apothecaries.[14]

One of the ways in which Sydenham's work came to the attention of future generations was through the writing and teaching of Herman Boerhaave (1668–1738). More than one-third of Boerhaave's students during his tenure as professor of medicine at the University of Leiden (1709–38) were British, and his doctrines dominated the new medical faculty at Edinburgh University through to the 1760s.[15] Since around one-third of the surgeons serving in the Army, Navy, and East India Company had received some training at Edinburgh,[16] it seems reasonable to suppose that many would have viewed the diseases of warm climates in a similar way to Boerhaave; at least on their arrival. This may help to explain the great emphasis they placed on observation at the bedside, as well as of the disease environment outside the hospital. Though by no means an uncritical admirer of Sydenham, Boerhaave was heavily indebted to the 'English Hippocrates' and followed him in paying close attention to the workings of nature. However, he thought that Sydenham's approach lacked a firm foundation in natural philosophy, and he was more explicitly indebted than Sydenham to the corpuscular theories of matter espoused by Boyle, seeking a basis for medicine in chemistry and mechanical philosophy.[17] In this he was by no means alone, and

[12] Cunningham, 'Thomas Sydenham and the "Good Old Cause"'.

[13] Cunningham 'The Transformation of Hippocrates'. The *Epidemics* was one of a number of Hippocratic texts that came to light during the sixteenth century; its case-study approach proved attractive to medical practitioners who sought to ground their work on observation of natural phenomena. See Siraisi, *The Clock and the Mirror*, 119–48.

[14] See Webster, *Great Instauration*; Cook, *Decline*; Cunningham, 'Transformation'; Pelling, *Medical Conflicts in Early Modern London.*

[15] Christie, 'The Origins and Development of the Scottish Scientific Community', 131.

[16] Chitnis, 'Medical Education in Edinburgh', 174.

[17] Lindeboom, *Hermann Boerhaave.*

by the 1680s, even the Royal College of Physicians had embraced mechanical philosophy, regarding Galenism as indefensible.[18]

As we shall see in some later chapters, the therapeutic legacy of Boerhaave consisted largely in a renewed emphasis on bleeding and other 'antiphlogistic' measures to clear obstructions of bodily vessels. In other respects, it was to reintroduce Sydenham to British practitioners, bringing greater respect for bedside observation and renewed interest in the environmental causes of disease.[19] But unlike Sydenham, Boerhaave also stressed the importance of observations made post-mortem and this aspect of his practice was taken up enthusiastically in the Indies.[20]

Although Boerhaave embraced mechanical philosophy, he had an abiding interest in chemistry and held opinions on the genesis of fever that resembled those of English physician Thomas Willis, especially the idea that putrefaction was a form of alkalescence.[21] Boerhaave's writings on putrefaction dominated accounts of the diseases of warm climates for much of the eighteenth century, particularly his opinion that bile was especially prone to corruption and that persons of plethoric disposition were most liable to suffer from putrid diseases.[22] A measure of his continuing relevance was that even a celebrated figure like William Cullen was criticized in the 1760s for deviating slightly from the Dutch master in his lectures to students in Edinburgh. As Cunningham has observed, the enduring popularity of Boerhaavian medicine lay in its attempt to reconcile different medical traditions, ancient and modern.[23] And yet, even his most ardent admirers recognized certain deficiencies in Boerhaave's work which needed to be supplemented by others.[24]

One such was Friedrich Hoffman (1660–1742), a slightly older contemporary of Boerhaave, who held the first chair in medicine at Halle. Hoffman's ideas and approach were similar to those of Boerhaave, as both attempted to find a new basis for medical practice in anatomy and physiology, and in chemical and mechanical philosophy.[25] Hoffman attempted to synthesize the best of the Classical tradition – particularly its clinical acumen – with insights from the New Philosophy, although mechanical analogies are less evident in his work than in that of many contemporaries.[26] However, it was Hoffman's statements about the relationship between climate and disease that had special relevance for practitioners in the Indies. Like Sydenham, Hoffman articulated the Hippocratic view that each climate, age, sex,

18 Brown, 'The College of Physicians'.

19 Smith, 'Medical Science'; Lindeboom, 'Boerhaave's Debt to British Science'.

20 James, *The Modern Practice of Physic*, vol. 1, 2.

21 Ibid., 80. Both Boerhaave and Willis ascribed many physiological processes to fermentation, but they differed on matters of detail, for example in explaining the precise nature of the chemical process causing nervous sensations. See Knoeff, *Herman Boerhaave*, 192.

22 James, *Practice of Physic*, 80–1.

23 Cunningham, 'Medicine to Calm the Mind'.

24 Ibid., iii.

25 See French, *Medicine before Science*, 233–6. Hoffman's worldview was based on a rational awareness of God, which could be revealed through the study of nature.

26 King, *Medical Enlightenment*, 181–200.

and season had its 'special diseases' and that climate exercised a profound effect upon human character. Similarly, he ascribed epidemics to different 'constitutions of the air', which affected the humours of the body and its solid parts through moisture, heat, and cold, and by carrying effluvia from decaying matter. Crucially, he identified heat as the quality of air most likely to be harmful to health and, like many tropical practitioners, claimed that the salubrity of air depended greatly on the position of the sun and the moon, attributing certain diseases to the moister, heavier, and denser air said to accompany a full moon.[27]

For most British physicians, this synthesis of ancient and modern wisdom became an article of faith, providing a bulwark against the reproaches of empirics and sceptical laymen. By stressing the accord between ancient and modern physicians, exponents of learned medicine hoped to counter accusations of confusion and dissension within their ranks. According to the physician John Barker, the work of Hoffman, Boerhaave, and other modern authorities conformed to a basic 'rule of practice' first espoused by Hippocrates: that is, to observe Nature and gently to assist her course.[28] The idea of a general rule of practice grounded in nature was one that appealed strongly to practitioners in the Indies. So, too, did many specific elements of the writings of Sydenham, Boerhaave, and Hoffman. But the majority of the practitioners who comprised the medical services of the Army, Navy, and East India Company were less concerned than Barker with questions of professional unity. They, too, invoked the spirits of ancient and modern authors but their exclusion from elite circles of power led them to make a virtue of dissent. The remainder of this chapter and those that follow provide an account of their critical engagement with European medicine and the formation of a relatively distinct branch of medicine in which they claimed unique authority and expertise.

British medical literature pertaining to the tropical colonies drew upon the scattered observations of European travellers (some of whom were from the British Isles) and a number of specifically medical texts written in the main by Portuguese and Dutch physicians who had worked in the East and West Indies during the course of the sixteenth and seventeenth centuries. The earliest European medical literature focusing on the tropics was concerned largely with India and the East Indies. From the mid-sixteenth century, Portuguese physicians and travellers, most notably Garcia da Orta (c. 1490–c. 1570), began to write about aspects of medical practice in colonies such as Goa.[29] Established in 1510, Goa was the principal Portuguese colony in India, but the Portuguese presence there also afforded European physicians the opportunity to venture further afield, including to the courts of Indian rulers

[27] Hoffman, *Fundamenta Medicinae*, 43–5. See also Barrett, *Disease and Geography*, 109–16.

[28] Barker, *An Essay on the Agreement betwixt Ancient and Modern Physicians.*

[29] Garcia da Orta (1490–1570) lived in India for about 36 years, from 1534 to his death in around 1570. His experience appears to have been limited to the west coast of India, being based in the Portuguese colony of Goa. See Boxer, 'Two Pioneers of Tropical Medicine'.

such as the Mughal emperors. It was at Goa, however, that the Portuguese established a considerable library of Indian and European books and manuscripts, not to mention the first printing press in the Indies, which was assembled in Goa in 1556.[30] Early Portuguese medical texts tended to concentrate on the therapeutic and other properties of Indian plants (together with a few other items), and their chief aim was probably to enlarge the therapeutic arsenal of those who practised in Europe. In so doing, they provided a critique of orthodox Galenic therapeutics, revealing its limitations and challenging accounts of certain drugs in classical Greek and Arabic texts. By contrast with later writers, da Orta said little about the role of climate and concentrated on types of behaviour conducive to health or productive of disease.[31] The malady known as *morxi* or *mordechi*, for instance – which bears a close resemblance to cholera or severe dysentery – was considered seasonal only in the sense of accompanying an abundance of fruit, which encouraged over-eating.[32] The same is true of Christophori a Costa's treatise on the spices and medicines indigenous to the East Indies, which followed much the same lines as da Orta's text and praised the latter as a 'rare and excellent genius'.[33] A Costa provided a concise summary of the materials described by da Orta with some additions, listing a variety of simples and spices and their various properties. Subsequent editions of his work carried additional comments and illustrations, but their focus remained sharply on *materia medica*, having little to say about aetiology.[34] Again, these works appear to have been intended as much for practitioners in Europe as those bound for the Indies, and it is probably significant that they were collected and edited by physicians who appear to have had no overseas experience.[35]

The lack of attention given to climate in these texts suggests that it is inappropriate to see them as landmarks of 'tropical medicine'.[36] In fact, there is little reason to suspect that climate or geography was central to the way in which medical practitioners understood diseases in the Indies at this time. Aetiology concentrated on the Galenic non-naturals rather than on the environment in a broader sense. Some Portuguese travel narratives did make reference to epidemics,[37] but most had little to say on the subject of disease,[38] and they often reflected on the absence from India of the pestilential fevers that ravaged

[30] Furber, *Rival Empires of Trade*, 325.

[31] Rather, '"The Six Things Non-Natural"'.

[32] Da Orta, *Coloquios*.

[33] A Costa, *Aromatum & medicamentum*, 4.

[34] A Costa (a.k.a. Cristivao da Costa, Cristobal Acosta, Christophile de la Coste, etc., c. 1515–92), was a physician and surgeon of Burgos in north-western Spain. The first edition of his work was translated into Latin by the Flemish botanist Clusius (Charles de l'Ecluse), who also translated da Orta's *Coloquios*.

[35] e.g. Colin (ed. and tr.), *Histoire des Drogues*. Colin was a master apothecary at Lyon and sought to augment European pharmacopoeia with drugs from the East.

[36] e.g. Boxer, 'Two Pioneers'.

[37] Zupanov, 'Drugs, Health, Bodies and Souls in the Tropics', 1–2, 38–9.

[38] De Castenada, *Historie of the Discoverie and Conquest of the Portingales*.

Europe.[39] When epidemics did occur, they were often attributed to decadence and immortality as much as environmental factors.[40] This broadly favourable or at least neutral view of the region's climate persisted well into the seventeenth century. Although medical and lay authors began to pay more attention to climate as a cause of disease, it was seen in terms of a divinely ordained balance between destructive and creative forces.[41]

According to most authors, the principal scourge of the East Indies was the dysentery, or 'bloody flux', which was by far the most fatal malady affecting Europeans.[42] The terrifying outbreaks of dysentery in European settlements spurred some medical practitioners to investigate further the causes of disease. Writing of an outbreak of flux among Portuguese troops during the siege of Columbo in 1588, the historian Manuel de Faria y Sousa observed that, 'The Doctors opening some that died of it, found their Entrails impostumated, which they said proceeded from Heat occasioned by Drought.' Afterwards, they were said to have employed cooling medicines to good effect.[43] In India, outbreaks of the disease known as *morxi* also prompted the dissection of some of those who died from it, the earliest case being the opening of a man who died from disease in Goa in 1543. The dissection was ordered by the governor of the colony.[44]

The practice of dissecting bodies with a view to discovering the nature of disease was still comparatively rare in Europe, but morbid anatomy seems to have been an important feature of European medicine in the Indies almost from the beginning. In the majority of cases, these early dissections are recorded by laymen rather than medical practitioners, but that began to change in the seventeenth century, as morbid anatomy began to figure prominently in medical texts. The first European practitioner to commit his observations on morbid anatomy to print was Jacob de Bondt, or Bontius (1592–1631), who was employed as head surgeon with the Dutch East India Company at Batavia (Jakarta).[45] Batavia was the main outpost of the Dutch East India Company in the East Indies and an important trading post, not only for spices – the main business of the Dutch Company in the region – but also for silver and silk. Europeans seem to have lived in Batavia much as they would in Amsterdam, wearing similar clothes and adopting similar lifestyles, few of which were conducive to health.[46] Sickness and death rates in the Dutch settlement were

[39] Harrison, *Climates*, 27.
[40] Zupanov, 'Drugs', 38–9.
[41] Terry, in *The Travels of Pietro della Valle*, 373.
[42] Chang et al., *The English Factory in Taiwan*, 608, 627.
[43] De Faria y Sousa, *Portuguese Asia*, vol. 3, 52.
[44] Zupanov, 'Drugs', 1–2.
[45] Bontius was the first head of surgery in the Dutch Company's Asian settlements. He worked at the hospital contained within the Company's bamboo fort; a brick-built structure being constructed some years after Bontius's death. See Bruijn, *Ship's Surgeons of the Dutch East India Company*, 97–8. He was educated at the University of Leiden.
[46] Furber, *Rival Empires of Trade*, 302–3.

consequently high and provided plenty of work for the Company's surgeons. However, as an important commercial centre, Batavia also presented considerable opportunities to surgeons wishing to purchase exotic medical substances, and those inclined to do so could easily enlist the help of Javanese practitioners. Indeed, in the seventeenth century, this was far from unusual.[47]

Bontius availed himself of all these opportunities. He took advantage of the high mortality during the siege of Batavia in 1628 to conduct post-mortem examinations of Europeans who had perished from diseases such as dysentery; his observations being set down in the last of the four 'books' – manuscripts sent individually to his brother in 1631[48] – that comprise *De medicina Indorum* (1642). The previous three books contain critical notes on da Orta's descriptions of plants and medical dialogues, as well as sections on diet and health, and on the medical method most appropriate to practice in the East Indies. The manuscripts which constitute *De medicina Indorum* offered guidance primarily to those practising medicine in the region. The third and fourth sections are particularly interesting in this regard because they represent the first attempts systematically to understand the diseases of the East Indies as clinical entities, in relation to the locality that produced them. *De medicina Indorum* thus contains detailed descriptions of a range of fevers, dysentery, hepatitis, cholera morbus, and barbiers – a disease resembling beriberi. Book III is divided into chapters describing these different types of disease, each beginning with an account of their symptoms, periodicity, and so forth.[49] The method employed in Bontius's medical works is fundamentally the same as in his observations on the flora and fauna of the East Indies.[50] Like da Orta, Bontius ascribed some of these diseases to individual behaviour, particularly over-indulgence in alcohol and fruits, but he dwelt longer than his predecessors on the relationship of disease to meteorological conditions. Barbiers, dysentery, and hepatitis were among the diseases that Bontius ascribed at least in part to the air of Batavia,[51] which often became unwholesome because of the action of heat and moisture in accelerating putrefaction, as was often said to be the case with epidemics of plague in Europe and Egypt.[52]

In this respect, Bontius's writings resemble those of Prospero Alpini (Alpinus) more closely than da Orta, and it is significant that later editions of *De medicina Indorum* were published alongside Alpini's *De medicina Ægyptiorum*.[53] Bontius's account of the relationship between climate and disease is similar to Alpini's, especially in its treatment of heat and putrefaction. However, *De medicina Indorum* is not as detailed as Alpini's treatise and does not digress into the relationship

47 Boomgaard, 'Dutch Medicine in Asia'; Cook, *Matters of Exchange.*
48 Cook, *Matters of Exchange*, 209.
49 e.g. chapter 14 of Book 3 on fever. See Bontius, *De medicina Indorum.*
50 Cook, 'Global Economies and Local Knowledge'.
51 Bontius, *An Account of the Diseases*, 2, 15.
52 Woodall, *The Surgion's Mate*, 326.
53 Alpini, *De medicina Ægyptiorum.*

between climate and human character. Like the Hippocratic text *Airs, Waters and Places*, Alpini made much of the effects of climate on the temperament and longevity of Egypt's inhabitants,[54] whereas Bontius's description of Batavia in relation to disease is much briefer and to the point. The health of the port, according to Bontius, depended largely on the direction of the wind: if it blew from the mountains across the stagnant water of the marshes close to the town, its air became impregnated with poisonous and foetid vapours, but if the wind blew from the sea it purified the air, while preserving the humours from putrefaction.[55] This account of putrefaction was consistent with contemporary European literature on fevers (as derived from the work of Jean Fernel, for example), and Bontius drew analogies between the effects of land winds in Batavia and Europe, particularly the dangers of mountain winds in Italy, France, and Spain.

In Book IV, Bontius moved from a description of the diseases of Batavia to a brief account of their pathology.[56] He had received an excellent training in anatomy at Leiden and he set about elucidating the nature and course of diseases by dissection, aided by two resident surgeons at the Dutch hospital.[57] From these dissections (nine are recorded), he drew inferences about the relationship of various organs to the symptoms of diseases and about which organs were most sensitive to the climate of the tropics. He was the first author to conclude that the liver was particularly liable to disease if Europeans spent too long in tropical climates; partly on account of that organ's sensitivity to heat and partly because of heavy consumption of alcoholic liquors.[58] The liver was to become central to the pathology of tropical diseases during the eighteenth century, when it was reckoned to be the seat of most ailments suffered by Europeans. Bontius's approach to the study of disease thus combined insights from pathology with close observation of the symptoms exhibited by patients at the Dutch East India Company's hospital in Batavia. Like some physicians in Europe, he saw morbid anatomy as a branch of natural philosophy; as one of several means of obtaining information about the nature of disease that might be useful in arriving at a cure. He did not, however, attempt to classify disease, insisting that 'The fevers of India were too erratic and irregular to be reduced to classes.'[59]

In its attention to the connection between locality and disease, *De medicina Indorum* set the tone for many works on the East Indies written in the seventeenth century. As commercial intercourse between Europe and Asia became more frequent, and as the countries of the East Indies were explored more extensively by Europeans, there was a growing tendency to differentiate between localities and their maladies. Sir Thomas Herbert's *Travels into Africa and Asia*

[54] Ibid., Book 1, chap. 12, 20ff., 35.
[55] Bontius, *Account*, 10–16.
[56] Bontius, *De medicina*, Book 4.
[57] Cook, *Matters of Exchange*, 194–5.
[58] Bontius, *Account*, 30.
[59] Ibid., 61.

(1638) was typical in this respect, taking into account such factors as the mineral content of soils and conditions of the atmosphere produced by heat and putrescence.[60] His account employed a Hippocratic vocabulary in which the air was ascribed anthropomorphic qualities such as benevolence and wholesomeness.[61] Most writers on the East Indies agreed on the medical dangers of the rainy season, for example, as well as of land winds, which blew pestilential vapours from swamps and marshes.[62] Indeed, such considerations were beginning to play a part in the selection of localities for European settlements and there was a distinct preference for elevated locations which would be both cooler and more distant from marshes and other sources of miasma.[63] Old Goa and the first European settlement at the port of Bandar Abass in Persia were abandoned for precisely these reasons.[64] While certain locations were considered altogether unsuitable, seventeenth-century authors generally believed that Europeans could adapt to tropical climates if they took sufficient care to avoid the worst localities and if they regulated their behaviour in such a way as to mitigate the adverse effects of climate. Provided this advice was followed, there seemed to be no reason why Europeans should not enjoy their health as much as at home.[65]

The advice given to those embarking for the East Indies was still very traditional and based on regulation of the non-naturals. Europeans were prescribed a regimen appropriate to their constitution and for each season of the year, the most common advice being to avoid excessive indulgence in alcohol, food, and sexual relations, all of which were said to weaken the constitution and render it more liable to disease. Some Europeans, particularly the Portuguese, also engaged in prophylactic bloodletting, in the hope that their plethoric constitutions would be renewed with blood that was thinner and better adapted to life in the tropics. British residents in the East Indies were rather less inclined to do this, although the practice was not altogether unheard of. Another means of acclimatizing oneself was to eat native foods and to adopt aspects of local dress, but even this was comparatively rare. The diet of Indians, for example, was reckoned by many to be insufficiently nourishing for Europeans.[66]

Most writers on the East Indies tried to make sense of the relationship between locality and disease by referring to the great authorities of classical antiquity, particularly the Hippocratic text *Airs, Waters and Places.* Although it was not a standard part of the medical curriculum, *Airs, Waters and Places* fascinated many philosophically inclined practitioners.[67] It posited a causal relationship between the

60 Herbert, *Some Years Travels*, 43.
61 Ibid., 40, 343–4; Bontius, *Account*, 110–11.
62 Ovington, *A Voyage to Suratt*, 61–3.
63 e.g. the location of the Carmelite monastery at Goa; see *Six Voyages de Jean Baptiste Tavernier*, 159.
64 Martin, *Mémoirs*, 424; Boxer, *Portuguese Society in the Tropics*, 31–2; Pearson, 'First Contacts'.
65 Harrison, *Climates*, chap. 1.
66 Ibid., 32–57.
67 Siraisi, *The Clock and the Mirror*, 128–9.

natural world and human characteristics, explained in terms of the humoral theory of disease. Thus localities exposed to cold, northerly winds tended to produce inhabitants that were sturdy and lean, with fierce temperaments and a tendency to bilious and ophthalmic diseases. Those accustomed to warm south-westerlies, by contrast, tended to be flabby and phlegmatic. The text also made specific observations on the peoples of Europe, North Africa, and Asia, although the latter are confined to the west and centre of the continent. The author's remarks are to some extent evaluative, with distinctions being drawn between the courage of different races, for example.[68]

European travellers in Asia tended to make similar generalizations, but from the end of the seventeenth century their observations were rendered increasingly in terms of the New Philosophy. John Fryer's *A New Account of East India and Persia* (1698) is a case in point. A Cambridge-educated physician, Fryer embarked on a lengthy tour of India in 1672, undertaken in the interests of the East India Company.[69] His main aims in writing were to counter some of the unfavourable descriptions given of English expeditions to India in French travel literature and to provide information useful for commercial ventures. Fryer also managed to convey a religious message and one aim of the book was to reclaim atheists, 'by leading them . . . to behold the Beauty, Order, and admirable Disposition of the Universe'.[70] Fryer's natural theology resembles earlier travel narratives in its providential ideas, but his specific intention was most likely to counter the atheistic implications of Hobbesian philosophy.[71] The order and regularity of the Newtonian universe was often used at this time to augment scriptural authority and was particularly attractive to latitudinarians, who adopted Newtonianism to naturalize their atomistic yet harmonious view of social order. It was an outlook shared by most fellows of the early Royal Society, and as a fellow himself, it is not surprising that Fryer took a similar view.[72]

In most respects, Fryer's *Account* differs little from previous travel narratives, not least in its treatment of the relationship between localities and health. Situations such as marshes and swamps are identified as unhealthy and productive of fluxes and fevers, as are certain seasons, especially the monsoons. As in earlier literature, the native inhabitants are said to be resistant to the effects of climate, whereas European newcomers are the most vulnerable, especially the young and plethoric. As he put it, 'we are here, as Exotick Plants brought home to us, not agreeable to the Soil . . . but to old Men and Women it seems to be more suitable.'[73] Fryer attributed the high incidence of malignant and putrid fevers in the least healthy settlements (such as Bombay) to rapid putrefaction,

68 'Airs, Waters and Places', in Lloyd, *Hippocratic Writings.*
69 Goodwin, *rev.* Carter, 'Fryer, John (*d.* 1733)', *DNB.*
70 Fryer, Preface, *A New Account of East India and Persia.*
71 See Shapin and Schaffer, *Leviathan and the Air Pump.*
72 Jacob, *Newtonians.*
73 Fryer, *New Account,* 68–9.

particularly during the monsoon. The atmosphere generated disease in two ways: firstly, by producing noisome particles which became suspended in the air; secondly, by impairing the body's vital processes, particularly digestion. For this reason, Europeans were liable to fluxes, dropsies, barbiers, gout, stones, and of course malignant and putrid fevers.[74] Yet the monsoon was not an unmitigated evil as far as health was concerned, for the rains had a cleansing effect. 'This City is very nasty by their [the Indian's] want of privies', he wrote, 'and their making every Door a Dunghill; yet never had they any Plague, the Heats evaporating, and the Rains washing this filth away.'[75]

The framework for Fryer's natural-historical account of disease was conventionally Hippocratic,[76] yet some his descriptions reveal the influence of the corpuscular theories developed by Boyle and others. Writing of the mountain air of the Western Ghats, for instance, Fryer wrote of 'the flowing Particles of the Atmosphere' which were cooler and purer than the hotter, stagnant air in the plains below.[77] Although there is no evidence that Fryer had read Boyle's *General History of the Air*, it is likely that he was familiar with it, as he was elected a Fellow of the Royal Society in 1697 and appears to have remained one for ten years.[78] It is also likely that Fryer knew the work of Sydenham and Hoffman, which also bore the imprint of particulate theories of matter. Like Hoffman and the Hippocratic writers, Fryer believed that effluvia suspended in the air were among the main causes of fever and like Hoffman and Boyle, he also emphasized the pathogenic affects of heat. Hoffman attributed the prevalence of fevers in Mediterranean countries to their hot summers, compared with the north of the continent.[79] Boyle also drew on evidence from those who had travelled in the East and West Indies to supplement his own observations on the adverse affects of weather on the human body.[80]

By the end of the seventeenth century, the works of Bontius and other practitioners who had written on the East Indies were fairly well known in Europe,[81] but the first authors who attempted to describe the diseases of the

[74] Fryer, *New Account*, 68.
[75] Ibid., 113.
[76] Ibid., 113–14.
[77] Ibid., 129.
[78] Hunter, *The Royal Society*, 149.
[79] Hoffman, *Fundamenta medicinae*, 44.
[80] Boyle saw the air as a diaphanous fluid consisting of three kinds of 'corpuscles': exhalations from terrestrial matter, magnetic particles, and 'elastical' particles. The latter were crucial to Boyle's notions of the effects of heat upon the air, likening them to the springs of watches that were coiled due to compression by an external force, but continually endeavouring to stretch themselves out. Heat was one of the most powerful agents which caused this expansion or rarefaction of the air. He illustrated these points with examples from the East Indies, among other places. Boyle, *The General History of the Air*, 44–5, 152–3, 245.
[81] It is evident, for example, that the descriptions of the East Indies found in Ramazzini's popular treatise on the relationship between climate and disease are drawn from the work of Bontius. See Ramazzini, *Health Preserved*, Book 1. His work on the atmospheric origins of epidemics was first published as *De constitutione anni M.DC.LXXXX* (1690).

West Indies did not refer to them. Their reference points were still, in the main, classical authorities such as Hippocrates and popular accounts of voyages of discovery. Dr Henry Stubbe's observations on the Caribbean islands are typical in this respect. Formerly a Parliamentarian, though not a Puritan, the idiosyncratic Stubbe (Stubbes) made peace with the restored monarchy and through the recommendation of the king's principal physician, Alexander Frazier, was appointed Charles II's physician to Jamaica in 1662, being granted £200 for expenses. Finding the climate disagreeable, Stubbe returned to England two years later and began to practise medicine in Warwick. Although his experience was limited, Stubbe recounted his observations on Jamaica and his voyage there to the Royal Society, his account being published in the *Philosophical Transactions* in 1668. Stubbe was profoundly dissatisfied at the lukewarm reception his works received at the Royal Society and he subsequently became an inveterate critic, satirizing its fellows and their work in a flurry of scurrilous pamphlets.[82] His account displayed similar preoccupations to contemporary literature on the East Indies and, in some measure, reflected the preoccupations of the Royal Society in its attention to the affects of air upon the human body:

> The Change of Climat [sic] and the effects of it are very sensible to our Bodies, as we approach the *Tropick*. There usually happened (as you may observe in *Purchas's* Voyages) sickness in our ships about that time; and as soon as the seamen pass the *Tropick*, they still use expressions of Joy by firing of Guns in testimony of their gladness for their safe arrival so far.[83]

However, Stubbe believed that the worst effects of the transition from temperate to tropical latitudes could be avoided by prophylactic measures, including bloodletting. Although bleeding seems to have been unpopular with the English in the East Indies, it was sometimes resorted to by seamen voyaging to the West Indian islands. Stubbe explained that bloodletting was necessary because English constitutions were naturally plethoric on account of the high proportion of meat in their diet. If not corrected, they would experience quickening of the pulse and dullness and oppression of spirits.[84]

Stubbe's account was concerned with far more than medicine, however, and the first treatise written specifically on the diseases of the West Indies did not appear until a few years later, in the form of Thomas Trapham's *Discourse of the State of Health in the Island of Jamaica* (1679). Trapham bore the same forename

[82] Feingold, 'Stubbe [Stubbes, Stubb], Henry (1632–1676)', *DNB*; Cook, 'Physicians and the New Philosophy'; Jacob, *Henry Stubbe*. Although Stubbe courted the Society for a brief period until the publication of his 'Observations', he had earlier been a critic of the Oxford Experimental Philosophy Club, most of whom were among the Society's founder members. See Webster, *Great Instauration*, 158–72. On the Royal Society, natural history and travel narratives more generally, see Carey, 'Compiling Nature's History'.

[83] Stubbe, 'An Enlargement of the Observations', 707.

[84] Ibid., 708.

as his father, who was an eminent surgeon closely associated with the parliamentarian cause during the Civil War. It was the elder Trapham who prepared the body of the executed Charles I for burial, quipping that he had 'sewn on the goose's head'. Later the same year, he was awarded an MB by Oxford University, which had been recently purged of Royalists, followed by an MD in 1658. Afterwards, he became Cromwell's personal surgeon on his Irish and Scottish campaigns and was appointed surgeon to the Savoy military hospital in London in 1651. He was prominent in local affairs and held several non-medical offices, including that of land-tax assessor. His greatest interest, however, was in religious affairs and he was a strident Presbyterian. Following the Restoration and the passage of the Test, Uniformity and Corporation Acts, Trapham was dismissed from his offices and appeared in court on a number of occasions for attending illegal assemblies.[85]

Trapham's son was also educated at Oxford (Magdalen) during the Interregnum, but did not study medicine there, proceeding to Leiden in 1663 and thence to Caen, where he took his medical degree. The fact that he did not remain in England after the Restoration suggests that, like his father, he found the atmosphere uncomfortable. This may also account for his decision to proceed to Jamaica in or about 1668, where he established a medical practice and became an active member of the island's assembly.[86] Apart from this, little is known of his time in Jamaica, except that he met his death in an earthquake which destroyed the island's first capital, Port Royal, in 1690. With so little information about Trapham's career, it would be foolish to speculate about any connection between his writings and his family background. However, his decision to migrate to Jamaica reminds us of the attractions of the colonies to Dissenters, including other medical practitioners.[87] Indeed, it will become evident that many of the foremost practitioners in India and the West Indies hailed from Dissenting backgrounds and were active in networks of Dissenting physicians and natural philosophers. As E. P. Thompson once cautioned, 'Dissent' can be a misleading term, as it covers so many sections and intellectual tendencies.[88] Quakers and Unitarians figure strongly among those whose careers are examined here, but in many cases it is impossible to identify sects with certainty, and we are left only with associations between individuals and occasional expressions of opinion. But however difficult it may be to identify in some cases, the links between colonial practice and the Dissenting tradition are strong and ought not to be overlooked.

Trapham's medical writings certainly display something of his family's uncompromising Presbyterianism, containing many digressions on providence and

[85] See Brod, 'Thomas Trapham'; Kupperman, 'Fear of Hot Climates'.

[86] Munk, *The Roll of the Royal College of Physicians of London* [hereafter, Munk's *Roll*], vol. 1, 345; *Journals of the Assembly of Jamaica*, 1821, 164.

[87] On the diaspora of Dissenting physicians more generally, see Birken, 'The Dissenting Tradition in English Medicine', 200–1.

[88] Thompson, *The Making of the English Working Class*, 28.

matters of morality and health, particularly the degeneracy of the Catholic powers and their colonies. His book is peppered with references to 'lazy Spaniards' devoted to vice and 'easie Pleasure', who had neglected the stewardship of their plantations. It was through their sensual indulgence with what Trapham termed 'the animal People' of the Indies that they had been infected with the pox, which had been communicated to Europe with the return of Columbus and disseminated there by Spanish troops. Trapham believed that the venereal poison originated in American Indians, like yaws in Africans, because they had coupled with beasts. The spread of the disease to the Spanish thus provided ample evidence of their unfitness to rule an empire, and he felt it his duty to warn his countrymen ('intending Conquerours' [sic]) 'to escape the same degenerating Pit of naturally necessary destruction'.[89] England had seized Jamaica from the Spanish in 1655 and in the years thereafter it developed rapidly into a sugar-based economy which generated enormous wealth for a few.[90] This bounty and the relative social freedoms of the island fostered lifestyles which many regarded as decadent. Trapham was clearly concerned about the moral downfall of the island's people, and it is rather ironic that he should have lost his life in an earthquake which many regarded as divine punishment for the godless ways of its inhabitants.

However, Trapham's main concern was to inform newcomers to the island about its natural history and to warn them of ills arising from its environment. He saw himself as a 'Samaritan', whose conscience dictated that he assist new residents in understanding the maladies of Jamaica and how to prevent and treat them.[91] Trapham believed that the two main features of tropical airs – heat and moisture – were complementary, the one mitigating the other. This fortunate outcome was attributed to the action of the two principal heavenly bodies, the fierce heat of the sun being softened by moisture, which was thought to derive from the action of the moon. Its influence loosened the 'saline bonds' of the sea, producing salty matter for the sea breezes which, in turn, refreshed the island by stirring its stagnating air. The movement of the sea breezes was, itself, thought to be due to the heat of the sun.[92] Trapham's *Discourse* was thus impregnated with the same providential ideas that dominated texts on the climate of the East Indies, the only peculiarity being that providence was in this instance gendered, acting through a balance between male and female principles. 'Male qualities', he wrote, 'can never be benign enough without amorous mixtures of female softness; thus Male and Female created He them, and they replenished the earth'.[93] Less poetically, Trapham added that the air of the island was full of nitrous matter, for the winds blew over large deposits of saltpetre, which helped to

[89] Trapham, *A Discourse of the State of Health in the Island of Jamaica*, 23–4, 112–13, 117.
[90] See Dunn, *Sugar and Slaves*.
[91] Trapham, *Discourse*, 2.
[92] Ibid., 5–6.
[93] Ibid., 13, 53.

preserve the body against putrefaction and which acted as a cooling stimulant.[94] The 'thick' but briskly moving air of Jamaica, softened and cooled by moisture and native minerals, rendered the island habitable and free from many of the worst ailments of Europe. The absence of plague was attributed to these qualities, as was the fact that fevers tended to be of the mild intermittent type, rather than the putrid or continued varieties. Smallpox and scurvy were seldom to be found and many diseases common in Europe seemed to diminish in severity.[95]

With its many references to *Airs, Waters and Places*, Trapham's *Discourse* resembles the writings of Bontius, Fryer, and others who described the diseases of the East Indies. However, his account of fevers was in some respects more traditional, harking back to the belief that they were produced by a combination of natural and preternatural heat.[96] According to Trapham, the most common maladies such as intermittent fevers or agues were due solely to the excessive heat of the tropics and not, as others believed, to the influence of some poisonous miasma. The island's heat was implicated in two ways: firstly, by producing an excess of what Trapham termed 'Choler' (yellow bile); secondly, by preventing a healthy discharge of this humour from the body.[97] But the agues of Jamaica were seldom fatal and this led Trapham to conclude that the physician ought to mimic the island's atmospheric equilibrium. Following the Hippocratic dictum that nature should never be forced but led, he insisted that 'Nature is the curer of all her diseases' and the physician but an 'observing Minister'. In this case, it lay to the physician simply to prescribe a cooling regimen, in order to remove the excessive heat.[98]

The writings of Trapham and others contributed to a growing interest in the effects of air on human health, especially in the august circles of the Royal Society, in which Boyle, Hooke, and others had already embarked upon similar investigations. By the 1680s, the meteorology of the tropics was being systematically investigated,[99] the most notable contribution coming in a presentation to the Royal Society by the astronomer Edmund Halley, who put forward an account of the trade winds, which, he thought, arose from rarefaction and cooling of the air. Halley based his account partly on his own experience of living in tropical regions and partly on those of navigators acquainted with the Indies.[100] The debts acknowledged by Halley and Boyle show that voyages of discovery, colonial expansion, and trade were providing English natural philosophers with important insights into the workings of nature.[101] The same was true of medicine. Correspondents from around the world sent their own observations back to England in the hope of

94 Trapham, *Discourse*, 17.
95 Ibid., 17, 68–9, 70–1.
96 Ibid., 77–8.
97 Ibid., 84.
98 Ibid., 79–80, 87.
99 Cosgrove, 'Tropic and Tropicality'.
100 Halley, 'An Historical Account of the Trade Winds'.
101 Shapin, *A Social History of Truth*, 194–6; Grafton, *New Worlds, Ancient Texts*.

having them discussed at the Royal Society and printed in its *Transactions*, and they were positively encouraged to do so. Letters were received from a range of learned gentlemen rather than just physicians, illustrating the extent to which non-specialists were able to participate in discussions of medical and philosophy. One such, from a clergyman, appeared in the *Philosophical Transactions* in 1693, describing the seasonal incidence of fever in the colony of Virginia. The letter noted the coincidence of endemic diseases such as fevers, fluxes, and dropsy with the onset of rainy weather in September, the bodies of settlers having already been weakened by the intense heat of summer. As in much contemporary literature on fevers, the proximate cause of these diseases was said to be a 'ferment' in the blood; the author concluded that 'Tis wonderful what influence Air has over Mens Bodies.'[102]

In such accounts it was assumed that the air was capable of moulding human bodies, even to the extent of determining their colour and texture, quite apart from their susceptibility to disease. In the East Indies, it was already common to attribute the differences between Europeans and native inhabitants, as well as between the different 'races' of Asia, to the effects of climate. These relatively fluid categories bore the imprint of *Airs, Waters and Places* but also harmonized with local ideas about the effects of climate on physical and mental characteristics.[103] The same was true up to a point for the Americas and the West Indies, but there was a distinct difference in the way in which African bodies were discussed, with hereditary differences featuring more prominently. In a letter to the Royal Society in 1675, Dr Thomas Towns claimed that:

> The Blood of the *Negro's* [sic] is almost as black as their skin. I have seen drawn forth the Blood of at least twenty, both sick and in health, and the supersicies of it all is as dark, as the bottom of any *European* Blood, after standing a while in a dish. So that the Blackness of *Negro's* is likely to be inherent in them, and not caused by the scorching of the Sun, especially feeling that other Creatures here, that live in the same Clime and heat with them, have as florid Blood as those that are in a cold Latitude.[104]

Although ideas about race mostly reflected the dominance of Hippocratic accounts,[105] other theories derived from antiquity proposed the propagation of blackness through lineal descent.[106] Towns's theory may be typical of the latter, but it may also presage a more systematic medical interest in the composition of African bodies, which was soon to base racial distinctions on clinical and

[102] 'A letter from Mr John Clayton, Rector of Crofton at Wakefield in Yorkshire, to the Royal Society, May 12 1688, giving an Account of several Observations in Virginia, and in his Voyage thither, more particularly concerning the Air', *Phil. Trans.*, 17 (1693), 781–95.

[103] Harrison, *Climates*, chap. 1.

[104] 'An Extract of Mr Listers, containing some Observations made at the Barbado's', *Phil. Trans.*, 10 (1675), 399–400.

[105] See Glacken, *Traces on the Rhodian Shore*, Part 3; Harrison, *Climates*, chap. 1; Goldenberg, 'The Development of the Idea of Race'; Floyd-Wilson, *English Ethnicity and Race.*

[106] e.g. George Best's *True Discourse of the Three Voyages of Discoverie* (1578). See Hannaford, *Race*, 166–7.

pathological observations.[107] Either way, physical difference was beginning to loom large in writings on disease and climate, the dominant idea being that European newcomers were vulnerable until their bodies had acclimatized.

One of the few people to challenge the medical lore of the West Indies was the physician Hans Sloane, who published the first part of a medical and natural-historical account of his voyage to Madeira, Barbados, Neves, St Christophers, and Jamaica in 1707. Sloane (1660–1753) arrived in Jamaica as a young man, taking up an appointment as personal physician to the Duke of Albemarle. Apart from the prospect of lucrative employment and high status as a physician to an aristocrat, Sloane was tempted by the prospect of discovering natural remedies, previously unknown in Europe. In this, he drew inspiration from the Ancients: 'This voyage seem'd . . . to promise to be useful to me, as a Physician; many of the antient [sic] and best Physicians having travell'd to the places where their drugs were brought, to inform themselves concerning them.'[108] Like earlier writers, Sloane was truly impressed by the abundance and variety of tropical nature, and saw it as indubitable evidence of a divine architect.[109] Yet the diseases of the West Indies were not as different as most medical practitioners on the islands insisted. 'I was told that the diseases of the place are all different, from what they are in Europe', he recalled, 'and to be treated in a differing method.' But Sloane claimed that he 'never saw a disease in Jamaica which I had not met with in Europe',[110] and was sceptical of the common belief on the islands in a 'seasoning fever': a kind of rite of passage through which European bodies became inured to the climate.[111]

Sloan was very much in a minority, however. Most of his contemporaries insisted on the peculiarities of warm climates and acted accordingly, easing their passage from one clime to another.[112] The framework for understanding these differences was beginning to show signs of change, with use of terms drawn from corpuscular and mechanical philosophy. But in essence it remained Hippocratic: it was fundamentally the same as *Airs, Waters and Places* in its emphasis upon the seasonality of disease and the ascription of moral qualities to climates and peoples, the latter being moulded to some extent by the former. The task of the physician appeared to be that of gently assisting Nature rather than intervening violently to thwart her. In the coming century, this situation was to change radically. The theological view of a divinely ordained balance within each climate was slowly abandoned in favour of a medicalized cartography which stressed the differences between, and similarities within, specific climatic zones.

[107] Saakwa-Mante, 'Western Medicine and Racial Constitutions'.

[108] Sloan, *Voyage*, vol. 1, i. On Sloan's collection, see Kniz, 'Curiosities, Commodities and Transplanted Bodies'.

[109] Sloan, *Voyage*, vol. 1, iii.

[110] Ibid., xc.

[111] Ibid., xcviii.

[112] Kupperman, 'Hot Climates', 215.

2

'Accidents of the air': Sydenham and Boerhaave in the tropics

In 1704, William Oliver, a physician and Fellow of the Royal Society, observed that there were three schools of thought concerning fever among practitioners in London. One held that fevers arose from obstructions of the body which blocked perspiration, causing particles that were normally expelled to be trapped within the body, disordering the humours. Another, which he labelled 'Cartesian', supposed the essence of fever to consist in a 'troubled and disturbed mixture of the blood' caused by the introduction of extraneous matter. These foreign particles were thought to obstruct the free passage of the humours through the body, leading to fever. The majority of practitioners, however, subscribed to Thomas Willis's view that some 'poisonous ferment' seized the spirits and that fever was essentially a struggle between the animal spirits and some 'venomous enemy'.[1] If Oliver is a reliable witness, it would appear that the majority of practitioners attributed fevers to an external cause, most likely some form of particle or poison. Indeed, the role of aerial particles in the causation of fever was widely acknowledged, even by those who expressly challenged the incorporation of mechanistic natural philosophy into medicine.

One such was the Cambridge-educated physician Edward Strotter, whose treatise *Criticon febrium* (1716) was intended primarily to demonstrate the abuses of mathematics in physic. Strotter was critical of mechanistic physicians and their works on fever, attacking, among others, Lorenzo Bellini, George Cheyne, and Archibald Pitcairne.[2] He was not averse to physicians drawing insights from mathematics and natural philosophy, but he was hostile to what he regarded as an 'affected Shew of Learning' that purported to place the truth of the author's argument beyond all doubt. Strotter's claims were more modest but, in common with some mechanists, he did make use of the Newtonian concept of gravity, and made references to particulate matter in the atmosphere and in the

[1] Oliver, *A Practical Essay*, 12–14.

[2] See King, *Philosophy of Medicine*, chap. 5; Cunningham, 'Sydenham versus Newton'; Guerrini, 'Archibald Pitcairne'; idem, 'Isaac Newton, George Cheyne and the "Principia Medicinae"'; Friesen, 'Archibald Pitcairne'.

blood. In this lay the essence of Strotter's own theory of fevers, which was that they were 'the mediate Product of some deprav'd State of the Blood, put into a Hurry from some external Accident of the Air'.[3]

The atmospheric conditions that gave rise to disease were clearly of growing interest to medical practitioners in Britain, most crediting Sydenham (via Boerhaave) with having revived this aspect of medicine. This was especially true of those who ventured to the East and West Indies, where practically all medical treatises from the 1720s acknowledged their debt to the 'English Hippocrates'. However, tropical practitioners were becoming increasingly aware of one another and, for the first time, those in the Caribbean began to draw on the slightly older corpus of literature pertaining to the East Indies. One early example is Richard Towne's treatise on the diseases of Barbados. Towne's life and career are scarcely documented, but it seems that he went to the island as a private physician, most likely engaged by the owner of a sugar plantation; he also appears to have been an acquaintance of Sloane, to whom his book is dedicated.[4] Like earlier writers, Towne paid homage to *Airs, Waters and Places* as the seminal work on the influence of the atmosphere on human bodies, but also acknowledged the contributions of more recent authors, including Alpini, Bontius, and Willem Piso (1611–78), who had written in emulation of Hippocrates on the diseases of South America.[5] But Towne was attempting to understand the relationship of climate to disease in a new way, using the concepts of mechanical philosophy, which seemed to offer a reliable basis for construing the relationship between cause and effect.[6] As noted earlier, some historians have also suggested that there was a close affinity between iatromechanical ideas of the kind exhibited by Towne and the Tory-Anglican worldview.[7] In this case, however, there is insufficient biographical information to enable us to establish such a connection. Moreover, there are so many exceptions to this generalization – the iatromechanical views of Whigs such as Richard Mead, for example – as to render claims for any exclusive religious or political affinity with mechanical philosophy problematic, to say the least.

Towne believed that tropical air affected health by acting directly upon the body, particularly the vascular system. Using a vocabulary reminiscent of Hoffman and Boerhaave, he argued that its 'additional *Moisture*, in Concurrence with the extraordinary *Heat* of the *Climate*, must render the Fibres of the Body more lax, abate the *Vigour* of the Circulation, encrease [sic] the *Viscidity* of the

[3] Srotter, *Criticon febrium*, 3–4, 80, 174.

[4] Towne, *A Treatise of the Diseases most frequent in the West-Indies*, iii.

[5] Piso was a physician and botanist who was based at the Dutch settlement in Brazil, 1633–44; see Cook, *Matters of Exchange*, 212–21. The first book of Piso's great work was headed, 'On Airs, Waters and Places'; see Piso, *De Indiae utriusque re naturali et medica*, 3–22.

[6] Towne, *Treatise*, 1.

[7] e.g. Jacob, *The Newtonians*; Friesen, 'Archibald Pitcairne'.

Blood, promote *sensible* and diminish *insensible Perspiration*'.[8] To this humid state of the atmosphere he attributed a wide range of maladies from fevers and dysentery, through to dropsy, elephantiasis, and general languor of the body. Fevers were the most common ailment and all Europeans who remained in the tropics for some time would be subject to a 'seasoning' fever, he warned. Referring to Sydenham's observation that fevers accounted for two-thirds of Mankind's ills, Towne asserted that the proportion was even higher in the West Indies.[9] However, he believed that Barbados posed little danger to Europeans once they had been seasoned, describing it as 'one of the most delightful Countries in the Creation'.[10] Drainage and cultivation had improved the health of the island's inhabitants, and the formerly endemic malady, dropsy, with its characteristic swellings and distended bellies, was less frequent than before. Towne attributed this to the clearance of much of the forest from the island, which had rendered its climate less moist.[11]

Other diseases, however, appeared to be only partly the product of climate, being aggravated by inappropriate behaviour. Dysentery and colic, for example, were common in sultry weather but attacked disproportionately those of bilious temperament or those who over-indulged in spirituous liquors, the latter tending to be black slaves or white servants.[12] This discrimination between the effects of climate on individual constitutions is found throughout Towne's treatise. Wet weather, he claimed, was generally agreeable to those with bilious temperaments, whereas warm weather suited persons of a moist, phlegmatic disposition.[13] This was a standard Hippocratic inference, but diseases such as elephantiasis – which affected mainly African slaves – posed a more difficult problem. Towne made the common observation that elephantiasis resembled leprosy and that black people were most liable to it after suffering from acute fever and other long illnesses. But unlike some other West Indian practitioners, he did not regard this susceptibility as being due to some innate propensity; rather, slaves were particularly liable to develop the disease because of their exposure to cold and damp, and their poor diet. For the same reason, the disease seldom occurred among white people and then only among those 'whose unhappy Circumstances have reduced them to Hardships but little inferior to what the *Blacks* are obliged to undergo'. He claimed that his explanation also accounted for the wide geographical distribution of the disease, which according to Lucretius and other classical authors had also appeared in North Africa and Egypt. Elephantiasis, in other words, was a disease typical of slave societies.[14]

Towne's text is, therefore, something of a hybrid. It is very traditional in its emphasis upon individual constitutions and the non-naturals but modern in its use of mechanical philosophy to account for the action of climate on human

[8] Towne, *Treatise*, 10–11. [9] Ibid., 19–20. [10] Ibid., 14.
[11] Ibid., 11.
[12] Ibid., 71, 114.
[13] Ibid., 7–8. [14] Ibid., 184–5.

bodies. Its prominent references to Sydenham mark it out from previous works on the diseases of hot climates and locate it at the beginning of a new genre of literature, in which practitioners invoked Sydenham and Hippocrates as symbols of empirical enquiry.

Henry Warren's treatise on pestilential fevers in Barbados is also typical in this respect, likening the malignant fever he experienced there in the 1730s to a fever described by Sydenham:

> I am of opinion, that this Fever is truly of the *Pestilential* Kind, and ought properly to be called by no other Denomination. It resembles very nearly (except in that the Condition of the Blood is not the same) the Pestilential Fever described by Dr Sydenham, which continued for some time after the Plague of *London*, and it is attended with many Appearances, peculiar to the Plague itself.[15]

Like Trapham and Towne, Warren appears to have worked in the West Indies as a private practitioner, probably on a sugar plantation, and like them, his observations of disease were solely ante-mortem. None of these three physicians drew insights from morbid anatomy, perhaps, like Sydenham, because they believed it could tell them little, or like Warren, because they feared the possibility of infection from corpses that had died from putrid diseases. Although they would have had the opportunity to dissect African slaves if they so desired, they would not have had the steady supply of bodies available to surgeons in the Army, Navy, and East India Company. As physicians, too, they may have shared the distaste shown by some of their colleagues for morbid anatomy, which some regarded as the province of surgeons.

In this sense, the approach taken by Trapham, Towne, and Warren differed from that of Bontius and the majority of practitioners who were later to study disease in the East and West Indies. But in other respects, there are close affinities, particularly their natural-historical interest in disease and the primacy of climatic factors in their writings. Indeed, references to Bontius in British West Indian texts suggest a growing affinity between practitioners in the East and West Indies and, in the coming decades, cross-referencing between the two regions became more common, as did comparisons with other warm climates, such as the Middle East and the Mediterranean.[16] This was one consequence of the increasing volume of commercial and naval traffic between these regions and the growth of military settlements in both India and the Caribbean. There was now a sense that hot climates, if not yet the tropics in particular, constituted a distinct disease zone. European travellers were also becoming accustomed to the idea that their

[15] Warren, *A Treatise concerning the Malignant Fever in Barbados*, 3.

[16] This appears to have occurred earlier in Dutch writings. Piso discusses the work of Bontius (which was clearly an inspiration) at the beginning of his natural historical and medical account of Brazil, although it is not extensively referenced in the remainder of the book. See *De Indiae*, Preface.

bodies would alter on reaching hot countries, 'paying tribute', as one traveller put it, to the change of the air by succumbing to a 'very painful purple fever'.[17]

From Sloane's remarks at the beginning of the eighteenth century, it is evident that most inhabitants of the West Indies already regarded their maladies as very different from those in Europe, to the extent that they required different forms of treatment. By the 1750s, such sentiments were also being expressed by military and naval surgeons, who normally remained in overseas stations for just a few years at a time. In an address to the Society of Naval Surgeons in 1751, the military surgeon George Cleghorn opened with the remark that, 'as many of you must be sensible, how little the best Information we can acquire in this temperate Climate, qualifies us for treating the Diseases which are frequent in warmer Latitudes', and called upon 'all who practise Physick in our Country to make proper Observations on the Sick, and communicate them to the Public, which should soon have a more exact and ample History of Diseases'.[18] In view of this, surgeons began to record not only the diseases that occurred in their stations but also the meteorological conditions that accompanied them, with a view to drawing inferences about the seasonality of disease. This is precisely what Cleghorn did on his arrival on Minorca in 1743, where he kept a daily diary of disease and weather until 1749, when his regiment left the island.[19]

Cleghorn used his observations to highlight points of contrast with the opinions of European authorities. His main object of study was the tertian ague of Minorca, the island's principal endemic malady. One of the European physicians whom Cleghorn criticized was Hoffman, who had carefully enumerated the fits in regular, distinct tertian fevers, according to the order in which they appeared. According to Cleghorn, the observations of Hoffman failed to accord with the fevers of Minorca, which appeared constantly to change their form, defying all attempts at classification. Fevers often mutated into other afflictions such as dysentery, in a manner similar to that described by Bontius and many Classical writers.[20] Indeed, Cleghorn maintained that the accounts of tertian fevers given by ancient authors such as Hippocrates and Caelius Aurelianus were more relevant to fevers on Minorca than the writings of the moderns.[21]

Such familiarity with the work of the ancients is to be expected from one who had shown unusual gifts for Classical languages as a child and who conducted a good deal of his correspondence in Latin. The works of Hippocrates and

[17] 'A Description of Tranquebar; from the Account of the Missionaries, printed at Halle', *Gentleman's Magazine*, 14 (1744), 661.

[18] Cleghorn, *Observations on the Epidemical Diseases in Minorca*, iii–iv.

[19] Ibid., vii–viii.

[20] Ibid., 145, 155.

[21] Ibid., 165–9. Caelius Aurelianus was a Roman physician and writer who probably flourished in the fifth century AD, although his dates are uncertain. He was widely considered to be second only to Galen and was best known for his translation from Greek to Latin of Soranus's *On Acute and Chronic Diseases*.

Classical authors were also discussed extensively at Edinburgh, where he received his education in medicine prior to entering the Army.[22] But these texts were to be regarded as guides and points of comparative reference rather than authorities slavishly to be followed. Cleghorn thus departed from the Hippocratic tradition, and from Sydenham, in his extensive use of morbid anatomy, to which he would have been introduced while studying medicine at Edinburgh under Alexander Munro Primus, a former student of Boerhaave.[23] He claimed to have dissected nearly a hundred persons who had died from fevers at the military hospital in Minorca and found in them characteristic signs of the disease, such as the darkening and corruption of organ tissues in the lower belly. The stomach and intestines were also typically overflowing with bilious matter and the spleen enlarged, sometimes weighing as much as four or five pounds, 'and so extensively soft and rotten, that it had more the Appearance of congealed Blood wrapt up in a Membrane, than of an organical part'.[24] From these observations, Cleghorn drew inferences about the tendency of fevers to rapid putrefaction in hot climates and about the importance of prompt treatment, particularly the purgation of rancid humours from the intestines.[25] These observations were of enduring importance, and Mathew Baillie's copy of Cleghorn's book, which was later deposited in the library of the Royal College of Physicians, contains annotations which indicate the value he placed upon it in preparing his seminal work on morbid anatomy. It is also significant that upon his retirement from the Army, Cleghorn chose to settle in Dublin, where he gave lectures on anatomy and was soon appointed the first lecturer in that subject at the university, afterwards becoming a professor. There, he amassed a considerable fortune from a private practice built on the reputation he gained from his book on fevers.[26]

[22] Cleghorn was born at Granton near Edinburgh, the youngest of five children of a farmer who died when he was three years old. He attended the local grammar school before being sent to Edinburgh to learn Latin, French, Greek, and mathematics. He entered the University of Edinburgh as a student of medicine in 1731, where he met the Quaker physician John Fothergill, with whom he later corresponded in Latin. He was appointed surgeon to the 22nd Regiment of Foot in 1736 and appears to have left the army shortly before settling in Dublin in 1751. He had a lucrative private practice in Dublin and divided his time between the city and his large farm in County Meath. See Moore, *rev.* Herrick, 'George Cleghorn (1716–1789)'; Higston Fox, *Dr John Fothergill*, 122.

[23] Cleghorn's interest in anatomy was already evident in his student days, when he, Fothergill, and several other members of a student medical society he had founded, conducted their own anatomical dissections in private accommodation. On Minorca, as well as conducting many autopsies, he pursued an interest in comparative anatomy, dissecting Barbary apes and comparing their anatomy to humans, and to the descriptions given by Galen and Vesalius. After returning from Minorca, Cleghorn attended the Windmill Street anatomy school run by William Hunter before moving to Dublin. See Hingston-Fox, *Dr John Fothergill*, 122; George Cleghorn to John Coakley Lettsom, Dublin, 30 April 1785, enclosing a brief autobiographical sketch for Lettsom's life of Fothergill, WMS 5370/16, WL.

[24] Cleghorn, *Observations*, 165.

[25] Ibid., 183–4.

[26] Moore and Herrick, 'George Cleghorn'.

While stationed in Minorca, Cleghorn corresponded on various matters relating to the fevers of the island with his fellow Edinburgh student and 'inseparable companion', Dr John Fothergill (1712–80). These letters formed the basis of Cleghorn's book, which was edited and revised by Fothergill after Cleghorn returned to Britain in 1749. Apart from illustrating the importance of Edinburgh medical training in forming the outlook of practitioners in the armed services, the connection between Fothergill and Cleghorn exemplifies the close links that existed between practitioners in the colonies and key Dissenting figures in British medicine. Fothergill came from an old Quaker family in Yorkshire and, before matriculating at Edinburgh, he was apprenticed to an eminent Quaker apothecary in Bradford. After remaining at Edinburgh to complete his MD – which was still relatively unusual – Fothergill sought further training at St Thomas's Hospital, London, before venturing abroad. On his return, he struggled as an unlicensed practitioner in London, but in 1744 became the first Edinburgh graduate to be examined and licensed by the Royal College of Physicians. While practising in London, he wrote *An Account of the Sore-Throat attended with Ulcers* (1748) and many papers, including several anonymous observations on the weather and diseases of London published in the *Gentleman's Magazine*. The latter appeared between 1751 and 1754, shortly after the appearance of Cleghorn's volume. Fothergill remained firm in his Quaker beliefs throughout his life and later became a respected adviser to Quaker members of the Pennsylvania assembly.[27]

There is no indication of Cleghorn's religious persuasion, but in view of his humble agrarian background, it is likely that he was a Dissenter of some kind. Cleghorn certainly had a strong sense of public duty and placed a great deal of emphasis upon moral probity, declaring honesty to be preferable to riches.[28] These were hallmarks of the Dissenting tradition. But whatever his religious beliefs, he shared a moral and philosophical outlook that was compatible with Fothergill's and through him was widely networked within British circles of rational Dissent. Fothergill did much to popularize Cleghorn's work and sent copies of his manuscript to correspondents.[29] The relationship between Cleghorn and Fothergill is also significant because both men were interested in the natural history of disease and its relationship with weather. As we shall see, such interests were common among practitioners from Dissenting backgrounds, although they were not exclusively the preserve of any particular denomination.

Cleghorn's career is instructive in another sense, too. It shows that experience gained overseas could boost the career of medical practitioners, particularly surgeons, whose star was already rising in Britain. First in Scotland (in 1722)

[27] Margaret DeLacy, 'Fothergill, John (1712–1780)'.
[28] Cleghorn, autobiographical sketch, WMS 5370/16, WL.
[29] e.g. John Fothergill to Dr William Cuming, 18 May 1751, in Corner and Booth (eds.), *Chain of Friendship*, 142–3.

and then in England (in 1745), surgeons seceded from barbers to form separate companies. These new bodies retained their old guild status, but surgeons now considered themselves members of a profession rather than a trade. Although they had yet to acquire the dignity which they sought, surgeons had undoubtedly risen in the public's estimation. Their practices appeared to be grounded on surer foundations than those of the feuding physicians, and a growing number had an impressive education in the arts and in physic, even if they did not leave university with a medical degree. Some, particularly those who had also trained as apothecaries, were beginning to make a living as general practitioners;[30] others had a year or two at Edinburgh before going on to practise as surgeons, returning later to obtain their MD, and some had studied at one of the teaching hospitals in London.[31] Thus, a growing number of surgeons also practised physic and some, like Cleghorn, acquired prominence as experts on disease. The medical services of the Army, Navy, and the East India Company were vitally important in this respect. They offered the prospect of rapid advancement through the acquisition of broad-based skills in physic and surgery: practical knowledge which could provide the basis for a lucrative private practice, hospital post, or university career.

Surgeons were not especially concerned about the English Royal College of Physicians, but on those occasions when they did cross swords, the former depicted the fellows of the College as effete and lacking practical experience. As we shall see, such claims were increasingly made in respect of fevers. However, this rhetoric obscures a more complex picture. Many physicians were also seeking to reform learned medicine in accordance with experimental philosophy, and there was very little difference in outlook between the most progressive physicians and their counterparts in the College of Surgeons.[32] The East and West Indies were thus important to reform-minded physicians for the same reasons as they were to surgeons. They provided additional data – such as that communicated in the Royal Society's *Philosophical Transactions* – as well as the chance to develop lines of investigation begun at home. The career of the Yorkshire physician William Hillary illustrates this nicely. Born into a prominent Quaker family in the North Riding, Hillary began his medical career as an apprentice to a Quaker apothecary in Bradford (perhaps the same man who took Fothergill as an apprentice) but left after seven years to attend Leiden University, where he became a student of Boerhaave. Graduating MD in 1722, with a thesis on intermittent fever, he later practised as a physician in Ripon, where he remained until 1734. During this time, he made observations on the weather and attempted to correlate meteorological conditions with the incidence of disease,

[30] Corfield, *Power and the Professions*, 153–4; Digby, *Making a Medical Living*, 107–15; Loudon, *Medical Care and the General Practitioner*.
[31] See Lawrence, *Charitable Knowledge*; Rosner, *Medical Education*.
[32] Vaughan, '"Improvements in the Art of Healing"'.

his findings being published in the second edition of his *Practical Essay on the Smallpox* (1740).[33] The first edition of this work (1735) also sets out his approach to disease, with a strong appeal to practitioners to employ natural-historical methodology. An historical approach was vital, he insisted, because most diseases had changed over time, with 'the different Climates, and changes of seasons and Constitutions of Years, the various Employments, and Ways of living'.[34]

After leaving York for Bath in 1734, Hillary practised among the rich and fashionable of the city and courted the patronage of the Earl of Chesterfield by performing a chemical analysis of a spring, grandiosely titled the Lincomb Spa. This publication resembles many other pamphlets produced from the early eighteenth century which purported to vindicate the therapeutic properties of spa waters. But in attributing its healing powers to the high proportion of air in the water, Hillary was demonstrating a consistent interest in the relationship between airs and health.[35] At this point in his career, Hillary was in touch with Fothergill in London, who possessed similar philosophical interests as well as being a member of the Society of Friends. He does not appear to have been happy in his position in Bath and was seeking Fothergill's help to find employment elsewhere, principally in the West Indies. Fothergill introduced Hillary to friends in London, who secured for him a place as a physician in Barbados. Hillary had apparently first considered moving to the larger and more populous island of Jamaica, but Fothergill and others had done their best to persuade him not to go there, on account of the island's reputation for poor health and loose morals. In Fothergill's opinion, Jamaicans were 'the most strongly disposed to sensuality of most people who have a claim to the title of Britons'. They had been corrupted by owning slaves, with whom they had become 'accustomed to libertinism . . . from a very early period'.[36] He thought Barbados an infinitely better option because the island was healthier and had several Quaker meeting houses; the inhabitants were also 'much more humane and polite than anywhere else, with a prospect of good employ'.[37]

When Hillary left for Barbados in 1746, he continued to develop his interest in medical meteorology, expanding the work that he had begun in Ripon. His detailed observations did not begin until 1752, owing to an accident which broke his barometer, but from that time until the late 1750s, he systematically recorded temperature, atmospheric pressure, and the level of moisture in the air. The first section of his *Observations on the Changes of the Air, and the Concomitant Epidemic Diseases in the Island of Barbados* (1759) selects details from these

[33] Booth, 'Hillary, William (1697–1763)'; idem, 'William Hillary, Pupil of Boerhaave'.
[34] Hillary, *A Rational and Mechanical Essay on the Smallpox*, 1.
[35] Hillary, *An Inquiry into the Contents and Medicinal Virtues of Lincomb Spa Water*, 24–5, 67.
[36] John Fothergill to Lt.-Col. Gilbert Ironside, Bengal, 22 December 1774, in Corner and Booth (eds.), *Chain of Friendship*, 432.
[37] John Fothergill to Alexander Fothergill, 11 September 1746, ibid., 118–19.

records, while the second comprises a treatise on the various diseases of the island, their causes, and their treatment. The evidence presented in the treatise was drawn overwhelmingly from Hillary's own observations and those of his friend Andrew Dury, who conducted similar investigations at a higher altitude. There are few references to the work of other practitioners, save Hippocrates and Boerhaave, except where Hillary found reason to depart from them. One of those singled out for criticism was Warren, as Hillary disagreed strongly with his conclusion that 'yellow fever' was a form of putrid bilious fever imported from Palestine to Marseilles (the plague of the early 1720s), and thence to Martinique and Barbados. Rather, Hillary insisted that the disease was indigenous to the island, being produced by peculiar meteorological conditions.[38]

Hillary insisted that all practitioners would do well to study nature with the diligence of Boerhaave and Hippocrates. Accordingly, he discouraged his readers from slavishly emulating his therapeutic advice, for each disease and each patient was likely to differ.[39] The conclusions reached by Hillary, however, largely echo those of previous writers, especially those concerning the vulnerability of Europeans newly arrived in tropical climates and the need for them to adapt by altering their manner of living.[40] Yet he envisaged the action of heat and moisture upon the body in a mechanical way, as befits a student of Boerhaave and in keeping with his earlier writings on smallpox, which are replete with descriptions of the body as a machine. In Boerhaavian fashion, he declared that tropical airs tended to 'relax' the fibres of the body and could cause chemical changes in the fluids which engendered putrefaction. The hot, moist air of the rainy season, he averred, gave a 'putrescent diathesis to the fluids', the blood in particular being much more 'lax, loose, and attenuated . . . than it is in England'.[41]

Hillary was one of the first to claim that a study of a particular locality (in this case, Barbados) might have relevance for other climates in the Torrid Zone, as he referred to it. This claim may account for the considerable popularity of a treatise which was otherwise quite specific; it went through several editions, the last being published in 1811.[42] However, the enduring appeal of the book also rested on its thorough-going empiricism. Although some later writers disagreed with Hillary on specific points and reckoned his work underdeveloped from a philosophical point of view, most acknowledged the value of his observations. The popularity of the work also, no doubt, contributed to his success as a practitioner on the island of Barbados, where he amassed the tidy sum of £6,000 before leaving for England in 1759.[43]

38 Hillary, *Observations on the Changes of the Air*, 144–5.
39 Ibid., Preface, 3; 'Treatise', Preface, 1.
40 Hillary, *Observations*, 1766 edn., iii, ix, xi.
41 Ibid., vii.
42 Hillary, *Observations*, 1811 edn.
43 Booth, 'Hillary'.

Another significant member of the circle of correspondents linked to Fothergill was Alexander Russell. Russell hailed from a well-to-do legal family in Edinburgh and met Fothergill and Cleghorn when he attended the city's university to study medicine. With Cleghorn and William Cuming, he had been a founder member of the student medical society, which Fothergill was invited to join in 1734. In 1740, Russell took up a position as medical practitioner at the Levant Company's factory at Aleppo in what is now Syria, where he worked for fifteen years. There, like Hillary and Cleghorn, he made a special study of regional diseases, climate, and natural history, and like Cleghorn, he found Fothergill's help invaluable. As well as being a sounding-board for ideas, Fothergill was able to provide him with books that could not easily be purchased overseas. This was a particular problem in small outposts such as Minorca and Aleppo, where men such as Cleghorn and Russell felt intellectually isolated. Russell appears to have sent Fothergill his 'trifling observations on the plague' from around 1746,[44] while the latter was still in Philadelphia. In due course, Fothergill urged Russell to put them into a book, which appeared in 1756 as *The Natural History of Aleppo*. In this book, Russell commented on all the diseases of the locality, including common endemic fevers, the local skin condition known as *mal d'Aleppo*, and, most significantly, the plague, which raged for three years during his residence in the city. Although he held the common view that plague was a contagious disease, like his younger half-brother, the physician-naturalist Patrick Russell, he believed that its incidence was modified significantly by climate and season. Russell kept detailed monthly records of temperature and rainfall and correlated these with fluctuations of disease, which brought him to the conclusion that extreme heat checked its progress.[45] Like many writers on tropical climates, Russell also mentioned a kind of mild seasoning fever, known locally as 'the goose', which affected Europeans soon after their arrival.[46] As might be expected, his discussion of these diseases and their treatment was informed by Cleghorn's work, which he cited on several occasions.

Russell's book was completed with Fothergill's assistance after he returned to Britain in 1755. After gaining an MD from Glasgow, Russell settled in London and obtained a licence from the Royal College of Physicians, soon being appointed Physician at St Thomas's Hospital. This is significant because Russell was among the first of a number of practitioners who returned from overseas to find employment in hospitals; a location in which they were able to put their expertise in dealing with fevers to good use. Fever was then widely recognized as a major problem in charitable hospitals for the poor, much as in institutions for the care of soldiers and sailors. Like medical practice in the colonies, hospitals afforded more opportunity to experiment with different therapies

[44] Russell to William Cuming, Aleppo, 26 November 1746, WMS 7544/10, WL.
[45] Russell, *The Natural History of Aleppo*, 226.
[46] Ibid., 140–1.

than conventional private practice. Russell himself experimented with a mysterious substance called the 'Root of the Mezereon' for the treatment of venereal disease, for example, while others made liberal use of Peruvian bark (cinchona) in the treatment of a wide range of complaints.[47] But work in hospitals for the poor was, in some cases, also an economic necessity, especially for practitioners – such as Russell – who were unable to enter the charmed fellowship of the Royal College. Like Fothergill, Russell was a member of the 'Society of Collegiate Physicians', a turbulent band of practitioners who pressed unsuccessfully for full voting rights for licentiates of the College.[48] His membership of this group suggests that he may have shared the reformist political inclinations of some of its members, the impetus for medical reform being stimulated in part by the contemporary movement for 'Wilkes and Liberty'.[49] But Russell's first-hand knowledge of plague and Mediterranean lazarettos drew him to the attention of the Privy Council: the body responsible for quarantine arrangements in Britain. The Council consulted Russell about the possibility of plague spreading from the Levant to Britain, and the Lords of the Council were so impressed by his knowledge that they asked him to draw up a plan for tackling the disease should it arrive in Britain. This was not completed before his sudden death from a 'putrid fever' in 1768, during which he was attended by Fothergill and another physician friend, William Pitcairn.[50] Although he was unable to complete this task, the fact that he was asked to undertake it provides an early indication of the status that some practitioners working overseas would obtain over the coming decades.

The careers of Hillary, Cleghorn, and Russell all indicate a link between medical meteorology and rational Dissent. Although the religious beliefs of Cleghorn and Russell are unknown,[51] they operated within and were nourished by a circle of rational Dissenters loosely centred on Fothergill. The connection between meteorology and Dissent becomes stronger still if one looks forward

[47] Lawrence, *Charitable Knowledge*, 223–99, 306.

[48] Ibid., 264. See also Vaughan, '"Improvements in the Art of Healing"', 241–56; Waddington, 'The Struggle to Reform the Royal College of Physicians'; Stevenson, 'The Siege of Warwick Lane'. The inaugural meeting of the Society also included the physician Dr Huck, who had corresponded with Dr John Pringle from the West Indies about yellow fever (see following chapter).

[49] Waddington, 'Struggle to Reform'. The 1760s was a time of increasing radicalization in British politics. John Wilkes became the figurehead of the more radical section of the Whig party which feared a return to royal absolutism. Wilkes had been imprisoned in the Tower of London for libelling the king and on his release campaigned loudly for freedom of speech, marking the start of a turbulent period in British politics which coincided with the storming of the Royal College of Physicians by some of its licentiates in 1768. The followers of Wilkes did not have a clear programme but it incorporated a range of issues including franchise reform and the abolition of slavery. On the broader political context, see for example: Cannon, *Parliamentary Reform*; Christie, *Wilkes, Wyvil and Reform*; Thomas, *John Wilkes*.

[50] Fox, *Dr John Fothergill*, 118, 120.

[51] There is some evidence to suggest that Russell's family was Anglican, as his mother was the daughter of the minister of West Calder, a Church of Scotland institution. See Boulger, *rev.* Wallis, 'Russell, Alexander (1714–1768)'.

slightly to the work of Joseph Priestley (1733–1804) and other radical chemists. It may be that the air served as a metaphor for a more fluid and less restrictive society, but there is no firm evidence that this was so, and any link between rational Dissent and medical meteorology probably lay more in a commitment to empiricism than in the content of medical theory. The medical analysis of airs was part of a more general attempt to base theory and practice upon hard facts. As such, it appealed to practitioners of a reformist inclination but also to those who wished to avoid controversy and the conjecture that gave rise to it. Thus, it comes as no surprise to find that meteorology appealed not only to Dissenters but to some elite physicians of a latitudinarian persuasion who sought to ground medical practice in science, as well as to find a naturalistic basis for their politics and religion.[52] As one historian of medicine has recently commented, religious heterodoxy, or at least toleration of a liberal interpretation of scripture, formed a linkage between Dissenters and some Anglicans with strong interests in mechanical and – to a lesser extent – chemical philosophy.[53]

A case in point is the heterogeneous group of physicians who pursued their interests in medical meteorology as fellows of the Royal Society: the Tory satirist and royal physician John Arbuthnot (1667–1735); the former Dissenter and student of Boerhaave John Huxham (1692–1768); and the Newtonian, Cambridge-educated physician James Jurin (1684–1750), who was to become the Society's president.[54] These eminent doctors followed the Baconian methods recommended by Sydenham and drew their inspiration from *Airs, Waters and Places* and Books I and III of the *Epidemics*. Not only did these texts suggest ways in which disease and weather could be profitably investigated, their emphasis upon observation was completely in accord with the irenic and inductive approach to knowledge espoused by the Royal Society.[55] As Andrea Rusnock has argued, these physicians developed a Baconian-Hippocratic methodology, the key elements of which were the acquisition of useful knowledge through accurate observation.[56] But as elite physicians they continued to venerate other ancient authors, not simply as commentators upon Hippocrates, but for their 'fine and useful Observations in all Parts of Physic', as Huxham wrote of Galen. Celsus, too, was described by Huxham as 'the Latin Hippocrates', while Alexander of Tallis was held in high esteem for following Hippocrates and for making useful observations of his own.[57] Like other contemporary writers, Huxham was

52 But latitudinarianism was, itself, closely intertwined with rational Dissent. See Gascoigne, 'Anglican Latitudinarianism'; Fitzpatrick, 'Latitudinarianism'.

53 Vaughan, '"Improvements in the Art of Healing"', 13–14.

54 See Furdell, *The Royal Doctors*, 238–42, 244–5; Ross, 'Arbuthnot, John (*bap.* 1667, *d.* 1735)'; Rusnock, 'Jurin, James (*bap.* 1684, *d.* 1750)'; Moore, *rev.* Hankins, 'Huxham, John (c. 1692–1768)'.

55 Shapin and Schaffer, *Leviathan and the Air Pump*; Shapin, *Social History of Truth.*

56 Rusnock, 'Hippocrates, Bacon, and Medical Meteorology at the Royal Society'.

57 Huxham, *An Essay on Fevers*, v–xi.

attempting to establish a long tradition of empiricism in medicine and to show that the profession was united by fundamental principles.

Huxham rarely cited the works of practitioners in the Indies, but he made numerous observations on disease and meteorology from his home in Plymouth. There, he also had the opportunity to examine sailors who had returned from the colonies with an assortment of exotic fevers. Huxham's opinions were thus valued by many who travelled to the Indies because they were based on first-hand observation as well as extensive knowledge of a range of ancient and modern authorities. Indeed, the nature of his inquiries and his methodology provided the template for some practitioners whose employment took them overseas. One such was the naval surgeon Robert Robertson, also elected to a fellowship of the Royal Society, who conducted meteorological investigations during voyages to Africa in the 1760s and 1770s.[58]

Although Huxham appears to have had few direct connections with the colonies, the work of his contemporaries Jurin and Arbuthnot was heavily indebted to observations made overseas. In his capacity as President of the Royal Society, Jurin actively sought such information and received letters from Europe and North America on the relationship between climate and health.[59] However, it is Arbuthnot's *Essay Concerning the Effects of the Air on Human Bodies* (1733) that provides us with perhaps the clearest indication of the significance of colonial observations on climate and disease. When Arbuthnot wrote his book, few European physicians were passionately interested in the influence of the atmosphere upon health. With the obvious exception of Sydenham, he could point to only a handful of other modern physicians who had conducted similar enquiries, most notably Bernadino Ramazzini of Modena and Padua, who had written about the diseases afflicting different parts of Europe, Asia, and Africa.[60] In view of the paucity of modern literature on the subject, the majority of the sources drawn upon by Arbuthnot were Hippocratic texts, recent works in natural philosophy, such as Stephen Hales' *Vegetable Staticks*,[61] and the writings of practitioners based overseas, particularly those of Bontius, which he cited with approbation.[62] It is also notable that Arbuthnot cited Halley's work on tropical climates, which he credited with helping to form the notion of the tropics as a distinct climatic zone.[63]

[58] Robertson, *Observations on Fevers*, ix. In emulation of Huxham, Robertson recorded data such as longitude, latitude, wind direction and strength, rainfall, atmospheric phenomena, and phases of the moon, and correlated these with observations on the sick list.

[59] e.g. Lining, 'Extracts of Two Letters'. See also Rusnock, 'James Jurin'; idem, *Vital Accounts*, 113.

[60] Ramazzini, *Health Preserved*, Book 1.

[61] Arbuthnot, *Essay*, 16.

[62] Ibid., 136.

[63] Ibid., 76. Apart from his work on winds, Halley computed the geometric relationship between latitude and heat.

Arbuthnot's main concern was with the effects of climate upon human character, and his work informed chapters fourteen to eighteen of Montesquieu's *L'Esprit des Lois* (1749), in which the latter famously speculated on the relationship of climate to political institutions.[64] Yet, as a physician, Arbuthnot also remarked upon the effects of air upon human health, particularly its relationship to epidemics. At the time of Arbuthnot's writing, there was mounting concern in Britain with so-called crowd diseases: the epidemics of fever associated with institutions like hospitals and prisons, as well as with rapidly growing cities. In all of these, the air seemed to be implicated as either a direct or an indirect cause of disease.[65] Of the atmospheric conditions considered by Arbuthnot, he placed particular emphasis on extremes of moisture and dryness, human bodies being 'intolerant of Excesses of any kind'. It is tempting to speculate that there was a strong affinity between such views and the distrust of enthusiasm so characteristic of Arbuthnot's Tory Anglicanism; there are also perhaps undercurrents of concern with social order in his writing on crowd diseases and their prevention. For example, Arbuthnot computed that: 'Three Thousand human Creatures living within the Compass of an Acre of Ground, would make an Atmosphere of their own Streams about 71 Feet high, which, if not carried away, would turn pestiferous in a moment',[66] which led him to conclude that: 'the very first Consideration in building of Cities is to make them open, airy, and well perflated.'[67]

There is an interesting and possibly significant analogy here with the reforms that would shortly be advocated by the likes of John Pringle and which began to be implemented in some military hospitals and naval vessels from the middle of the century. For many writers – medical and lay – disease was becoming synonymous with indiscipline. Newly formed populations, be they in industrial towns or standing armies, were unknown quantities and threatened to destabilize the old order. The political dangers of the crowd thus found a parallel in the incipient threat of disease; a threat which emanated from dark, teeming spaces not unlike those of the colonial tropics. Indeed, by the turn of the nineteenth century, the heat and filth of the tropics would become a potent metaphor for the pathogenic conditions generated by industrialization and international commerce.

Although some of the epidemic diseases afflicting Britain did not appear to correspond to seasons, it was generally agreed that their cause lay in some noxious quality of the air. One of the most prominent, but also controversial, texts on this subject was that of the young physician John Barker (1708–49).[68] Having

[64] Harrison, *Climates*, 93–4; Glacken, *Traces*, 562–7.
[65] e.g. Huxham, *Essay*, 54–73; idem, *Observations on the Air*.
[66] Arbuthnot, *Essay*, 16–17.
[67] Ibid., 17.
[68] Barker was the son of a Derbyshire physician and was educated at St Thomas's Hospital, London and at Wadham College, Oxford, where he matriculated in 1728, and graduated BA in 1731, MA and MB in 1737, and DM in 1743. He practised medicine in Salisbury from 1737 to

studied an epidemic of fever at Salisbury, he concluded that air could act directly and indirectly to cause fever. It acted directly by bracing or relaxing the solids; by condensing, dissolving, or rarefying the blood and other humours; by heating or cooling the body; or by stopping perspiration or causing it to be increased too much. Such influences were usually remote rather than immediate causes of illness, however, merely predisposing individuals to disease. Epidemic influences, by contrast, were capable of affecting the body immediately, although their nature remained obscure. None of this was particularly new, but in Barker's work the action of the air upon the human body is described in a way that differs markedly from most of his contemporaries. Whereas the air appeared to act indirectly upon the body by affecting the humours, epidemic influences acted upon the nerves and were thus capable of rapidly prostrating any individual unfortunate enough to be exposed to them.

The prominent role which Barker gave to the nervous system probably owed much to the influence of Malcolm Flemyng, a student of Boerhaave and a teacher of physiology based in London.[69] Boerhaave had written about the nervous system but it did not occupy such a prominent place as it did in Barker's aetiology of fever. However, as we shall see in the following chapters, interest in the anatomy and physiology of the nervous system intensified and it began to figure far more prominently in literature on fevers, initially prompted by the work of Albrecht von Haller and the Scotsman Robert Whytt, but later, and more profoundly, by the teachings of William Cullen, John Brown, and Erasmus Darwin.[70] But these were signs of things to come and by no means typical of the way in which fevers were understood around 1750. At that time, both in the colonies and in Britain, the dominant paradigm for explaining fevers was still essentially humoral, although key concepts such as putrefaction had been elaborated and refined in terms of chemical or experimental philosophy. Practitioners who had experienced disease in the colonies played an important role in this process through their keen attention to the causes of disease, both within and outside the body. Although they were not yet sufficiently numerous to dominate medical debates in Britain, their interventions were increasingly significant. The works of Cleghorn and Hillary are particularly important as they show that experience overseas could confer distinct professional advantages, both in terms of status and material benefits. Their reputation rested on painstaking observations

1746, during which time he became involved in a public dispute over the nature and treatment of an epidemic of fever which swept southern England. His published works all defended his views on the fever. In 1746, he became a member of the Royal College of Physicians and moved to London to become physician at the Westminster Hospital, and in September the following year he was appointed Physician to the Army in the Low Countries. He died at Ipswich in 1749. See Austin, *rev.* Herrick, 'Barker, John (1708–1749)', *DNB.*

69 Barker, *An Inquiry into the Nature, Cause, and Cure of the Present Epidemick Fever*, 11, 14.

70 Smith, 'Concept of Typhus', 131; Lecture Notes of Robert Whytt, 'Of the Cause of Fevers', 1761, 4–6, RCPE; French, *Robert Whytt*, chap. 4; Meier, '"Sympathy"'.

and it was the accuracy of their data that assured their continuing relevance through to the nineteenth century. In seeking an experiential basis for medical knowledge, Cleghorn and Hillary were following in the footsteps of Trapham in the West Indies and Bontius in the East. All insisted on the distinctiveness of tropical climates and on the need to modify or reject the teachings of European authorities. In this respect, the works of Hippocrates, Sydenham, and Boerhaave served as exemplars and guides rather than canonical texts.

It is striking that some of the most prominent writers on the diseases of hot climates were from Dissenting sects or operated within Dissenting circles: Trapham and Stubbe in the seventeenth century, and Hillary and Cleghorn in the eighteenth. Both the latter had a strong affinity with other Dissenting practitioners who made similar studies of disease in Britain. They were seeking a new basis for medical knowledge in which professional authority was derived from a close study of nature rather than solely from knowledge of texts. But the natural-historical method was one to which some elite physicians were also committed and observations made in the colonies informed the work of Arbuthnot and Jurin, among others. The transactions of the Royal Society, and less formal circles such as Fothergill's, made the work of colonial practitioners known to a growing body of enthusiasts who were also investigating the relationship between disease and meteorological phenomena. But those with experience of working in hot climates tended to regard the Torrid Zone as a unique environment in which disease appeared in markedly different forms. The following chapters will show how such observations coalesced to form a self-referential and relatively distinct body of literature on the diseases of warm climates, but one which had great significance for British medicine as a whole.[71]

[71] See Arnold, 'Introduction', in Arnold (ed.), *Warm Climates*, 7–8.

3

The medicine of warm climates

The distinctiveness of warm climates from a medical point of view rested primarily on two observations. First, that putrefaction was accelerated in tropical latitudes by the abundance of heat and moisture. This, and the lush vegetation of the tropics, appeared to be the source of the ubiquitous miasmas which caused Europeans to sicken and often to die. Second, the tropical climate sapped the resistance of newcomers, leaving them vulnerable to such vapours. It was only after a year or so, when Europeans had become 'seasoned' to their new abode, that they could entertain any hope of health and longevity. By the mid-eighteenth century, these ideas were firmly entrenched as part of the folklore of European settlements in the East and West Indies but, from the middle of the eighteenth century, this local knowledge began to coalesce in a new corpus of medical literature devoted to the diseases of hot climates. For the first time, medical practitioners began to write about the diseases of all warm climates, seeing a substantial degree of similarity between them. This development was stimulated by a conflagration of nearly global proportions: the Seven Years War (1756–63). The war saw European troops dispatched in large numbers to tropical locations in the Americas and the East Indies and lent greater urgency to medical investigations. A posting overseas provided military and naval surgeons with the opportunity to observe new disease environments and to conduct investigations of a pathological nature. Their post-mortem examinations appeared to reveal the imprint of the tropics within and seemed to offer conclusive proof of a distinctive pathology characterized by rapid putrefaction.

Medical practitioners working in colonial hospitals differed considerably from most of their professional colleagues in Britain, who had less inclination or, at least, fewer opportunities to pursue morbid anatomy.[1] Historians may have underestimated the interest in morbid anatomy in Britain before 1815,[2] but legal restrictions undoubtedly limited the number of bodies available for dissection.

[1] Maultiz, *Morbid Appearances*, 3, 109–16; idem, 'Channel Crossing'; Bonner, *Becoming a Physician*, 148–52.

[2] Exceptions include: Bateson '"Open up a few corpses"'; Keel, *Médecine Clinique*; idem, 'The Politics of Health'; Lawrence, *Charitable Knowledge*.

Even in the most progressive medical schools, such as Edinburgh, medical students rarely had the opportunity to perform dissections themselves.[3] But this is not to say that students were uninterested in anatomy; quite the reverse. A high standard of anatomical knowledge was required of those examined at Surgeons' Hall prior to their appointment to the Army, Navy, or East India Company.[4] As well as being useful for future employment, many students at Edinburgh and the London surgical-anatomical schools acquired a real taste for anatomy during their studies. This could rarely be satisfied in civilian practice at home, but the military and naval hospitals of the East and West Indies provided surgeons with an unparalleled opportunity to pursue their interests. The high death rate of Europeans overseas meant that there was no shortage of cadavers for dissection, and there were no legal or customary obstacles to prevent it. The only constraints on dissection were the rapid deterioration of bodies in hot climates, the fear that putrefying corpses might spread infection, and occasionally concern about the effects of dissection upon the morale of European soldiers.

The post-mortem dissections conducted in colonial hospitals were exploratory in nature and aimed to elucidate diseases which defied classification or treatment. They thus had more in common with the pathological investigations of Revolutionary Paris than the didactic autopsies conducted in 'proto-clinics' like the Vienna or Edinburgh infirmaries.[5] As a result, pathological investigation occupied a far more important place in colonial medicine than in Britain. It became the foundation of aetiology and therapeutics in the tropics long before British doctors ever dreamt of walking the wards in Paris. This is not to deny the significance of Paris medicine but to recognize that Parisian methods and concepts were grafted onto an already vibrant British tradition in morbid anatomy. Indeed, some of the greatest advocates of Paris medicine were surgeons who had gained analogous experience in the colonies.

A TENDENCY TO PUTREFACTION

In the mid-eighteenth century, medical literature in Britain dwelt on the so-called putrid or pestilential fevers that ravaged ships, gaols, and other confined spaces. These 'crowd diseases' appeared to be putrid in the sense that their symptoms evinced signs of bodily corruption such as foul odours, and because their external or exciting cause was attributed to decay.[6] For the many practitioners who followed Sir John Pringle (1707–82), putrid diseases constituted a distinct class

[3] Lawrence, 'Ornate Physicians and Learned Artisans'; Risse, *Hospital Life*, 261–71.

[4] This can be inferred from the primers that were produced for students in the second half of the eighteenth century; e.g. Gentleman of the Faculty, *Anatomical Dialogues*.

[5] Foucault, *The Birth of the Clinic*, 126–8.

[6] Corbin, *The Foul and the Fragrant*, chap. 6; Riley, *The Eighteenth Century Campaign to Avoid Disease*, 97–100; Pickstone, 'Dearth, Dirt and Fever Epidemics'.

comprising largely of pestilential fevers but also diseases which exhibited degeneration and decay, scurvy and leprosy being the most obvious examples. Like the fevers associated with ships and gaols, scurvy was becoming more common as the length and frequency of voyages increased, and, together, these diseases posed a grave threat to Britain's military and naval efficiency.

Pringle's interest in putrid diseases developed during his time as a physician with the Army in Continental Europe during the War of Austrian Succession (1740–8). There, the British Army lost thousands of men to dysentery, typhus, and other fevers which Pringle attributed to poor hygiene, pestilent locations, and adverse weather – all of which accelerated putrefaction. Pringle's *Observations on the Diseases of the Army* (1752) was a turning point in military medicine, partly because it offered practical advice that could be implemented by any commander who had a mind to do so. More fundamentally, the book differed from the bulk of medical literature which still attributed military diseases to individual behaviour, such as 'irregularities in diet', rather than to environmental factors. Pringle was very much aware of this difference and made a point of emphasizing it.[7]

Pringle's work on military diseases developed in tandem with a broader philosophical interest in the nature of putrefaction, which he pursued after leaving the Army in 1748. In that year, Pringle settled in London, where he established a successful private practice, becoming physician-in-ordinary to the Duke of Cumberland, presumably on the strength of his military connections. The following year, he had several essays published in the *Philosophical Transactions*, all of which were closely related to his forthcoming book on military diseases. The first dealt with the fevers of gaols and hospitals; the others with substances that accelerated or retarded putrefaction. One of these – entitled 'Experiments on Septic and Antiseptic Substances, with remarks on their Use in the Theory of Medicine' – won the Royal Society's prestigious Copley medal. Pringle had been a Fellow of the Society since 1745 and was to become its president in 1772, a post he held until 1778. During this time, he encouraged others to work on putrefaction, as well as pursuing other lines of investigation, in electricity, for example. He also played a major role in the development of pneumatic chemistry, highlighting the medical uses of the different types of air (gases) identified in experiments by the Dissenting natural philosopher Joseph Priestley (1733–1804).[8] He shared Priestley's religious outlook and had Unitarian sympathies, even though he did not openly espouse these beliefs. Priestley also undertook experiments which furthered some of Pringle's ideas about

[7] Pringle, *Observations*, 1757 edn., 86.

[8] Golinski, *Science as Public Culture*, 106–9; Blair, 'Pringle, Sir John (1707–1782)'. On Priestley, see Schofield, *The Enlightenment of Joseph Priestley*; Anderson and Lawrence (eds.), *Science, Medicine and Dissent*; Schaffer, 'Priestley's Questions'.

putrefaction, showing, for example, how air impregnated with noxious effluvia extinguished the 'vital principle' within it.[9]

Pringle's putrefactive theory of disease was fundamental to the theory and practice of medicine over the next few decades, especially in the colonies. At its heart was the idea that most intermittent and remittent fevers were caused by 'putrid effluvia' emanating from marshy grounds.[10] In addition to these fevers, there was another class of fevers which were often termed 'malignant' or 'pestilential', which acquired the property of contagion when experienced in confined spaces. These diseases generally arose from the corruption of animal bodies or from the breath of the sick.[11] Pringle's lectures to the Royal Society in 1750 communicated the results of a series of experiments in which he attempted to elucidate the process of putrefaction causing the latter class of diseases. He concluded that digestion was not possible without some degree of putrefaction but that putrid diseases were produced by an excessive amount. The prevention and cure of such diseases therefore seemed to lie in slowing the process until it was no longer pathological. Acids of various kinds – including those given off by the process of fermentation – appeared to be the best antidotes to putrefaction, or 'antiseptics' as Pringle termed them. Other antiseptic substances included Peruvian bark, camphire, and all astringents.[12] As well as being significant for work on fevers, these experiments had a major impact on the treatment and prevention of other supposedly putrid diseases, including scurvy. They inspired, for example, the work of naval practitioners such as David MacBride, who took Pringle's theory a step further, using insights from the pneumatic chemistry of Black, Priestley, and others. Fermentation, he argued, generated the 'fixed air' that was necessary for the cohesion and vitality of healthy bodies.[13]

As he was developing his ideas about putrefaction and its relationship to disease, Pringle maintained a regular correspondence with practitioners working in the Indies. One common theme in their letters is the difference between fevers encountered in the tropics and those in Europe. To a man, Pringle's correspondents were united in considering tropical fevers more violent and fatal than those at home, although they acknowledged that their symptoms resembled fevers in Europe. The great intensity of these fevers was usually attributed to environmental conditions such as marshy and low-lying situations, and heavy and prolonged inundations; all of which were conducive to putrefaction.[14] Pringle's

[9] Priestley, 'Observations'; idem, 'On the noxious Qualities of the Effluvia of Putrid Marshes', 90–4.

[10] Pringle, *Observations*, 1810 edn., 164.

[11] Ibid., 254–5.

[12] Pringle, 'Some Experiments on Substances Resisting Putrefaction'.

[13] Carpenter, *The History of Scurvy*, 85.

[14] Extract of a letter from Mr James Stevenson, Surgeon to the East India Company factory, Notall, 10 December 1752, vol. 1, f. 1; letter from Mr Blair, Guadeloupe, February 1761, vol. 6, f. 222, Papers of Sir John Pringle, RCPE.

correspondents placed special emphasis upon the relationship between disease and uncultivated ground, 'improved' land being seen as more healthy because dense vegetation blocked refreshing breezes and left an abundance of putrefying matter.[15] Another common observation was that newcomers were most at risk from disease, especially those who refused to modify their intemperate habits.[16]

However, one of the most significant aspects of the correspondence between tropical practitioners and Pringle is that it demonstrates the growing importance of morbid anatomy. Morbid anatomy had been rejected by some physicians, notably Sydenham, but other practitioners claimed that it afforded important clues to the causes of disease. In the infirmaries of Vienna and Edinburgh, morbid anatomy was primarily intended as an aid to disease classification. The number of dissections that could be performed in British medical schools was also limited and the situation did not improve significantly until the Anatomy Act of 1832.[17] In the colonies, where there were no such constraints, surgeons insisted that dissection could provide vital information about the nature of the deadly diseases that faced British forces in the Indies, much as Pringle had opened the bodies of deceased soldiers when confronted with the ravages of dysentery and hospital fever in Flanders, in the 1740s.[18] Towards the end of the Seven Years War, Pringle learned that Dr Huck in the West Indies had instructed his surgeons to dissect the bodies of soldiers who had died from yellow fever. These dissections revealed that their stomachs were full of a black humour similar to that which had been vomited before death, and that their gall bladders were distended and livers damaged. The information from these autopsies was used to determine a more suitable course of therapy.[19]

By the 1760s, post-mortem investigations of yellow fever were common and were beginning to figure prominently in literature on the disease. James Makittrick's Edinburgh MD thesis of 1764 was one of the first to describe the pathology of yellow fever in detail, based on the author's own post-mortem dissections in the West Indies.[20] The form and substance of his work was replicated in many subsequent dissertations but not necessarily his conclusions. Whereas Makittrick considered yellow fever to be a distinct disease, and dwelt upon the differential diagnosis of fevers,[21] Huck did not consider it so. As far as he was concerned, it was merely a variety of common autumnal fever, rendered more putrid by the tropical climate and the inhalation of 'bad air' in transport

15 Extract of a letter from Mr Hall, factor to the East India Company at Fort Marlborough, Sumatra, 1753, vol. 1, f. 3, Pringle Papers, RCPE.

16 Extract of a letter from Dr Temples, Jamaica, July 1763, vol. 7, Pringle Papers, RCPE.

17 Maulitz, *Morbid Appearances*, 138–9; Richardson, *Death, Dissection and the Destitute.*

18 Pringle, *Observations*, 212–22, 265–9.

19 Annotations on Hillary's *Observations*, 2 October 1762, vol. 5, ff. 339, 431, 539, Pringle Papers, RCPE.

20 Makittrick, *Dissertatio medica*, 6–7.

21 Ibid., 11–23.

ships and hospitals. There was also a good deal of disagreement about the cause of the disease. A substantial minority considered yellow fever to be contagious, as it often appeared in epidemic form. But most practitioners, including Huck and Makittrick, thought that it was due to a putrescent quality of the atmosphere.[22] Makittrick, for instance, drew an analogy with MacBride's work on scurvy, suggesting that humid, stagnant, and corrupt airs were lacking in fixed air, which was vital to human health.[23]

It is easy to see why Pringle would have been interested in such observations, but the subject was even more pressing for practitioners in the tropics, where there was 'so great a tendency to putrefaction', as the Madras surgeon Gilbert Pasley put it, and where the ventilation of hospital wards was considered even more essential than in Britain.[24] The newly annexed territory of Bengal was thought to be far worse in this respect than the Company's southern factories. As Fleming Martin, Chief Engineer at Bengal, wrote to his father, 'from what I have seen, the best constitutions in the most moderate persons are a poor match against a fever or other disorders in this country'. He continued, 'no man here is without complaints, and life and death are so suddenly exchanged, that medicines have not time very frequently to operate before the latter prevails. This is generally the case in malignant fevers, which are here termed *pucker* [sic] *fevers*, meaning (in the native's language) strong fevers.'[25]

Putrefaction loomed large in works issuing from the pens of most East India Company surgeons, James Lind's Edinburgh MD thesis on the putrid remitting fever of Bengal (published in 1776) being an oft-cited example. James Lind (1736–1812) – who is often confused with his more famous kinsman, the naval surgeon of the same name – arrived in Bengal after first practising surgery in Glasgow.[26] He was well connected in philosophical circles, being a close friend of the engineer James Watt, a cousin of the chemist James Kier, and an acquaintance of Erasmus Darwin. All were members of the Lunar Society of Birmingham, which, like the medical services of the Company, Army, and Navy, drew many – though by no means all – of its members from Dissenting backgrounds.[27] Lind decided to seek employment with the Company in 1763 after completing courses of lectures in geometry, science, and medicine at Edinburgh

[22] Annotations, vol. 5, f. 430, Pringle Papers, RCPE. See also Section II, chapter 5, infra.

[23] Makittrick, *Dissertatio*, 23–6.

[24] G. Pasley to Surgn. Samuel Spolt, 3 April 1771, Madras Public Consultations, No. 191, 5 April 1771, P/240/31, APAC, BL.

[25] 'Letter to Mr Dacosta, Librarian, &c., to the Royal Society, from Mr William Martin, containing an Extract of a Letter from his Son at Bengal, on the Heat of the Climate', *Phil. Trans.*, 57 (1767), 217–18.

[26] Douglas, *The Genealogy of the Family of Lind*, 4, 7; Lind, *Sketch for a Medical Education*, 5–6.

[27] Uglow, *The Lunar Men*. A few of the Lunar Society's members, such as Thomas Day and Richard Edgeworth, had been educated at Oxford. The society also had a less obviously dissident tone than some of the provincial literary and philosophical societies that were established later in the century. See Langford, *Polite and Commercial People*, 660–2.

University. He wrote excitedly to Watt about his intention to visit the East and of travelling from India to China, which was still venerated as a source of ancient wisdom. Shortly afterwards, Lind left Edinburgh for London, where he completed another course of study in chemistry and anatomy, before joining the Bengal Medical Service as an Assistant-Surgeon. In December 1765, he departed for India, taking with him an electrical machine (the subject of much of his correspondence with Watt),[28] a sextant ('I have turned longitude mad', he declared), a telescope, and a microscope.[29]

When Lind arrived in Bengal, he collected meteorological data avidly, just as Cleghorn and Hillary had done in Minorca and Barbados, correlating these with clinical observations. He returned to Britain in 1767 in ill health, whereupon he resumed studies at Edinburgh, gaining an MD in 1768 which was later published in English as *A Treatise on the Putrid and Remitting Marsh-Fever, which raged at Bengal in the year 1762.* In Edinburgh, he continued his astronomical work, publishing a paper on the transit of Venus in the *Philosophical Transactions of the Royal Society* in 1769. The following year, he was made a Fellow of the Royal College of Physicians of Edinburgh, and in 1772 he made a voyage to Iceland with Joseph Banks and other natural philosophers, serving as the party's astronomer.[30] By now, Lind had acquired a considerable reputation as a natural philosopher and physician, and was prominent in Edinburgh and London society, as is evident from his appointment as a royal physician. On settling in Windsor, he continued to develop his numerous interests in natural philosophy and was elected a Fellow of the Royal Society in 1777. There, Lind tutored the radical poet Percy Bysshe Shelley in natural philosophy while the latter was at Eton, and he appears as the 'Old Hermit' in Shelley's *Revolt of Islam* and as Zonaras in the fragment *Prince Athanese.* It has also been claimed that Lind's experiments with electricity – which replicated Galvani's experiments with frogs – provided the inspiration for Mary Shelley's Dr Frankenstein.[31] At the same time, Lind resumed his correspondence with Watt, which had lapsed for some years, and their discussions ranged widely from hot-air ballooning to the construction of a pneumatic machine designed to cure Mrs Lind of cancer.[32]

Pneumatic chemistry – which informed much of what had been written on putrefaction in the second half of the eighteenth century – was 'widely perceived as tied to radical reformist tendencies'. Critics of radicalism, such as Edmund

[28] The bulk of the correspondence concerns either electricity or steam power, e.g. Watt to Lind, Glasgow, 6 November 1764; 30 November 1764; 5 October 1768; Lind to Watt, Edinburgh, 3 September 1765, Papers of James Watt (1736–1819), JWP C1/15, Birmingham City Archives [hereafter, BCA].

[29] Lind to Watt, Edinburgh, 29 October 1763; London, 9 December 1765, JWP C1/15, BCA.

[30] See von Troil, *Letters on Iceland*; Lind, *Treatise.*

[31] Goulding, 'The Real Doctor Frankenstein?'; Copper, *rev.* Wallis, 'Lind, James (1736–1812)'.

[32] Watt to Lind, Birmingham, 20 September 1783; 26 December 1784; 25 February 1795; 18 March 1795; 10 August 1796, JWP C1/15; Lind to Watt, 7 August 1796, JWP W/9, BCA.

Burke, likened the mobs of revolutionary Paris to wild gases that had broken loose, while similar metaphors were employed by the champions of reform. The fact that many practitioners in the colonies were drawn to pneumatic chemistry underlines the importance of Dissent and Dissenting networks to our story and, more generally, to the development of new languages and practices surrounding the air in the late eighteenth century. However, Lind was quite cautious in this respect. Although he believed that pneumatic chemistry could be useful in the treatment of a number of diseases, he did not wish publicly to be identified with its more extreme advocates such as Thomas Beddoes and his followers, whom he labelled a 'set of Miscreants'.[33]

In Lind's *Treatise*, and in his career more generally, we can see many of the hallmarks of medicine in the East and West Indies: the preoccupation with the link between environment and disease, observation based on meticulous record-keeping, and a willingness to challenge received wisdom in British medical circles. The importance of Edinburgh looms large, as do connections with Dissenting physicians and natural philosophers. In a manner similar to William Hillary, Lind seems to have been attracted to the colonies not only by the prospect of professional advancement but by intellectual curiosity. Employment with the East India Company offered Lind the prospect of enlarging his investigative canvas and of contributing to philosophical discourse in Britain. As we shall see in later chapters, these channels often led to the Lunar Society and to some of the medical and philosophical societies established in British provincial towns. We see consistent lines of enquiry, too, especially an interest in how atmospheric phenomena might affect human health; investigations which were increasingly informed by the pneumatic chemistry of Priestley and others. Lastly, Lind's career shows that experience gained overseas could contribute significantly to one's reputation as a physician or natural philosopher, opening doors to the Royal Society and the royal household, if not to the Royal College of Physicians.

A similar trajectory, though not as socially exalted, can be seen in the career of Lind's cousin and namesake, the naval surgeon James Lind (1716–94). Lind was also born in Edinburgh and began his career as a surgical apprentice, though in Edinburgh rather than Glasgow. Like his younger cousin, he attended lectures at Edinburgh University before joining the Royal Navy in 1738. He served in the Navy for ten years, mostly in the English Channel, before returning to Edinburgh, where he graduated MD in 1748, with a thesis on venereal disease. Afterwards, he appears to have practised in the city and was elected a Fellow of the Royal College of Physicians of Edinburgh in 1750; he was also a member of the Philosophical and Medical Society of Edinburgh and was elected a Fellow of the Royal Society of Edinburgh in 1783. After leaving the Navy, Lind wrote two books which established his reputation as one of the foremost writers on naval medicine: his *A Treatise of the Scurvy* (1753) and *An Essay on the Most*

[33] Levere, 'Natural Philosophers in a Coffee House', 138.

Effectual Means of Preserving the Health of Seamen in the Royal Navy (1757). The publication of the latter seems to have secured his appointment as Physician to the Royal Naval Hospital at Haslar in 1758. It was there that Lind encountered many sailors who had been sent back to Britain after contracting diseases in hot climates, particularly the West Indies; an experience which induced him to write a sequel to his previous work on the health of seamen, aimed precisely at those who encountered hot climates.[34] Although he never visited the countries that he wrote about in this book, his clinical experience at Haslar, together with an extensive knowledge of relevant literature and network of correspondents, led many to regard it as authoritative. Indeed, Lind's *Essay on Diseases Incidental to Europeans in Hot Climates* (1768) became a standard work of reference for half a century. It went through many editions (the last in 1811) and was translated into German, Dutch, and French. As in the case of his earlier publications, the *Essay* owed its influence to its comprehensive, methodical approach to the subject, rather than to patronage. As one of his biographers notes, Lind was not well connected at the Admiralty and had little taste for politics.[35]

Previous authors on the diseases of the East and West Indies had cited each other, but they tended to focus on a particular locality. Lind's *Essay* was the first attempt to synthesize this knowledge and make it applicable to all hot countries, considering them to be epidemiologically distinct from temperate lands and requiring different methods of preservation and treatment.[36] Like previous writers, Lind remarked that hot climates were more deadly to Europeans because of the combination of extreme heat and moisture. He concluded that the fevers of hot climates tended to be putrid in nature; not only in the sense understood by the Ancients – that is, distinguished by pungent or putrid odours – but in that they were attributable to a process akin to the decay of corpses.[37] Bodily putrefaction, according to Lind, was usually caused by exposure to putrid effluvia, which could have an almost immediate effect on newcomers to the tropics. 'A few of the Sailors', he recalled, 'are sometimes at first seized with Fluxes, which denote a Disposition in the Air to Putrefaction, and to beget a malignant Fever of the remitting, or intermitting Form, most frequently of the double tertian Kind. This Fever, which is the genuine Produce of Heat and Moisture, is the Epidemic between the Tropics, upon the Coast of *Guinea*, and in *Jamaica*; and is the autumnal Fever of all Hot Countries.'[38]

The malign influences that pervaded tropical airs appeared not to affect all persons equally, however. Lind followed previous writers in believing that women and the middle-aged had a better chance of avoiding disease than young males

[34] On Lind at Haslar, see Lloyd and Coulter, *Medicine and the Navy*, vol. 3, 215–19.
[35] Bartholemew, 'Lind, James (1716–1794)'.
[36] Lind, *An Essay on Diseases Incidental to Europeans in Hot Climates*, 6th edn., 91–4.
[37] Ibid., 10, 12.
[38] Lind, *An Essay on the Most Effectual Means of Preserving the Health of Seamen*, 2nd edn., 49.

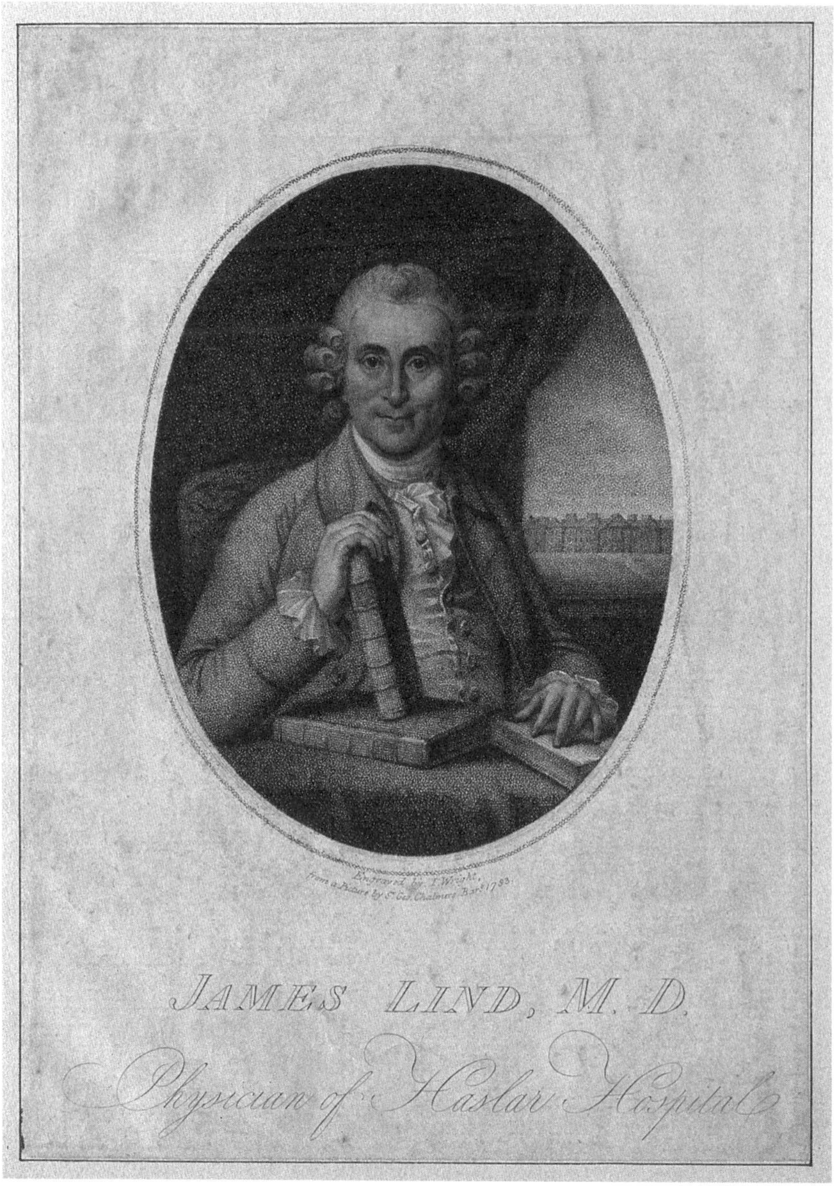
Engraved by I. Wright,
from a Picture by Sr Geo. Chalmers Bart 1783.
JAMES LIND, M.D.
Physician of Haslar Hospital

I.1. James Lind, MD

because their constitutions were less plethoric.[39] In this sense, Lind's *Essay* followed a very traditional, Hippocratic line of reasoning. Its novelty lay, rather, in its broad geographical canvas. It was a text for an imperial age, born of a war fought on three continents and of the East India Company's expansion as a territorial power.[40] But Lind's *Essay* was not simply the product of economic necessity; at its heart was a conviction in the unity of hot climates, an idea which had emerged from the work of Halley, Arbuthnot, Hillary, and others. It is therefore significant that Lind identified climate as *the* principal factor in the high mortality of Europeans, rather than their supposedly dissolute lifestyles. As he put it, 'the most abstemious and temperate persons often die soon, in unhealthy climates, as well as the irregular and debauched'.[41] Lind's *Essay* thus stands as a landmark for much the same reasons as Pringle's *Observations on the Diseases of the Army*: not only in terms of their comprehensiveness and practicality, but because both ascribed the majority of diseases to environmental causes rather than individual behaviour.

Like Pringle, Lind offered detailed advice on how to choose the most salubrious locations for military camps and settlements. Europeans in the tropics were warned to look out for a distinct alteration in the temperature of the air at sunset (the harbinger of 'chill'), and for fogs, swarms of flies, corrosion, and rapid decay of flesh (all signs of putrescence).[42] Even though a strict regimen provided no guarantee of good health, sensible precautions such as light diet and clothing were also beneficial.[43] In Lind's view – which reflected the conventional wisdom of the tropical colonies – it seemed likely that Europeans could become acclimatized given a few years' residence, by which time they would become exempt from the most deadly diseases.[44] His belief in the influence of the environment on human bodies was sufficiently strong to enable him to conclude, with Arbuthnot and Montesquieu, that it was 'Upon the soil, the temperature of the climate, the colour, strength, and activity, the constitutions and health of the inhabitants greatly depend.'[45]

Another key exponent of the putrefactive theory was John Clark (1744–1805), a surgeon on the Indiaman, *Talbot*, who later came to apply insights gained in the colonies to his practice in Britain. Like many of the Company's surgeons, Clark came from a humble background, being the son of a tenant farmer in Roxburghshire. After attending grammar school in Kelso, he went to Edinburgh University to study divinity (he was a Unitarian) but afterwards switched to medicine, only to leave because of ill health the following year. After a surgical apprenticeship in Kelso and further medical studies at Edinburgh and London, he took up an appointment as a surgeon in the Company's Marine service in 1768.[46] Clark resided in India between 1768 and 1771 and appears to have

[39] e.g. Lind, *Essay on Diseases*, 98–9, 107–8. [40] Ibid., 8.
[41] Ibid., 4. [42] Ibid., 149. [43] Ibid., 257.
[44] Ibid., 218–19. [45] Ibid., 226.
[46] Maehle, 'Clark, John (*bap.* 1744, *d.* 1805)'.

visited most of the Company's settlements. His chief concern was with the putrid fevers of the subcontinent, a class of maladies which he understood in similar terms to the Linds. These fevers were characterized by symptoms such as foetid breath, haemorrhage, and offensive stools, which betrayed a process of decay similar to the decomposition of dead animal matter;[47] according to Clark, 'all dangerous diseases of hot climates, particularly fevers, depend[ed] upon a putrescent disposition of the fluids'. Clark's mode of investigation resembled previous works on the diseases of hot climates in its invocations of Hippocrates and Sydenham, and it is particularly reminiscent of Hillary, Lind of Windsor, and Cleghorn, all of whom kept meticulous records of meteorological conditions alongside their medical case books.[48]

Clark's observations were regarded as very reliable and attracted the attention of his superiors in the East India Company's medical establishment, who commissioned him to write a book on the subject. In it, he employed the standard three-fold division of intermittent, remittent, and continued fevers, which he distinguished primarily on the basis of their symptoms. He placed less emphasis upon morbid anatomy than many colonial surgeons, maintaining that 'Dissections throw no light into the proximate cause of disease, as they only shew its effects.'[49] But the symptoms of Indian diseases did not provide reliable evidence for their classification, for they could easily mutate into one another. Indeed, all appeared to be varieties of the same disease.[50] These views echo aspects of William Cullen's nosography, in which the varieties of fever were specific to time and place. But what struck writers on the diseases of hot climates was the rapidity with which they could mutate from one form to another. One author thus concluded that: 'There appears to be an intimate connection between them [fevers], for they are frequently combined together, often interchange with each other, and it rarely happens that one is epidemic without the other. They would seem to depend on the same cause, perhaps differently modified.'[51] In other words, any form of fixed classification was useless.

It is tempting to see a connection between Clark's Unitarian beliefs and his belief in the unity of fevers. But as we have just seen, other practitioners working in the tropics took a similar view and we can safely assume that only a few of them would have been of the same religious persuasion as Clark.[52] If the Dissenting tradition can be said to have left its imprint on colonial practice, it was probably most evident in a general distrust of established authorities and a

[47] Clark, *Observations on the Diseases of Long Voyages to Hot Countries*, 122.

[48] Ibid., 53.

[49] Ibid., 134–5.

[50] Ibid., 118. Clark was one of several empirically minded writers on fever who found Sydenham's legacy ambiguous, in that it led some practitioners needlessly to replicate varieties of fevers, different species arising from different states of the atmosphere. See Bynum, 'Cullen and the Study of Fevers', 144.

[51] Hunter, *Observations on the Diseases of the Army in Jamaica and on the Best Means of Preserving the Health of Europeans in the Climate*, 15.

[52] See also Robertson, *Essay on Fevers*.

strongly empirical orientation. What mattered most to surgeons working in the colonies was not how a disease ought to be labelled but what caused it, and in crude terms at least, the answer seemed clear: putrefaction. Clark maintained that effluvia from rotting matter could easily induce fever in persons whose bodies were already predisposed to putrefaction by long residence in a tropical climate. It was no accident that the most deadly fevers in India afflicted the Company's servants in Calcutta, which was located just a few miles from a major source of putrefaction: a large salt-lake. 'As soon as the rains are over', he noted, 'the lake subsides, and leaves on the ground an abundance of mud, slime, prawns, and other fish, which soon putrefy with the heat of the season, and occasion very noxious exhalations.' There, in the rainy season, putrid remitting fever and dysentery prevailed and were very often fatal, especially to newcomers.[53]

Although other parts of India were considered unhealthy during the rainy season, Bengal had the unenviable reputation of having the worst climate on account of the preponderance of low-lying marshes and swamps in the Ganges delta.[54] Kenneth Murchison, surgeon of the Indiaman *Fox*, wrote memorably about the 'Founts of Putrefaction' that he encountered there and their effects upon health.[55] With the possible exception of Batavia, Calcutta was generally thought the least healthy of all European settlements in the East Indies.[56] Madras, by contrast, was a veritable paradise; its situation was 'dry, flat and pleasant', as was much of the Coromandel Coast, where the dryness of the land enabled rainwater to be absorbed or evaporated.[57] But the healthiest part of India was said to be the south-western coast of Malabar, as refreshing sea breezes cleansed the atmosphere for up to six months of the year.[58]

Although the Indian climate was clearly something to be feared on occasion, it was generally believed that even the most unpromising environments could be transformed by improvement of the land. Like Lind, Clark saw cultivation as the key to healthy settlements; a conclusion which was compatible with the East India Company's new role as a territorial power.[59] It also harmonized with Clark's Unitarian beliefs and with the Dissenting tradition more generally, which stressed Mankind's potential for improvement in conformity with the laws and design of a benevolent God.[60] The doctrine of Improvement was now

[53] Clark, *Observations*, 45, 51.

[54] e.g. Henry Smith, Cawnpore, to his sister, 2 February 1773; Smith, Dinapore, to his father, 23 February 1773; F 76/IV/590–602, Herefordshire Record Office; Diary of Kenneth Murchison (1751–96), Surgeon to the Indiaman Fox, 1772–3, Bengal Medical Service, 1776–84, entry of January 1777, 13, MSS Eur. G.52, APAC, BL.

[55] Diary of Kenneth Murchison (1751–1796), entry of January 1777, 13, MSS Eur. G.52, APAC, BL.

[56] White, *Dissertatio medica.*

[57] Clark, *Observations*, 39.

[58] Ibid., 34–5.

[59] Ibid., 130–1.

[60] See Wood (ed.), *Science and Dissent.*

perhaps the dominant ideological force behind British imperialism,[61] and, as noted earlier, the Company's establishment at Bombay had already begun to drain and cultivate areas around the European settlement with the express purpose of rendering it more salubrious.[62] Clark also recommended various measures to improve the health of those sailing on ships to India. While putrid remitting fevers were generally regarded as miasmatic diseases, Clark reckoned that they could occasionally become contagious in cramped conditions, in which people were exposed to the putrid breath of the sick.[63] For this reason, he insisted that the air on board ships in the tropics ought to be kept as cool and pure as possible, and that the sick ought not to be crowded together. In keeping with Pringle's notion of antiseptic substances, Clark also recommended that Europeans in India eat a diet high in vegetable matter in order to combat the 'putrescent disposition of the fluids' in hot climates, and follow a regime of personal cleanliness and gentle laxatives.[64] If newcomers heeded this advice and took care to arrive at healthy times of the year, they might become acclimatized to their new abodes, particularly if they spent their first year in India in one of its more salubrious locations.[65]

After Clark left the East India Company, he returned to Britain and took an MD from St Andrews before moving to Newcastle upon Tyne, where he built a large practice. In that city, he joined the congregation of the Unitarian chapel in Hanover Square, whose minister was William Turner, the principal founder of the Newcastle Literary and Philosophical Society.[66] The Society promoted many aspects of philosophical and technological improvement, and Clark was the driving force behind a number projects for the betterment of the city, including smallpox inoculation (prior to the advent of vaccination) and the establishment of the Newcastle Dispensary in 1777. As Physician to the Newcastle Infirmary from 1788 and a member of the city's Medical and Physical Society, he also played a key role in that hospital's extension and prepared the way for the creation of a separate fever hospital in 1804. Clark believed that the creation of this 'house of recovery' within the Infirmary would do much to stem the rising incidence of fevers in Newcastle and Gateshead, which he attributed to overcrowding and squalid living conditions among the poor. 'Every removal of a fever [case], to the House of Recovery', he argued, 'will on an average prevent four cases of fever – nay often will suppress the Contagion at once.'[67] His

61 Drayton, *Nature's Government.*

62 Raynal, *Philosophical and Political History*, vol. 2, Book 3, 108–9.

63 Clark, *Observations*, 133.

64 Ibid., 149, 240.

65 Ibid., 346–8.

66 Orange, 'Rational Dissent and Provincial Science'.

67 Clark to Mr J. Airey, Secretary to the Infirmary, undated, 1802, Reports and Correspondence of the Committee for Promoting an Institution for the Cure and Prevention of Contagious Fevers', Hospital Archives 58, Special Collections, Robinson Library, University of Newcastle [hereafter, U of N].

arguments in favour of a fever hospital drew explicitly on the experience he had acquired in military and naval hospitals, and on the East India Company's ships. On their outward voyage, these vessels were normally crammed with what Clark referred to as 'military recruits picked up from jails, or enlisted from the refuse of society in populous and manufacturing towns' who often brought fever onto the ships. Sloth and squalor on board added to the problem, and remittent fevers picked up from unhealthy harbours *en route* meant that vessels often arrived with many of their original crew dead or dying. Clark's two voyages to the East gave him the opportunity of 'making observations on febrile contagion', during which he witnessed its 'limited sphere' – the fact that such diseases were contagious only in confined and poorly ventilated spaces. From this, he deduced the power of ventilation and cleanliness in checking the progress of fever, and by these means was successful in preventing its ravages on board the vessels in which he travelled, as well as in hospitals once he had landed. And, as he emphasized to the Committee considering the creation of a fever hospital for Newcastle and Gateshead, the same means had proved highly effective in Britain, where he had always managed to prevent the spread of contagion in schools and other such institutions by ventilation, cleanliness, and separation of infected patients.[68]

One of the children who attended one of the boarding schools mentioned by Clark was the daughter of the Liverpool physician Dr James Currie (another authority on fevers), who was sufficiently confident in the measures taken by Clark to allow his daughter to remain there during an outbreak of scarlet fever.[69]

It was Clark's intention that the fever hospital would be accompanied by the establishment of a Board of Health with powers to remove cases of contagious fever to the hospital and fumigate houses where such had occurred. Patients at the Infirmary or presenting at the Dispensary with symptoms of contagious fever were to be automatically transferred to the new institution. None of these proposals was particularly contentious, but the location of the hospital was. Another local physician, Dr Ingham, was among those who favoured the establishment of a hospital in a more remote location, stating that an institution for contagious fevers located centrally was likely to be opposed. Clark countered this on grounds of economy and efficacy, claiming that such an institution abutting the Infirmary would protect the hospital and the most populous areas. Ultimately, Clark's scheme was the one favoured by the committee considering the proposals, and it was decided to appeal to local clergy (Anglican and Dissenting) to raise money for the establishment.[70] It was opened in 1804, the donations being large enough to construct 'a noble and commodious building'.[71]

[68] Clark to Governors of the Newcastle Infirmary, 16 June 1802, Hospital Archives 58, U of N.

[69] Ibid.

[70] 'Report of the Committee for promoting an Institution for the Cure and Prevention of Contagious Fevers, in Newcastle and Gateshead' (1802), Hospital Archives 58, U of N.

[71] 'Report of the State of the Institution for the Cure and Prevention of Contagious Fever in Newcastle and Gateshead, for the Fourth Year, ending April 30, 1808,' Hospital Archives 58, U of N.

Clark died shortly after the hospital was opened and so was unable to play a part in its work, but it operated much as he had wished, accepting poor patients from the surrounding area, while the committee ensured that their houses were 'purified'.[72] The establishment of this institution, like that of other fever hospitals in Britain, owed a good deal to enlightened self-interest, as the Committee considering the proposal declared in its final report, it 'will rescue the poor, and secure the middle and higher ranks of society from contagion'.[73] But popular concerns over the spread of contagion meant that the hospital's establishment, or at least its location, was not a foregone conclusion. It thus seems reasonable to conclude that Clark's overseas experience proved persuasive; after all, it was on these grounds that he presented his case to the committee and to the public at large. As in his published work, he made extensive use of anecdotal evidence of the causes of fever and the methods that appeared to prevent it, with occasional reference to epidemiological statistics.[74] Clark also enlisted the support of prominent military and naval authorities on fever such as Lind of Haslar and Cleghorn, as well as civilian hospital physicians such as James Currie of Liverpool and John Ferriar of Manchester. The controversial pneumatic physician Thomas Beddoes also backed the proposal. This demonstrates that colonial practitioners were part of a wider constituency of reform-minded medical practitioners, for whom hospitals provided the key to medical progress. In fact, Clark felt that most of the important medical advances of the previous fifty years had either occurred in hospitals or had arisen from observations made in them.[75]

During his time in Newcastle, two further editions of Clark's *Observations* were published by popular demand, one with minor additions in 1780, the last, posthumously, in 1809. In the intervening period, Clark's book became widely cited in works on the diseases of hot climates, perhaps second only to Lind's *Essay*.[76] However, there are some significant differences between the first and final editions of Clark's *Observations*, and it appears that his work at the Newcastle Infirmary and Dispensary induced him to retreat from some of his earlier assertions about the distinctiveness of diseases in tropical countries. In the third edition of his *Observations*, Clark declared that 'The opportunities the author has had of making observations, in different parts of the globe, convince him that diseases, in every climate, are respectively the same.'[77] In view of this, he argued, the treatment and prevention of fevers should be basically the same in all climates; something which he tried to indicate in an amended title.

Like other surgeons who had returned from overseas, Clark was attempting to demonstrate the relevance of his work to a much broader constituency, not simply in an attempt to improve his professional standing, but also perhaps to

[72] Ibid., 3. [73] 'Report of the Committee', U of N, 3.
[74] See also Troehler, 'Quantification'.
[75] Clark, *A Collection of Papers*.
[76] e.g. Fontana, *Osservazioni*, 5. [77] Clark, *Observations*, 1809 edn., iv.

enable him to comment on matters of general public concern. As it happened, the appearance of the third edition followed soon after the disastrous campaign at Walcheren, which resulted in the evacuation of over 6,000 men to England, most of whom were suffering from the endemic fever of the Zealand marshes.[78] Presciently, he had identified one of the main failings of the Army in respect of health: the reluctance of combatant officers to take responsibility for the prevention of disease. These matters had been left entirely to surgeons, who lacked the power to implement the measures they thought necessary. According to Clark, they had often been 'foiled in preventing the prevalence and mortality of diseases, not only by the obstinacy and prejudices of the men, but also, not infrequently, by the inattention or neglect of their superiors'.[79] Thus putrid diseases had regularly wreaked havoc in the Company's armies, and at Onore, for instance, an outbreak of disease led to the desertion of many of the Company's soldiers to the armies of its adversary, Tipu Sultan.[80] In order to remedy this, Clark proposed that 'regulations of health' be given to all officers and that they should be 'made responsible for carrying them out'.[81] This recommendation placed Clark in the vanguard of those who sought to reform military medicine,[82] although it took more than a century for anything of the kind to occur.

The East India Company's growth as a territorial power, and the consequent expansion of its military medical establishment, meant that it eventually became the main source of publications on the diseases of warm climates. The former Company surgeon Charles Maclean left his readers in no doubt of this when he observed that the great size of East India Company's medical establishment fostered a particularly independent cast of mind.[83] In the 1780s, however, a growing number of influential treatises were also produced by practitioners attached to the Army and Navy in the Caribbean, as well as in the warmer parts of North America during the War of American Independence. One of the most significant of these was Benjamin Moseley, who came to Jamaica as a surgeon-apothecary after receiving an education in medicine at one of the London hospitals and in Paris. In Jamaica, he held the post of surgeon-general, and worked at the island's military hospital. He spent the best part of twelve years on the island, although he was engaged in military expeditions elsewhere. After returning to England in 1784, Moseley attempted to ingratiate himself with high society by acquiring the trappings of a physician, obtaining an MD from St Andrews in 1784 and becoming a licentiate of the Royal College of Physicians in 1787. Following a short Continental tour, he established a private practice in London that attracted many rich and

[78] This figure is taken from Blane, *Select Dissertations*, 95.
[79] Clark, *Observations*, 1809 edn., vii.
[80] See Forbes, *Oriental Memoirs*, vol. 4, 145–54; Cruso Papers, 163, MSS Eur. E.151, APAC, BL.
[81] Clark, *Observations*, viii.
[82] Ackroyd et al., *Advancing with the Army*, 33–4.
[83] Maclean, *Practical Illustrations*, xiii.

fashionable patients; through one of these – Lord Mulgrave – he gained the post of Chief Physician to the Royal Military Hospital, Chelsea, later becoming personal physician to the Duke of York.[84] Most of his works were written after he left the West Indies and abound in references to modern and ancient authorities in the manner of a traditional physician.[85] Yet Moseley had more in common with military surgeons than with most metropolitan doctors, stressing the primacy of experience over tradition ('tyrant custom') and the importance of observation. Like other colonial practitioners, he was also fond of invoking Hippocrates and Sydenham, seeing the latter as marking the beginning of modern medical practice.[86]

Moseley's hostility to doctrine extended to modern fads and systems, particularly the application of mechanical philosophy to medicine. Following Newton, he observed, it had become fashionable to 'purge and vomit mathematically' and for practitioners to have 'a perfect acquaintance with everything but nature'; a reference to the speculations of Richard Mead and other heavily mechanistic physicians.[87] So too with the systems of the great nosologists, the volume of whose writings, he quipped, was inversely proportional to their experience of disease. 'And thus', he wrote, 'diseases are created, and cures performed, which have only had existence, like BERKELEY's matter, "because they were perceived by the ideas".' Moseley's aim was quite different: to produce a 'repository' of his accumulated knowledge, a genre of medical writing that had recently been revived by his colleague Sir George Baker (1722–1809), President of the Royal College of Physicians.[88] The result was his *Treatise on Tropical Diseases* (1787), which went through four editions, the last in 1803.[89]

Although it concentrated on the West Indies, Moseley's *Treatise* also drew upon medical literature on the East Indies, which enabled him to make generalizations about all tropical diseases; indeed, his title is the first in which the term 'tropical diseases' appears. Although one ought to be wary of placing too much emphasis upon a single title, it is significant because it establishes Moseley's text as part of a new genre of medical literature that had a distinct focus upon the diseases of warm climates. Thus, in addition to frequent citations of Hippocrates, Sydenham, Bacon, and Ramazzini, Moseley acknowledged, among others, Bontius on the Dutch East Indies; Cleghorn on Minorca;

[84] Brunton, 'Moseley, James (1742–1819)'. Mulgrave was a naval officer who had served in the Caribbean during the American War; he occupied a number of minor offices in the Pitt administration, including joint Paymaster-General (in 1784) and Controller of the Navy (in 1788). See Rodger, 'Phipps, Constantine John, second Baron Mulgrave in the peerage of Ireland and Baron Mulgrave in the peerage of Great Britain (1744–1792)'.

[85] Moseley's *On Hydrophobia, its Prevention and Cure* is the best example of his affected style.

[86] Moseley, *A Treatise on Tropical Diseases*, 2nd edn., v.

[87] Ibid., viii. [88] Ibid., x. [89] *London Medical Journal*, 2 (1782), 86–94.

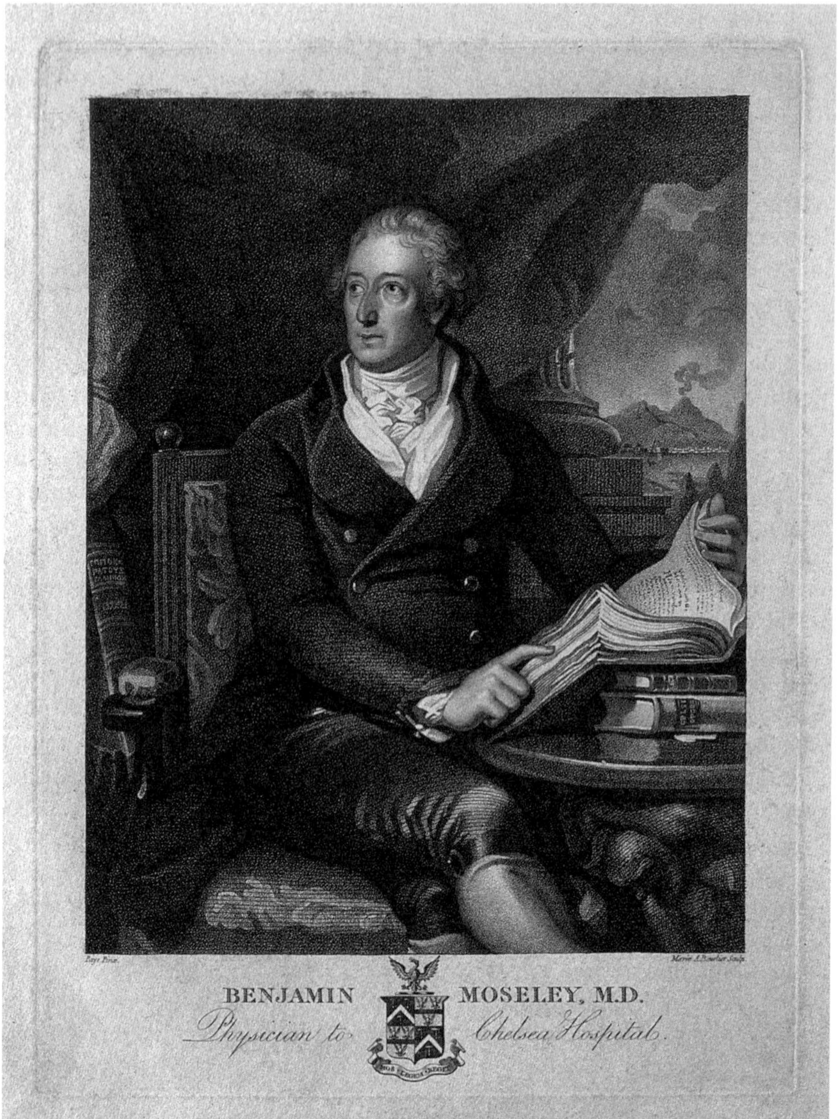

I.2. Benjamin Moseley, MD

Trapham, Towne, and Hillary on the British West Indies; Chévalier on the French West Indies;[90] and Rouppe on the Dutch West Indies.[91]

Like other literature on the diseases of warm climates, Moseley's *Treatise* was lavish with advice about how to assist acclimatization; on how to recognize unhealthy localities and on the kinds of constitutions most suited to warm climates. In all these respects, his *Treatise* mirrors other contemporary works, most notably that of John Hunter of Jamaica, whose book on the diseases of that island was published a year after the first edition of Moseley's. In choosing localities, both Hunter and Moseley stressed the advantages of elevation and dryness, hospitals, and barracks ideally being as far as possible from the 'pernicious vapours' which were the cause of 'obstinate intermittent fevers, diseases of the liver, and putrid diseases'.[92] Both were quite optimistic about the prospects for European health in the islands, believing that Europeans could thrive if they took proper precautions.[93] However, they acknowledged that some adapted more easily than others, supposing acclimatization to be easier if the subjects were not too young and plethoric, and that women were more likely to adapt than men on account of losing blood through menstruation.[94] However, like Clark in India, both Hunter and Moseley insisted that the prospects of newcomers would be better if the Army were to send troops to the West Indies at the coolest and healthiest times of the year.[95]

Of the two writers, Hunter seems to have been the more optimistic about the long-term prospects for Europeans in the West Indies, believing that Europeans would not simply become inured to the diseases of the islands but actually grow blacker over many generations, rendering them better fitted for life under a hot sun; a view which rested on the theory of climatic 'degeneration' espoused by the French naturalist Buffon (1749–1804). Like Buffon, Hunter believed that white men had 'degenerated' from an original black race; a conclusion which he reached partly by analogy with animals: black animals occasionally had white offspring (albinos) but never vice versa.[96] Opinions such as Hunter's were probably viewed sceptically by many long-term residents of the West Indies, who could see little change in families that had emigrated there from Europe

[90] Chévalier was the author of a treatise on disease among French soldiers on the island of Martinique. See Narvaez et al., *Memoire pour Chévalier Chirurgien-major, au Régiment de la Martinique, et Apothicaire en la Ville du Fort Royal.*

[91] Louis Ludovicus Rouppe (1729–1780), author of *De morbis navigantium.*

[92] Moseley, *Treatise,* 39; Hunter, *Observations,* 15.

[93] Moseley, *Treatise,* 69; Hunter, *Observations,* 24: 'the human frame acquires by habit a power of resisting noxious causes... Hence Europeans, after remaining some time in the West Indies, are less liable to be affected by the causes of fevers than on their first arrival.'

[94] Moseley, *Treatise,* 413–15; Hunter, *Observations,* 25.

[95] Hunter, *Observations,* 28; Mosley, *Treatise,* 119–20.

[96] Hunter, *Inaugural Disputation on the Varieties of Man.* See also recollection of Hunter's theory in Commonplace Book of Thomas Thomson, Deputy Inspector-General of Hospitals, entry of 20 June 1808, Martinique, WM 4781, Western MS, WL.

several generations before. However, the supposedly slow process of any such adaptation provided some basis for the belief, as did occasional reports of apparently spontaneous changes of colour.[97]

Another important respect in which Moseley differed from other writers on the diseases of the West Indies was in his lack of attention to morbid anatomy. Dissection was still conducted regularly in the West Indies, as we learn from Thomas Cawley, a surgeon at the general hospital constructed at Kingston, Jamaica, during the American War. There, he dissected soldiers of the 83rd, 92nd, and 93rd regiments, most having died from flux (dysentery). From August to January 1780, some 249 patients were admitted to the hospital under Cawley's care, of which 117 had contracted fevers and 93 fluxes; 31 fever patients subsequently died, as did 51 of those with fluxes. Similar mortality rates were recorded by other surgeons, which provided them with more bodies than could be dissected in the short time necessary before the corpses began to putrefy. Perhaps in a reference to Clark's *Observations*, Cawley remarked:

> It is commonly objected to dissections, that they demonstrate effects rather than causes; but if we consider that the proximate cause of dysentery is secondary, or produced by an invisible, unintelligible, remote cause, which by none of its qualities is subject to our senses; and farther, that our chief aim in curing this disease consists in attempt to obviate the effects, it follows, that the farther knowledge we acquire by dissection of such effects in every stage of the complaint, the nearer we are likely to arrive at a rational and successful method of cure.[98]

From his dissections, Cawley concluded that the internal membrane of the rectum and colon were the true seats of the disease and that, while the remote cause of dysentery remained obscure, the constancy of its pathological signs suggested that it was likely to be caused, 'in all cases and climates', by the same specific poison.[99]

It is curious that Moseley did not mention these investigations in his work on dysentery, although it may be that he was unaware of them, having been attached to the expedition to San Juan (in present-day Nicaragua) in the same year. His neglect of morbid anatomy was also matched by a strident rejection of the doctrine of putrefaction. Some British physicians, notably Francis Milman, had already criticized the putrid theory of disease, but it still commanded assent among most practitioners in the tropics.[100] Moseley was therefore departing from received wisdom when he wrote that opinions about the tendency of fevers to putrefaction in hot countries were 'not founded on practice, however they may seem to agree with theory'. According to Moseley, the endemic remitting fever of

[97] e.g. Fisher, 'Account of a Remarkable Change of Colour in a Negro'.
[98] Cawley, 'An Account of the Dysentery', 344.
[99] Ibid., 360–1.
[100] Milman, *An Enquiry*. Milman disagreed with Pringle that scurvy arose from putridity of the blood and explained it, instead, in terms of diminishing nervous power.

the West Indies showed no putrid symptoms, and had its seat in the nervous rather than in the digestive system.[101] The absence of plague in the West Indies also seemed to suggest that the putrefactive tendency of its climate was less marked than many other countries. Moseley believed that the sea breezes, which he saw as largely acidic in their chemical constitution, neutralized and broke up the more malignant atmospheres.[102] The nervous theory of fevers emerging from a number of European medical schools seemed better able to account for the diseases he had encountered in the West Indies. He believed that the 'greater relaxation and debility of the nervous system in tropical climates' rendered the body susceptible to the most trivial change of air.[103] Furthermore, abandoning the putrefactive theory meant letting go of many potentially harmful customs and practices:

> The ridiculous notion that people are to die of putrid diseases in hot climates, unless they keep up their spirits, and embalm their bodies, by the assistance of an additional quantity of wine, strong liquors, and living well, as it is vulgarly called, has caused the death of thousands. Another almost equally pernicious practice, from the same notion of putrefaction, among new-comers, is, to devour great quantities of fruit, and to drench themselves with acid drinks: but if they escape a flux, they destroy the tone of the stomach, and are soon left without either appetite or digestion.[104]

This sceptical note heralds the emergence of a new paradigm in the medicine of warm climates. From the 1790s, a growing number of practitioners followed Moseley in attributing disease not chiefly to putrefaction or accumulations of bile, but to depleted energy. The essence of these theories was the notion of nervous debility; whether caused by the immediate action of an oppressive atmosphere or gradual exhaustion due to prolonged exposure to enervating climates. In the last few decades of the eighteenth century, the principal source of these ideas was William Cullen (1710–90), who occupied chairs at the University of Glasgow (1744–55) and then at the University of Edinburgh (1755–89), where, as Professor of the Institutes of Medicine, he taught many of those who joined the medical services of the Army, Navy, and East India Company.[105] Cullen believed that the remote cause of fevers was generally a poison that acted on the body's nervous system, weakening the heart and vasculature so that blood was not propelled around the body with its usual force. This produced a cold sensation in the skin and the extremities of the body, which in turn caused the heart to increase its action, producing the characteristic symptoms of chills followed by excessive heat and sweating. In the case of most tropical fevers, this poison appeared to be an 'infective' agent rather than a 'contagious' one. Contagious fevers were said to be caused by a specific poison directly communicated from person to person, whether by touch

[101] Moseley, *Treatise*, 84. [102] Ibid., 73. [103] Ibid., 52.
[104] Ibid., 69. [105] Bynum, 'Cullen, William (1710–1790)'.

or by the breath of the sick. The newly afflicted person suffered from the same disease as the person from whom it had been conveyed. Infectious diseases, by contrast, were derived solely from the atmosphere: from the inhalation of poisonous particles suspended in it. The latter were thought to emanate from marshes and other places in which putrefying matter abounded. The precise nature of this infective poison or poisons remained obscure, and the diseases resulting from it – unlike contagious diseases – could differ depending on the intensity of the poison and other factors. In making these observations, Cullen appears to have drawn upon the studies made by Cleghorn and Lind and upon his own experience as a surgeon on a ship which had sailed to the West Indies. It was in Porto Bello that he acquired an interest in the relationship between climate and disease and he went on to make several observations that harmonized with those of tropical practitioners. He believed that heat increased the 'Tendency to Putrefaction in animal Fluids' and that it was 'the leading Circumstance in the Production of Marsh Effluvia'.[106]

Cullen's views on fever show a gradual transition from the putrefactive paradigm which had dominated for much of the eighteenth century to one based on nervous physiology. In his writings and teachings, the two theories were by no means incompatible but, increasingly, the latter came to dominate. This growing preoccupation with neural function was evident not only in medical theory but in many spheres of intellectual life, especially at the Scottish universities. It may be attributed, in part, to the great popularity of Lockean epistemology, which grounded knowledge in the impressions made by objects upon the senses. But it also provided a convenient way of understanding a world which seemed to be more closely connected than ever before. Just as the Newtonians of the early eighteenth century had applied the laws of mechanics to bodily and social realms, so the proponents of nervous physiology began to consider society as an immense organism connected by nerves.[107]

The contours of this new nervous society will be exposed more clearly in Parts II and III of this book, but for now it will suffice to show how nervous physiology affected the way in which medical practitioners began to write about the maladies of the tropics. Emblematic of this shift were the works of William Lempriere, who had been an apothecary to the British Army in the West Indies during the 1790s. Lempriere stood in a long line of medical practitioners who insisted on the uniqueness of tropical disease environments and the need for medical practice to be based on close observation of local phenomena. His main aim was to 'remove the prejudices, or correct the erroneous systems which the young or inexperienced practitioner may have imbibed, previous to his arrival

[106] Lectures on Fevers, c. 1770, 167–8, Cullen Papers, 29, RCPE.

[107] Figlio, 'Theories of Perception'; Lawrence, 'The Nervous System and Society'; Rousseau, *Nervous Acts*, 35.

in a tropical climate'.[108] Having eleven years' experience of working in warm climates, Lempriere believed that he was in a strong position to offer practical advice not only to young military surgeons but also to civilian practitioners who might find themselves in the West Indies. Like the majority of those who had resided in these parts, he attributed the majority of diseases there, including the deadly yellow fever, to exhalations from marshes. Putrefaction, stoked by a humid climate, was almost invariably the culprit, he maintained.[109] And yet the 'impurities' to be found in tropical airs appeared to act disproportionately on those who possessed a 'certain idiosyncracy, or constitution'.[110] He was referring not only to the commonplace assumption that certain races appeared to be less affected by fevers, especially yellow fever, but to an individual's nervous temperament. One of the great predisposing factors in fever, according to Lempriere, was fear; those of a sensitive disposition being more liable to succumb to noxious influences than persons made of sterner stuff. During his recent experiences with the Army in Jamaica, he had found that dread of the climate had been 'very conspicuous among the troops' and that this made it more likely that they would both contract fever and suffer badly from it.[111]

The impressions, real and imagined, which foreign locations could make upon the nervous system fascinated Lempriere even before he went to Jamaica. Shortly before he was posted there, he wrote an account of a visit he made to Morocco, where he had been engaged to treat the son of the emperor. Like many eighteenth-century travel narratives, his account contrasted enlightened Europe with the prejudices, inertia, and cruelties of an oriental despotism. But it also bore the imprint of a new literary and aesthetic sensibility which was itself derived from nervous physiology. In addition to the standard features of such narratives, Lempriere dwelt on some of the seedier sides of life in the Moorish realms: the forbidden delights (as well as the iniquities) of the harem and the sexual opportunities awaiting European travellers. The picture he paints is at once exotic, titillating, and dangerous, the journey being experienced through the impressions it made upon the senses of the author.[112]

By the time he had completed his second work, on the diseases of Jamaica, Lempriere was sufficiently encouraged by the success of his earlier works to put pen to paper once more, this time extolling the benefits of the spa waters of the Isle of Wight, where he was employed as Physician at the Army Depot.[113] Like his earlier works, this account began with a description of the topography of the island and its benefits to health, as well as the 'grand and sublime'

[108] Lempriere, *Practical Observations on the Diseases of the Army in Jamaica*, vol. 1, x.
[109] Lempriere, *Practical Observations*, vol. 2, 4.
[110] Ibid., 9–10.
[111] Ibid., 11–12.
[112] Lempriere, *A Tour from Gibraltar to Tangier.*
[113] Lempriere, *Report on the Medicinal Effects of an Aluminous Chalybeate Spring.*

prospects to be viewed along the more rugged parts of the coast.[114] The impressions which its climate and Romantic scenery made upon those recovering from illness were highly beneficial, he claimed, not least upon those who had returned from tropical parts, as many of his military patients had. Like the spa waters themselves, which he subjected to rigorous trials in the island's military hospital,[115] they acted to stimulate constitutions which had been enervated by protracted residence in tropical climates. These therapies worked as a 'tonic' which refreshed the 'vital principle' that had been denuded by chronic complaints such as fevers and dysentery, or simply by nervous exhaustion.[116] As we shall see, such claims became increasingly common, not only in respect of invalids returning from the tropics, but for the growing number of valetudinarians who had succumbed to the ills of modern society. It was among such people, as well as former denizens of the tropics, that erstwhile colonial practitioners could expect to build a lucrative private practice.

[114] Lempriere, *Medicinal Effects*, 5.

[115] On the Isle of Wight, Lempriere subjected the waters to a trial among sixty military patients suffering from fevers contracted in the West Indies or at Walcheren. He claimed success in thirty-six of these cases within three weeks. Eight were obliged to give up taking the water for various medical reasons, but the rest made a progressive recovery while continuing to take it. Lempriere had previously conducted a similar trial with spa waters on fifty patients at the military depot at Trinidad, apparently with equally beneficial effects. In both cases, the waters had what he termed a 'tonic' effect. Ibid., 56–7, 66, 88.

[116] Ibid., 51–2.

4

Pathology, physiology, and race

As we saw in the last chapter, the post-mortem investigation of disease had been a prominent feature of medicine in colonial hospitals since the middle of the eighteenth century. Although the results of pathological investigations in the colonies were beginning to filter through to the profession in Britain by the 1790s the work of morbid anatomists in the colonies was soon eclipsed by a fashion for all things French, not least pathological anatomy as developed by Parisian practitioners such as Bichat.[1] But the precise impact of Paris medicine is difficult to determine. While some British practitioners made efforts to distribute and popularize the latest developments in European medicine, they had already begun to transform their understanding of disease and of the relationship between the human body and its environment. For many colonial practitioners, Paris medicine was not an exemplar slavishly to be followed but a vindication of the type of hospital-based medicine which they and their predecessors had been advocating for many years. They were by no means uncritical of French authors and believed that there was no substitute for their own observations. In the colonies, too, morbid anatomy was often oriented towards local problems, not the least of which was the perceived vulnerability of Europeans and the closely related question of differences between races. Medical ideas and practices in the colonies thus continued to be marked by a degree of difference from Europe, though perhaps less starkly than before.

THE PATHOLOGY OF RACE IN BRITISH INDIA

The idea that different races had evolved slowly to fit their environment was an important theme in the writings of the naval surgeon James Johnson, who was to become one of the foremost authorities on the diseases of tropical climates. Johnson's career provides us with an excellent illustration of a surgeon-apothecary who rose from humble origins to the pinnacle of the medical profession. Like many of his contemporaries, he saw the armed forces as a vehicle for professional

[1] On the rhetorical aspects of this, see Warner, 'The Idea of Science'.

advancement, punctuating periods of naval service with bouts of intensive study, making use of all the medical opportunities the service presented. A sketch of his early career is instructive because it shows the prominence of dissection in his surgical training at the London anatomy schools; training that would encourage him to seek the signs of disease within the body and not only in symptoms. Fortunately, Johnson's early career is well documented, owing to a long and detailed obituary written by his son in the *Medico-Chirurgical Review* in 1846; a journal which Johnson founded and edited until shortly before his death.[2]

Johnson was born in 1777, in County Derry, the son of a poor farmer. At the age of fifteen, he was apprenticed to a surgeon-apothecary in County Antrim and remained there for two years until transferring to another surgeon-apothecary in Belfast. Johnson then set off for London to further his medical career, securing a position as an apothecary's assistant. After regular attendance at lectures in surgery and anatomy, he passed an examination at Surgeon's Hall in 1798, and was appointed surgeon's mate in the Navy later that year. In his first year in the Navy, Johnson travelled to Newfoundland and Nova Scotia, availing himself of every opportunity to study cases in naval hospitals. On returning to London in 1799, he again threw himself into his studies, passing a second examination at Surgeon's Hall in 1800, which enabled him to find employment as a full surgeon on board another naval vessel sailing to Gibraltar. On his return, Johnson attended the Great Windmill Street anatomy school and placed himself under two surgeon-anatomists, Messrs. Wilson and Thomas. He acquired great skill as a dissector and was allowed to prepare the subjects for his teachers' lectures. Within a few months, Johnson was giving daily demonstrations in anatomy. In 1801, he applied again to the Naval Medical Board for a ship, with a strong recommendation from Wilson to the effect that Johnson had 'actually lived in the dissecting-room of Great Windmill Street during the last six weeks'. He was accepted and gained employment on a sloop serving in the North Sea, but found himself without employment following the peace of 1802. Having already impressed the eminent naval physician Sir Gilbert Blane with his knowledge and enthusiasm, Johnson was soon appointed to the *Caroline*, the ship in which he was to travel to the East Indies. *En route*, the Caroline anchored off Madeira and the coast of Brazil, where Johnson had the opportunity of studying a range of diseases. From South America, the vessel rounded the Cape and steered to Ceylon, and thence to Madras and Bengal, anchoring in the Hughly at the end of September 1803. From here, the *Caroline* set sail for Rangoon, returning to Bengal in November. It was there that Johnson had his first

[2] 'A Sketch of the Life, and Some Account of the Works, of the late Dr James Johnson,' *Medico-Chirurgical Review and Journal of Practical Medicine*, n.s. 3 (1846), 1–48. Most of the following biographical information is obtained from this source and the *DNB*.

encounter with the deadly remittent fever of the Ganges delta, which claimed the lives of many seamen in the Company's ships and those of the Royal Navy.

With Bengal as its base, the *Caroline* was sent on various missions in the East Indies: to the Andaman Islands, to the Malay coast and the Spice Islands, to Coromandel, and to China. In November 1805, suffering from persistent dysentery, Johnson left Bengal for England, where he arrived in January 1806. Soon after his arrival, Johnson wrote an account of his travels in the East – the *Oriental Voyager* (1807) – and, despite his shattered constitution, returned to dissection and lecturing. The prize money that he had obtained during his three years' service enabled him to enter as a student at Guys and St Thomas's, where he formed the acquaintance of the eminent surgeon Sir Astley Cooper. In the autumn of 1806, Johnson returned to Northern Ireland to marry and shortly afterwards obtained a post attending prisoners of war at the naval depots at Plymouth and Portsmouth, where he made a careful study of their diseases. In 1808, he was appointed to the *Valiant* in which he saw a great deal of active service in the Channel before being sent on the disastrous expedition to Walcheren, infamous for the loss of many soldiers to fever. After quitting the *Valiant*, he turned his notes on disease into what became his principal work – *The Influence of Tropical Climates on European Constitutions*, which was first published in 1813. The book went through six editions, the last of which was revised with the help of another old India hand, James Ranald Martin. One of the distinguishing features of the work was its grounding in pathological anatomy and its use of recent experimental work in physiology.

In 1814, shortly after the publication of the *Influence*, Johnson's reputation was such that he was appointed personal physician to the Duke of Clarence, the future William IV. His association with the Duke later led to his being appointed Physician Extraordinary to the King, in spite of the fact that he was not a member of the Royal College of Physicians. Johnson had, however, procured an MD from Aberdeen the year before, which entitled him to call himself a physician, if not to enter the charmed circle of the London College. On leaving the Navy, he decided to make a career in medical journalism, founding and editing the *Medico-Chirurgical Journal* (later named the *Medico-Chirurgical Review*) in 1816. Its first incarnation was as a monthly journal and it was devoted to reviewing British and foreign medical literature. It was the first journal of its kind, and it provided Johnson with a substantial income. This was a time when medical practitioners in Britain were becoming more interested in developments in France, and particularly in pathological anatomy as practised in Paris.[3] Indeed, the *Journal/Review* was one of the main organs through which the British profession came to know about pathological anatomy and its associated clinical practices. It has been claimed that Johnson studied for a time in Paris, perhaps

[3] Maultiz, *Morbid Appearances*; Warner, 'The Idea of Science'.

learning pathological anatomy there,[4] although there is no record of this in the obituary written by his son. His knowledge of French pathological anatomy may have been obtained entirely through the books that he reviewed. Nevertheless, in becoming a champion of Paris medicine, Johnson had found a way of promoting the kind of medicine that he himself had been practising for the last two decades.

Johnson's most influential work, *The Influence of Tropical Climates*, was published before he left the Navy and, although his fourteen-year naval career was punctuated by short breaks, he appears to have spent these studying or demonstrating anatomy and surgery in London. The first two editions show more than a nodding acquaintance with the literature of French pathological anatomists, but the emphasis on pathological anatomy grew out of his London training and his experiences in India, where he had the opportunity to conduct post-mortem examinations on a regular basis. Like many of his predecessors in India, Johnson placed great emphasis on excessive (or sometimes deficient) biliary secretion as a cause of many diseases including hepatitis, dysentery, cholera, and certain types of fevers. He found evidence of vitiated bile wherever these disorders occurred, appearing in post-mortem dissections as a mass of black or dark-green fluid.[5] Other sure indicators of bilious fever were inflammation of the small intestine, turgesence in the venous system, and engorgement of the viscera with blood. From the appearance of the organs after death, Johnson also hoped to find some means of treating the deadly remittent fever of Bengal. Describing one of the first fatal cases he experienced whilst moored in the Hughly, Johnson recalled that he 'had the body conveyed to a convenient place, in hopes dissection might afford some clue to my future efforts. On laying open the abdomen, I was surprised to find the liver so gorged . . . with blood, that it actually fell to pieces handling it.'[6] The dissection impressed upon his mind the importance of venesection as a means of reducing inflammation and engorgement; a practice that had been condemned by most previous writers on the diseases of tropical climates.[7] Johnson persisted in this course of action throughout his time in India and was later credited with reintroducing the practice of bloodletting in fevers to India, although he continued to use bleeding in conjunction with, and as precursor to, calomel.[8]

Like most of his predecessors in India, Johnson believed that bilious disorders were endemic among Europeans because their bodies were poorly equipped to cope with the country's extreme heat. Bodies that were not accustomed to such a climate, he claimed, suffered from increased secretion of bile, which became

[4] Maultiz, *Morbid Appearances*, 162.
[5] Johnson, *The Influence of Tropical Climates*, 1815 edn., 22–4.
[6] Ibid., 41–2.
[7] Ibid., 43.
[8] Goodeve, 'A Sketch on the Progress of European Medicine in the East', 147. These matters are discussed in greater depth in Section II.

vitiated when it was too copious to be used up in digestion. However, unlike previous writers, Johnson differentiated between the regions of India in which climate contributed more or less to hepatic derangement. Liver diseases, he insisted, were more common in Madras than Bengal because the latter had some remission from heat during its 'tropical winter'.[9] Unlike the London physician Dr William Saunders, who was, indebted to earlier British Indian authors, he argued that hepatic derangements occurred solely because of exposure to heat and not from an 'indigenous and local poison'; that is, a particular kind of miasma.[10] They were to be found to a greater or lesser extent across the tropical world, including the West Indies, from which Saunders claimed they were absent.[11] This was a small difference, perhaps, but one that illustrates the ways in which nervous physiology lent itself to more generalized notions of tropicality.

According to Johnson, heat alone was sufficient to cause hepatic derangement because a 'sympathy' existed between the skin and the liver: between perspiration and biliary secretion. Thus, when a European arrived in India and began to sweat profusely, his biliary secretion also increased. The notion of nervous sympathy had existed for over a century and was now in vogue again, due to the work of Xavier Bichat. The Parisian doctor was cited by Johnson, but he criticized him for misunderstanding the relationship between climate and internal secretions. Whereas Bichat had insisted that a cold, damp atmosphere made internal secretions more abundant, Johnson maintained that the reverse was true.[12] Johnson's notion of sympathy was also more restricted than that of Bichat, who saw this principle operating not only through the nervous system, but also in what he termed the 'cellular system', connecting similar tissues within the body.[13] Unfortunately for Europeans in India, there was little that could be done to counteract this tendency, for, while they might become acclimatized to a certain extent, complete adaptation was impossible. Johnson warned repeatedly that European constitutions were fundamentally unsuited to tropical climates and that Europeans would 'degenerate' if they remained in India too long.[14] Indians, by contrast, rarely appeared to suffer from hepatic disorders: the reason, according to Johnson, being the gradual adaptation, over many generations, of their cutaneo-hepatic systems. Johnson went so far as to suggest that Indians owed their 'sallow tints' to an active, though no longer pathological, biliary secretion. He added that this was 'quite conformable with the wisdom of Providence, and to the unceasing exertions of Nature, in remedying what she cannot entirely prevent'.[15]

9 Johnson, *Influence*, 2nd edn., 251–64.
10 Ibid., 251.
11 Ibid., 264.
12 Ibid., 265–8.
13 Bichat, *Anatomie Générale*, vol. 1, 82–3, 167.
14 Harrison, *Climates*, 103–4.
15 Johnson, *Influence*, 2nd edn., 355–6.

Johnson's theory of racial characteristics recalls that of Blumenbach, who argued that the 'black races of mankind' were 'afflicted with a permanent hereditary jaundice' which had emerged over many generations of exposure to hot climates.[16] It was also similar in certain respects to that of Rev. Dr Samuel Stanhope Smith, who had earlier attributed the colour of Indians to the superabundant secretion of bile and its secretion on the surface of the body.[17] But Johnson's explanation differs in that it emphasized the 'sympathy' between perspiration and biliary secretion. Also notable is his insistence that certain races were uniquely adapted to certain climates, which appears superficially to anticipate the racial doctrines of later theorists such as Robert Knox, who embraced Cuvier's opinion that no alteration or change had taken place in any animal – including man – since the earliest times. But, unlike the Cuverians, Johnson was prepared to admit that very gradual changes had occurred in the structure of plants and animals in response to climatic conditions.[18] He believed that it was possible for man to adapt to a new climate but only after *many* generations: a theory which Johnson lifted from Darwin's *Zoonomia.*[19] Herein lay the main distinction between Johnson and most of his predecessors, not least the military surgeon John Hunter of Jamaica, who believed that the human body could become fully acclimatized to a new climate within a single lifetime.[20] Just as medicine was now based on internal as well as external manifestations of disease, differences between human beings were increasingly seen as deep-seated and hereditary. Johnson was predisposed by his intensive training in anatomy to look for such differences, in much the same way as he was disposed to search within the body for knowledge about disease.

As a naval surgeon, Johnson had few opportunities to undertake comparative work and to observe the morbid anatomy of Indians; far fewer, at any rate, than most military and civil surgeons in India. It is impossible to say how frequently the dissection of Indian soldiers was conducted or in what circumstances, but there are occasional references to it around the turn of the century. In his account of the Egyptian campaign of 1801, James McGrigor mentions the dissection of soldiers, including sepoys, who had died of plague, noting that

16 Blumenbach, 'On the Possibility of Casual Mutilations in the Bodies of Animals', 1–2.

17 Johnson, *Influence*, 2nd edn., 336. See Smith, *An Essay on the Causes of the Variety of Complexion and Figure in the Human Species.* Smith (1751–1819) was a Presbyterian minister and seventh president of the College of New Jersey. He worked for a time as a missionary in Virginia and was critical of those, like Thomas Jefferson, who took a low view of the accomplishments of African-Americans. He considered climate to be one of three factors (the others being social organization and modes of life) that gave rise to differences in complexion and argued against rigid racial classification as exhibited by the work of Kames. His book was based on a lecture given to the Philosophical Society of Philadelphia in 1787.

18 Knox, *The Races of Man*, 86–7, 107, 215.

19 On Darwin's evolutionary theories, see King-Hele, *Erasmus Darwin.*

20 See Harrison, *Climates*, chaps 1 and 2; idem, '"Tender Frame of Man"'. There is no indication that John Hunter of Jamaica was related to the more famous London surgeon of the same name.

they were among the first morbid anatomical examinations of the disease.[21] One prominent military surgeon who grounded a theory of racial distinction on patho-physiological observations was James Annesley, the author of *Researches into the Causes, Nature, and Treatment of the More Prevalent Diseases of India.* This book went through two editions, the first in 1828, the second in 1841, and was widely read by the military surgeons for whom it was intended. Annesley had many years' experience in India and rose to become president of the Madras Medical Board. This post added greatly to the authority of his work, and his research on Indian diseases led to his being elected a Fellow of the Royal Society. Unfortunately, little is known about Annesley's training, but it is likely that he was a surgeon-apothecary rather than a physician. He probably studied at one of the London anatomy schools and, like Johnson, set great store by post-mortem examinations. He had no doubt that pathological anatomy could elucidate the causes of disease, as is shown in his treatment of cholera: a disease which had attracted a good deal of attention in India after it became epidemic in 1817. Annesley believed that cholera was essentially a disease of the nervous system and that diminution of nervous power was its proximate cause, usually resulting from an electrical charge of the air. The appearance of thick, black blood in most cases of cholera suggested to him that there had been a complete collapse of the body's circulatory powers, such as might occur if the body were subjected to a powerful electrical shock.[22] As we saw earlier, the electrical theory of cholera was well known in India,[23] but Annesley appears to have been the first to combine it with pathological anatomy.[24] His dissections also led to him to diverge from received wisdom about the cause of fevers. Whereas previous writers believed that most Indian fevers were caused by excessive bile, he insisted that the increased secretion of bile was a consequence rather than a cause of these diseases.[25]

In the 1820s and 1830s, putrid and bilious theories of disease were giving way to the conviction that fevers were caused by a disorder of the nervous system. This shift had begun in the West Indies in the 1790s but was now articulated with increasing force in India. In 1837, Henry Hurry Goodeve, Professor of Anatomy and Medicine at the recently founded Calcutta Medical College,[26] felt

[21] M'Gregor, *Medical Sketches*, 141.

[22] Annesley, *Researches*, 492–500.

[23] See, for example: Ainslie, *Observations on the Cholera Morbus*; Orton, *An Essay on the Epidemic Cholera of India.*

[24] Goodeve referred to Annesley's 'excellent work' on cholera. See his 'Sketch on the Progress of European Medicine in the East', 149.

[25] Annesley, *Researches*, 538.

[26] H. H. Goodeve (1807–84) became an MRCS in 1828 and took an MD at Edinburgh the following year. He became an Assistant-Surgeon in the Company's Bengal service in 1831 and a surgeon in 1848; he retired in 1853. After retirement, Goodeve went on to become an FRCS in 1844, MRCP (Lond.) and FRCP (Lond.), both in 1860. He was best known as Professor of Medicine at the new Calcutta Medical College (founded 1835) and as author of *Hints on Children in India* (1844). Crawford, *Roll*, 103.

able to dismiss the labours of previous generations of British practitioners in India who had been obsessed by bile and putridity, attributing to them every disease they encountered. 'Never was there a more complete mistaking of effect for cause', he believed, 'or a better illustration of the forcing [of] all facts to accommodate themselves to one theory.'[27] These vestiges of the humoral theory, as Goodeve saw them, had been superseded in India by what he termed 'rational medicine'.[28] He saw James Johnson as beginning this shift away from outdated nostrums, his work resting on the principles of nervous physiology. In the case of cholera, for example, Johnson had ridiculed the view that the disease was due to excessive bile, insisting that it arose as a result of the suppression of bile produced by a derangement of the bile duct which 'sympathized' with disordered circulation in the skin. But it was Annesley's 'excellent work', as Goodeve described it, that had done more than any other treatise on cholera to provide a rational account of its aetiology and pathology.[29]

With William B. O'Shaughnessy, Professor of Materia Medica at the Medical College, Goodeve was Secretary of the Calcutta Medical Physical Society, which had been founded in 1822, principally to allow members of the Presidency medical establishment to discuss matters such as medical topography, the relationship of meteorological phenomena to disease, and the investigation of native remedies. However, the society and its transactions, which were published from 1825, also served to familiarize Anglo-Indian practitioners with recent developments in European medicine, including Parisian pathological anatomy and physiology. By 1835, the Calcutta society had 367 ordinary members, 6 honorary members, including Sir Gilbert Blane, and 21 corresponding members, which included Continental Europeans and Indians. Similar societies were formed in Bombay, in 1837, and in Madras, a year later.[30] According to Goodeve, such organizations had given the profession in India a new lease of life. 'Within the last twenty or fifteen years Anglo-Indian medicine has advanced with rapid strides', he claimed, 'The immense improvements which have taken place in the medical sciences in Europe have doubtless contributed to this desirable end; for even in these distant regions do we feel... the influence of scientific discoveries at home.'[31]

The developments to which Goodeve referred represented a new phase in Anglo-Indian medicine, fostered by fledgling professional societies and the first college of European medicine, which was founded in Calcutta in 1835. The Medical College was established during the reforming administration of the

[27] Goodeve, 'Sketch', 133.
[28] Ibid., 125.
[29] Ibid., 149.
[30] *Transactions of the Medical and Physical Society of Calcutta*, 7 (1835), v–vi. The transactions of the Madras society attracted 144 subscribers for its first volume: *Madras Quarterly Medical Journal*, 1 (1839), xxii.
[31] Goodeve, 'Sketch', 152.

Governor-General William Bentinck, and was intended to provide instruction in Western medicine to Indians and Europeans through the medium of the English language. This superseded the short-lived Native Medical Institution, founded in 1822, which taught aspects of European and Indian traditional medicine (*Ayurveda* and *Unani*) side by side. The passing of this NMI is often said to mark the victory of 'Anglicism' over the hitherto dominant philosophy of orientalism, and the beginning of a new phase in British rule in which the colonial state sought to bring India into conformity with the dictates of reason and political economy.[32] Together with the establishment from the 1790s of hospitals and dispensaries intended for the use of the Indian poor, the new medical college in Calcutta, and those shortly to be founded in Madras and Bombay, enlarged the scope of Anglo-Indian medicine, which had hitherto been concerned largely with Europeans.[33] The colleges also provided a firmer institutional basis for various kinds of medical investigation, and Goodeve readily acknowledged the important contributions made to the study of diseases by the new generation of Anglo-Indian practitioners. Annesley's work on cholera was also taken seriously by medical practitioners in Britain, and reviewers applauded his painstaking observations and its grasp of recent medical theory.[34]

But this new generation of self-proclaimed 'scientific' practitioners did not have everything their own way. Goodeve had only arrived in India in 1831 and O'Shaughnessy in 1833, and some old India hands thought they still had much to learn. Frederick Corbyn, the editor of the *India Journal of Medical Science*, declared that:

> each and all of these gentlemen may be thoroughly acquainted with the principles of Cullen; they may be well versed in the arguments and subtleties of Brown and Darwin; embued [sic] with the doctrines of revulsions of Broussais, familiar with French pathology; fresh from the theatre of Anatomy and Chemistry; . . . but when they came to India their knowledge is bounded. Here they are to receive and to afford instruction![35]

He insisted that 'only those who have seen disease in India in all its various shapes and characters on the Indian constitution, are able to point it out, and to discover remedies for its removal'.[36] It was a familiar refrain and one that was to be heard frequently for the rest of the century. As Charles Morehead, editor of the *Transactions of the Medical and Physical Society of Bombay*, put it in 1838, 'to be slavish imitators of the doctrines, and systems of the European schools, is to shew, that we do not estimate our position here, at its true value to science'.[37]

[32] Bala, *Imperialism and Medicine in Bengal*; Alavi, *Islam and Healing*; more generally, Stokes, *English Utilitarians*.

[33] Arnold, *Colonizing the Body*, 54–60; Kumar, *Medicine and the Raj*, chaps 1–2.

[34] Review of Annesley's *Sketches of the Prevalent Diseases of India* (1825), *Medico-Chirurgical Review*, 4 (1826), 89.

[35] Editorial, *India Journal of Medical Science*, 1 (1836), 187.

[36] Ibid., 188.

[37] Editorial, *Transactions of the Medical and Physical Society of Bombay*, 1 (1838), ix.

The reformist rhetoric of Goodeve did, indeed, mask important continuities with the past, not least the perceived connection between meteorological conditions and human health. In Anglo-Indian medical literature of the 1820s and 1830s, the diseased body was still regarded as a microcosm of the environment, much as it had been a century before. The only difference was that the body's relationship to external phenomena was now construed in terms of nervous physiology rather than humoral imbalance. Environmental influences that depressed the body's vital powers had what Annesley termed a 'malignant or disorganizing' effect on the organs.[38] This could include inflammation of various membranes, accumulations of rancid bile, and so forth, depending on the constitution of the individual, his or her particular circumstances, and the nature of the epidemic influence. As Margaret Pelling has noted for England, the 1820s and 1830s brought a renewed emphasis upon physiology and process, owing partly to the influence of the French physician Broussais. This did not altogether sideline pathological anatomy, with its tendency to localize disease in particular organs, but it did lead to a modification of contemporary doctrine. Organic lesions now tended to be seen as 'secondary affections' or complications of a generalized febrile state induced by some external influence.[39]

One such influence was the noxious vapours that seemed to arise from decaying matter. As Annesley put it, 'There is, perhaps, no practitioner who has had any extensive experience of the diseases of warm climates . . . who is not fully aware that the majority of the most prevalent maladies within the tropics . . . are chiefly owing to the exhalations from marshy situations and from vegetable matter in a state of composition.' Although miasma arose in marshy situations in all climates, the intense heat and abundant rain of the tropics appeared to accelerate putrefaction and hence to increase susceptibility to diseases such as fever.[40] Annesley's writings abound with references to decay, dissolution, and degeneration: environmental, bodily, and social. He argued that atmospheric conditions arising from heat, moisture, soil, and vegetation were 'the most productive, although the more remote causes of national character – of advancement in all the arts, sciences, and refinements of life in some countries, and of moral and physical debasement in others. In one [Great Britain] their beneficent operation may be traced in the freedom, prosperity, and greatness of its inhabitants; in another [India], their noxious influences are manifest in the degenerate and debased condition of the species, whose wants, habits, enjoyments, and desires, seldom surpass those of higher animals.'[41] The enfeebled and degenerate state of the Indian body was thus, according to Annesley, a function of a

[38] Annesley, *Researches*, 555.
[39] Pelling, *Cholera, Fever and English Medicine*, 15–16.
[40] Annesley, *Researches*, 11.
[41] Ibid., 9.

degenerate and decaying society; as he put it, 'One of the chief effects of a high temperature is to hasten the decomposition of organized bodies.'[42]

These ideas recall the works of Robert Orme and other eighteenth-century writers on India, who sought to account for and justify British dominion in similar ways, not to mention those of Enlightenment conjectural historians like Adam Ferguson, who attributed human progress in large part to climatic influences.[43] But Annesley's work differs in one important respect: climate was now described as a *remote* influence (as in Johnson's works) and it was the accumulated effects of climate, passed on through countless generations, that most concerned him. Both he and Johnson should therefore be regarded as 'weak transmutationists', who allowed for a gradual, almost imperceptible, accretion of acquired characteristics over many generations. For all practical purposes, the basic distinctions between races were fixed, limiting the prospects for adaptation to different environments.[44] Each climatic zone, according to Annesley, was 'peopled by a particular and an appropriate race, of a different constitution and character, and calculated to pass their existence in such situations without having their lives materially shortened, or being more frequently subject to disease'.[45] For good or ill, Indians and Europeans bore the indelible imprint of their climate and, while Indians appeared to be inured to the effects of miasma, Europeans seemed to have an 'inherent predisposition to be affected by this cause'.[46]

It has already been suggested that pathological anatomy induced some of its practitioners to see racial differences as deep-seated rather than as surface phenomena, and post-mortem dissections offered what Annesley regarded as firm evidence of racial differences. Fevers appeared to manifest themselves differently in Indian and European bodies: they were more likely to appear as extreme debility in natives and less likely to attack the abdominal viscera than in Europeans.

As we shall see Part II, this belief had important implications for therapy because the weaker constitutions of natives seemed to warrant greater care in depletive treatments such as bloodletting.[47] In cholera, too, there were apparently subtle differences in racial pathology. In Indians, 'the disease generally terminated rapidly, the powers of life being readily overpowered', there being more evidence of congestion in the vascular system, whereas, in Europeans, there was a more violent response to the disease and more appearance of capillary action, as one might expect from their supposedly stronger constitutions.[48] Other writers

[42] Ibid., 29.
[43] Harrison, *Climates*, chap. 2.
[44] By 1830, the same was apparently true of the French tropical colonies also. See Jennings, *Curing the Colonizers*.
[45] Annesley, *Researches*, 1st edn., vol. 1, 63–4; 2nd edn., vol. 1, 24.
[46] Annesley, *Researches*, 2nd edn., vol. 1, 43.
[47] Ibid., 584–5.
[48] Ibid., 492.

claimed to find similar differences in respect of cholera, although not necessarily the same as those observed by Annesley. Surgeons S. W. Lister and T. Evans, attached to the 46th Regiment of Native Infantry, argued that European pathology was distinguished by the fact that the head was more likely to be affected sooner and more severely than among Indians, whereas Indians experienced more severe congestion of the chest.[49] Either way, there was an implicit hierarchy. For Lister and Evans, the mental superiority of Europeans appears to have been a source of vulnerability, in much the same way as their bodily vigour was for Annesley. But Annesley acknowledged that the weakness of Indians arose as much from the circumstances in which they lived as from innate characteristics. This was especially true of periods of dearth, for insufficient nourishment weakened the body, leaving it less able to withstand the debilitating effects of miasma.[50]

It is impossible to say how far Annesley attributed different pathological signs to nature or nurture, although his generalizations about race and environmental adaptation suggest that he believed certain characteristics to be unvarying across generations. This was also the opinion of the civil surgeon William Twining, who attributed the apparent differences in disease in European and Indian bodies to both lifestyles and constitutional peculiarities. William Twining (1790–1835) was Assistant-Surgeon at the Calcutta General Hospital, and during his time at the hospital he conducted numerous post-mortem examinations which formed the basis of his two books: *Clinical Illustrations of the More Important Diseases of Bengal* (published in Calcutta in 1832 and again in 1835) and *A Practical Account of the Epidemic Cholera* (1833), which is essentially a summary of the former publication intended for those facing cholera in Britain. During his time in Calcutta, Twining established a reputation as a forward-looking practitioner familiar with all the latest developments in European medicine, including pathological anatomy and physiology. He disseminated this information through the Calcutta Medical and Physical Society, of which he became Secretary, until his untimely death in 1835.[51] Goodeve later celebrated Twining as the most

[49] Lister, 'Report of Cholera in the 46th Regiment', 15.

[50] Annesley, *Researches*, 2nd edn., 521. See also Harrison, *Climates*, 170–4; Pickstone, 'Dearth, Dirt and Fever Epidemics'.

[51] Obituary of Twining, *India Journal of Medical Science*, 2 (1835), 376. Twining (1790–1835) died in Calcutta after rupturing a blood vessel whilst assisting an injured man. He was born in Nova Scotia and afterwards appears to have returned to Britain, where he trained as a surgeon (most probably in London). Twining joined the Army Medical Department in 1812, and in 1814 was promoted to Assistant-Surgeon. In 1821, he was sent to Ceylon to serve the Governor, Gen. Sir Edward Paget, from where he accompanied him to India. In 1824, he was appointed Commander-in-Chief of the British Army in the region. After his arrival in India, Twining joined the Bengal Army as a Surgeon and eventually took charge of the Calcutta General Hospital. He played a prominent role in the newly formed Calcutta Medical and Physical Society. See 'Obituary' cited above, and Crawford, *Roll*, 86.

prominent Anglo-Indian practitioner of his day and his *Clinical Illustrations* as 'indisputably the most valuable treatise on the subject hitherto published'.[52]

The importance of post-mortem examinations was emphasized throughout Twining's work. The introduction to *Clinical Illustrations*, for instance, draws attention to the great advantage of being able to examine the state of the internal organs soon after death, before the onset of post-mortem degeneration.[53] His treatise on cholera also began by stating that it was based on extensive post-mortem examinations.[54] He appears to have been greatly encouraged in this line of investigation by two of his superiors at the Calcutta General Hospital: Drs William Russell and John Turner, successively its chief medical officer. Twining wrote of Turner's 'anxiety to facilitate and promote every useful pathological inquiry, and to apply the strictest results of that inquiry to practice'.[55] True medical knowledge, he believed, was only to be gained through the 'laborious and accurate observation of facts',[56] and his observations led him to question a number of widely held views about the causation and treatment of certain Indian diseases. For example, Twining used post-mortem evidence to question the primacy of hepatic disorders as a cause of dysentery. He was unable to find in the majority of cases who died from dysentery (Indian or European) any mark of disease upon the liver.[57] Twining also used morbid anatomy to inform therapeutics, which he modified depending on what appeared to be distinct racial traits in pathology. This was to become a major feature of teaching and research at the Calcutta Medical School over the next two decades and one that many Indian students found equally fascinating.[58]

But while morbid anatomy was still central to the study of fevers in India, some medical practitioners were sceptical that it could yield much information about disease. The military surgeon Samuel Dickson cautioned 'That the study of morbid anatomy has given rise to a class of medical materialists who, hoping to find the origin of every disorder made manifest by the scalpel, are mistaking effects for causes'. Dickson followed 'the celebrated Brown' who had warned his disciples not to look for the causes of disease in dead bodies.[59] The relationship between neo-vitalism and anti-materialism was by no means clear-cut, however. Nervous physiology could lend itself just as easily to materialism or a kind of fatalistic naturalism: the medical equivalent of *laissez-faire* or Malthusianism.[60] But the principle of life, or *vis medicatrix naturae*, was often seen as God-given;

52 Goodeve, 'Sketch', 154–5.
53 Twining, *Clinical Illustrations of the More Important Diseases of Bengal*, vi.
54 Twining, *A Practical Account of the Epidemic Cholera*, xi.
55 Twining, *Clinical Illustrations*, ix–x.
56 Ibid., xxiv.
57 Ibid., 3.
58 Harrison, 'Racial Pathologies'.
59 Dickson, *The Fallacy of the Art of Physic*, 6–8.
60 Jacyna, 'Immanence or Transcendence'.

and, in working with nature, the wise physician was paying heed to 'a principle inherent in the constitution, originally stamped upon it by the Creator that gave it being, for the integrity of the functions that constitute life'.[61]

Thus, before practitioners attempted to speculate on the changes that took place in disease, Dickson insisted that they should acquaint themselves with physiology, or the basic principles governing human health.[62] He articulated the new conviction that 'The *post mortem* appearances found in the bodies of fever patients, are simply the occasional evidence of the inflammatory *effects* of the disease on different organs of the body, various and uncertain . . . '. The biliary theory was a case in point but so, too, was the more recent work of Broussais and his British counterpart Clutterbuck, who attributed the cause of fevers to local inflammation.[63] What mattered to Dickson, and to most of those indebted to Cullen's rebellious pupil John Brown, was the state of 'general irritation' that existed in the patient, which arose from the action of various external stimuli upon the nervous system.[64]

Having spent some years in southern India with the Royal Regiment, Dickson applied these insights to explain a wide range of diseases, not merely fevers, but also cholera, dysentery, hepatitis, and diseases that occurred almost exclusively among Indians, such as elephantiasis. In his discussion of cholera, Dickson revealed an establishment that was divided in its opinions over the seat of the disease on the basis of their post-mortem observations, some locating it in the inflammation of the brain, others in some particular state of the stomach, intestines, or liver (commonly, accumulations of bile). Others, like Dickson, insisted that such changes were merely the effects of nervous derangement;[65] a conclusion that he had reached after having performed experiments on a living dog, in which he had induced every symptom of cholera by injecting different substances into its veins.[66] But, like most other writers on cholera, Dickson attributed this derangement in human beings to certain states of the atmosphere, such as those charged with electricity. In line with Brunonian thinking, he also suggested that cholera, and even plague, were nothing more than varieties of remittent fever, all of which were caused by particular forms of epidemic influence.[67] These influences affected individuals disproportionately depending on whether they were abstemious or weakened by debauch, fatigue, and fear.[68] Indeed, he claimed that, 'The best preventive of cholera is severity of mind' and condemned the 'present panic' that existed on the subject in Britain, which had

[61] Norton, 'Intermittent Fever', 5.
[62] Ibid., 3; idem, *On the Prevalent Diseases of India*, vii.
[63] Dickson, *Diseases*, 96.
[64] Dickson, *Art of Physic*, 6.
[65] Dickson, *Diseases*, 2.
[66] Ibid., 20–1.
[67] Dickson, *Art of Physic*, 23, 31–2.
[68] Dickson, *Diseases*, 51.

recently experienced its first visitation of the disease. 'The higher ranks', he felt, should ignore the bulletins and reports on the disease which served only to cause public alarm, and 'make men selfishly alive to what God will take from them at his own time'.[69]

THE ANATOMY OF FEVER IN THE WEST INDIES

In the West Indies, morbid anatomy had been firmly established in hospital practice since the 1750s, and most surgeons posted to the islands with the Army and Navy during the Revolutionary and Napoleonic Wars continued to take advantage of the opportunities presented to them. The principal subject of their investigations was yellow fever, which claimed thousands of lives on St Domingue in the 1790s. Although the disease had spread to the Mediterranean coast by 1800, the West Indies was still the best place to make post-mortem observations. As Edward Doughty remarked in his treatise on yellow fever, practitioners who witnessed yellow fever in Spain were often forbidden from dissecting the bodies of those who had died from it. Having been stationed with the Army in Jamaica for eight years before being posted to Spain, Doughty noted that 'Everyone who died of the disease at Up-Park Camp [Jamaica], in 1802, was opened. This task, by choice, fell to my share; the other medical gentlemen occasionally assisted, and always one or two of the orderlies.'[70] But this was not the case in Cadiz, where Doughty had been posted after the beginning of the Peninsular War. The head of the Army Medical Department in Spain was Sir James Fellowes, who apparently attempted to prevent his surgeons from dissecting the bodies of British soldiers who had died from yellow fever. Unlike Doughty, Fellowes believed that the disease was contagious and that it might be spread by dissection; he also declared that dissection might have a depressing effect upon morale.[71] This was not normally a consideration in general hospitals, in which the dead patients had been removed from their regiments, but carrying out a dissection amidst a soldier's former comrades was quite another matter. However, Doughty suspected that the real reason for avoiding dissection had more to do with local opinion: 'the Spanish practitioners had such an aversion to anatomical enquiry, from their dread of contagion, and Sir James was on terms of the most social intimacy with them'.[72] While this may have been true of physicians in Cadiz, some Spanish practitioners did conduct a limited number

[69] Ibid., 79.
[70] Doughty, *Observations and Inquiries into the Nature and Treatment of the Yellow, or Bulam Fever*, 49.
[71] Ibid., viii, ix.
[72] Ibid., 100.

of dissections of yellow fever cases during other outbreaks,[73] as did other Mediterranean practitioners.[74]

With restrictions placed on post-mortem investigation in the services away from the colonies, most surgeons that were dispatched to the West Indies took full advantage of the freedom that their posting offered to dissect those who died from yellow fever. Their object in doing so was to elucidate the proximate causes of the disease – which viscera were most affected and how – and through this to gain knowledge of its remote or exciting causes.[75] It was also widely believed that pathological investigation would give practitioners a better idea of which treatments were likely to be successful.[76] It is therefore unsurprising that most Edinburgh MD theses written by surgeons returning from the West Indies contained a chapter on the pathological signs of yellow fever. It is not always clear whether the descriptions are the result of first-hand observation or simply a summary of existing knowledge, but in most cases it is likely to be an amalgam of both, as references are sometimes made to other works, presumably in order to corroborate their findings.[77] These MD theses tend to be rather derivative, but surgeons continued to stress the vital importance of seeing for oneself and testing the theories of others.

George Pinckard's observations on diseases of the West Indies exemplify this outlook. Describing the autopsy of a soldier who had died of yellow fever in the hospital at Stabroek, Demerara, Pinckard recalled that:

> The body was examined, with a view to ascertain the changes produced by the disease, but the appearances were not precisely such, as from conversing with other practitioners, and reading a variety of authors, we had been led to expect. The stomach was found to be the organ which exhibited the strongest marks of derangement.[78]

He later concluded that:

> From experience, and examination of the diseased appearances, I may hope for more accurate elucidation, and perhaps be enabled to arrive at some general maxim, which, in vain, I have looked for in the discordant opinions of the ingenious men who have devoted their pens to this great – this interesting, and most important subject.[79]

Pinckard was one a number of military practitioners in the West Indies who counted themselves as supporters of the nervous theory of Brown. These included Hector M'Lean, who wrote of the Brunonian doctrine that, 'by no means free from errors, it is the most comprehensive and enlightened that has yet

[73] De Arejula, *Breve descripcion de la fiebre amarilla padecida en Cadiz*, 423–32.
[74] Tommasini, *Reserches pathologiques sur la fièvre de Livourne*, 9–31.
[75] Clark, *Treatise on the Yellow Fever*, 19–20.
[76] M'Cabe, *Military Medical Reports*, v–vi.
[77] e.g. Steel, *De febre insularum Indiae occidentalis*, 8–11; Playfair, *De febre flava calpensi*, 8–9.
[78] Pinckard, *Notes*, vol. 2, 226.
[79] Ibid., 324.

appeared.'[80] As followers of Brown, they opposed the prevalent notion that fevers were caused by derangement of the biliary system and were inclined to be sceptical of elaborate theorizing. However, there was less uniformity of opinion among military and naval practitioners in the West Indies than among their counterparts in India. While this could be seen as an advantage, some contemporaries believed that the relatively limited time practitioners spent in any one station in the West Indies militated against the steady accretion of medical knowledge. Just as Charles Maclean had stressed the advantage conferred by the size of the East India Company's medical establishment, the Army surgeon Colin Chisholm envied its stability, which provided a repository of knowledge, particularly about the pathology of tropical diseases. 'Such ignorance can scarcely exist in the East Indies', he wrote,

> where a permanent establishment of medical, civil and military staff is constantly maintained; the members of which are well educated, intelligent and experienced men, and who readily communicate their knowledge to the newly arrived young surgeons. These, after being kept at certain stations until they acquire all the advantage such communication necessarily presents to them, practice; and in turn succeed to important stations, possessed of the accumulated experience of their predecessors: and thus instead of any deficiency or deterioration of tropical medical science, there is a constant increase and improvement. In fact the most valuable part of the medical practice of the West, has been derived from the East, and that at no very remote period.[81]

Chisholm embraced the biliary theory of fever of which some of his West Indian contemporaries, notably the Brunonians, were already highly critical, and deferred to Indian practitioners such as James Johnson. His rather limited pathological investigations tended to reinforce received wisdom about the bilious nature of yellow fever.[82]

In the early 1800s, morbid anatomy began to figure in a number of debates over the nature of yellow fever, not least its existence as a disease distinct from other forms of fever. Pathology therefore carried a heavy weight on its shoulders because the identity of yellow fever had a bearing on controversies over whether it was contagious and whether measures such as quarantine were necessary; a subject to which we shall return in the final section of this book. These political implications help to explain the vehemence with which some practitioners contested each other's descriptions of the post-mortem signs of yellow fever, a case in point being the dispute between the eminent naval physician William Pym and the military physician Edward Bancroft, who served with the Army in the West Indies before becoming Physician to St George's Hospital in London and a Fellow of the Royal College.

80 M'Lean, *Enquiry*, 57.
81 Chisholm, *A Manual of the Climate and Diseases of Tropical Countries*, iii–iv.
82 Ibid., 37, 185.

In his *Observations on the Bulam Fever* (1815), Pym endorsed Chisholm's view that yellow fever was a distinct disease propagated by a specific contagion, which had, in turn, definite symptoms and pathognomic signs. According to Pym, the fever was 'attended with a peculiar inflammation of the stomach, which, in most cases that prove fatal, terminates in gangrene, or in a diseased state of that internal or villous coat of that organ. . . .'[83] But Bancroft found Pym's description rather vague, there being no indication of in what this 'peculiarity' consisted.[84] His own descriptions of post-mortem signs, by contrast, were very detailed and closely correlated with pre-mortem symptoms. According to Bancroft, 'When the bodies of patients, in whom the affection of the head formed the principal feature of the disorder, have been inspected after death, the integuments of the brain have generally been found more or less inflamed, especially near the temporal bones; the vessels of the dura mater, and of the pia mater, were not infrequently observed to be very turgid with blood.'[85] He explained that these signs 'account[ed] sufficiently for the occurrence of those symptoms, and for the fatality that so often attends them, as well as for the derangement of mind, and the extreme feebleness of the limbs, which are the frequent consequences of this disorder in those who escape with life'.[86] Bancroft did not deny that there were forms of fever that affected the stomach more than the brain, but disputed the claim that these morbid appearances were unique to yellow fever, claiming that many cases of remittent fever displayed similar signs.[87]

The other major dispute concerning yellow fever in which pathological evidence featured strongly was its bilious origins. Some writers had begun to challenge bilious explanations of yellow fever as early as the 1790s, and did so partly on the basis of their post-mortem findings.[88] The main challenge to the biliary theory in the West Indies now came from a feisty young surgeon called Robert Jackson and his supporters among serving and former members of the Army Medical Department. Jackson and his followers believed that the nervous system played the central role in the causation of disease. Their basic conviction was that yellow fever, like other fevers, arose from hyper-stimulation of the nervous system and could be caused by excessive heat or any stimulant that 'exalts the irritable power'. As in Brown's system, which it resembled superficially, the nature of disease depended on the degree to which the nervous system was excited, so that various forms of fever, together with dysentery and some other complaints were but different manifestations of the diseased state of the body.[89] Jackson set himself against the biliary theory partly on account of the regularity

[83] Pym, *Observations upon the Bulam Fever*, 5.
[84] Bancroft, *A Sequel to an Essay on the Yellow Fever*, 25–6.
[85] Bancroft, *An Essay on the Disease called Yellow Fever*, 17.
[86] Ibid., 18–19.
[87] Bancroft, *Sequel*, 27.
[88] M'Lean, *Enquiry*, 33.
[89] Jackson, *A Sketch of the History and Cure of Febrile Diseases*, 3, 8.

of symptoms in febrile patients (which did not seem to accord to any supposed accumulation of bile) and because it mistakenly regarded excess bile as a cause rather than a consequence of disease.[90]

Most of Jackson's supporters believed that pathology was the essential basis of all medical theory and practice. James M'Cabe, for example, set about challenging those defenders of biliary theory who rested their case on the presence of excessive bile in the bodies of fever patients which had been opened after death. Although putrid bile was often present, so too, for example, was dark, venous blood in vessels of the brain, lungs, and intestines. His observations convinced M'Cabe that the chief cause of the disease was not the accumulation of bile but over-stimulation of the circulatory system, which ultimately led to its collapse, congestion of the blood vessels, and local inflammation.[91] He explained that 'the excitement of fever is followed by a general collapse or exhaustion of the system, during which the vitality of every part of the body is lowered in a degree proportioned to the previous excitement.... In the last stages of a fever... the vital principle may be exhausted to such a degree, that the forces which afterwards occasion the total evolution of the elementary principles of the body, may already begin to effect their general decomposition.' This morbid process explained the failure of the circulation, the congestion of blood, and also the failure of the body to deal properly with bilious secretions. It was the inability of the body to retain bile within the normal vessels which explained both the abundance of bile in many cases dissected and the yellowish appearance of the skin, into which it had seeped.[92]

Another writer who followed Jackson and M'Cabe in denouncing the biliary theory was Charles Powell, a former Army surgeon who had spent seven years in Antigua after completing his surgical training in London, in 1805. The works of Jackson figure prominently among those consulted by Powell, who listed them among his main influences.[93] Powell concurred that yellow fever was largely the result of heat acting upon the nervous system of persons who were not yet inured to the climate of the West Indies. Its effects were to oppress the circulation, leaving blood vessels distended, and also to over-stimulate the liver into secreting an excess of bile, which poured into the intestines and stomach. However, this bile was merely a symptom and not a cause of fever, there being nothing in bile that produced either putrefaction or fever.[94]

As will become evident in Part II, such opinions were to have a marked effect upon medical practice in the tropics and in Britain itself, permitting a return to bleeding as the primary treatment of fevers. Among military practitioners, the

[90] Jackson, *Treatise on the Fevers of Jamaica*, 11, 158–9.
[91] M'Cabe, *Military Medical Reports*, 17–20.
[92] Ibid., 26–32.
[93] Powell, *A Treatise on the Nature, Causes, and Cure, of the Endemic, or Yellow Fever of Tropical Climates*, 55.
[94] Ibid., 6–7.

role of Jackson is particularly noteworthy. Though of a fiery disposition, he seems to have inspired considerable loyalty among some of his subordinates, and it would seem from reviews that his works on fever were well received.[95] Like Twining and his colleagues in Calcutta, Jackson and his supporters believed that nervous physiology had supplanted the theory of putrefaction, with its roots in the 'exploded doctrine of humoral pathology'.[96] Practitioners in the East and West Indies were self-consciously turning their backs on the past; on what they regarded as outdated dogma and superstition. As *The Medico-Chirurgical Review* stated in 1825, there was 'a nearer approach to unanimity of doctrine and uniformity of treatment, at the present than at any former period since the dogmas of the schools gave way to clinical observation, pathological research, and unshackled discussion'.[97] This may have been wishful thinking, as the *Review* was a fervent advocate of 'progressive medicine and surgery'. Nevertheless, nervous theories of disease now underpinned the theory and practice of most of those who wrote on tropical fevers in the early 1800s, as did morbid anatomical observations.

As might be expected, pathological research had an important bearing upon the development of ideas about race and susceptibility to disease. Many eighteenth-century works on the diseases of the West Indies expressed the opinion that persons of African origin, or creoles, were less susceptible to fevers than Europeans, and that newcomers were generally less prone to disease than those who had resided in the Caribbean for a number of years. Cutting across this were differences attributed to gender and age, for example, with older persons and women generally deemed less susceptible to the adverse effects of the climate than young men, on account of their less plethoric constitutions. However, comparatively few authors insisted that any immunity enjoyed by Africans was the result of an innate disposition. Writing in 1791, Robert Jackson insisted that their comparative freedom from disease was merely due to length of residence in hot climates and that Europeans could acquire the same immunity from yellow fever after a year or two in the West Indies. But this was not true of remitting fever, he argued, which continued to attack all those exposed to miasma.[98]

In the early 1800s, most writers on fever upheld received wisdom on seasoning and acclimatization. Hector M'Lean, for instance, noted differences between the British and French, which he attributed, not to any essential difference in constitution, but to longer residence in the region and different habits of life. 'The French inhabitants were chiefly composed of people born in St. Domingo', he explained, 'and supported by that gradual adaptation to the climate, which

[95] Review of Robert Jackson's *Remarks on the Epidemic Yellow Fever* (1821), *Medico-Chirurgical Review*, 2 (1825), 485–506.

[96] M'Cabe, *Military Medical Reports*, 25.

[97] Review of works on fevers by William Burnett, Thomas Mills, Charles Maclean, R. Wade, and William Stokes, *Medico-Chirurgical Review*, 2 (1825), 3.

[98] Jackson, *Treatise on the Fevers of Jamaica*, 249–51.

habit confers on the natives of the most unhealthy regions.' The English inhabitants of the island, by contrast, 'were strangers from northern climates, and little habituated to any warm region'.[99] The French possessed other advantages, too. 'The manner of life in old France, or its colonies, was not calculated to form that irritable, sanguine, plethoric habit, in which the effects of inflammation are particularly felt', he added: their 'sober plan of life' abjured large quantities of meat and strong liquor, and embraced a hygienic regime which kept their bodies cool and clean. The latter entailed regular bathing in tepid water, which cleansed the skin and allowed it to breathe, as well as any measures calculated to keep them as cool as possible. The British took the opposite course, being prone to debauchery and careless of exposing themselves to the sun.[100]

The persistence of such ideas is also evident in the numerous testimonies collected by the French physician Nicolas Chervin during his visit to the West Indies and America in 1817–22. As an opponent of the theory that yellow fever was contagious, the statements which Chervin obtained from over 500 practitioners all offered various degrees of support for his contention that it was primarily a climatic disease that affected newcomers disproportionately. Most attributed this susceptibility to the greater 'vigour' of Europeans and the plethoric nature of their constitutions.[101] However, some felt that the immunity of residents could be lost if they were removed from the West Indies for any length of time. Dr John Thurston of St Christopher's testified that:

> I have never found it to affect creoles who from their birth have resided in the island, unless evidently brought on by intemperance or some other such immediate cause. But I join Doctor Jackson in affirming that they become susceptible of this fever after remaining for any considerable time in Europe or America, upon their return home.[102]

Many of the medical practitioners who gave statements to Chervin had conducted post-mortem investigations of yellow fever and Chervin himself performed hundreds of autopsies on yellow fever cases on Guadeloupe, for example. However, there is no indication that he or any of his contacts believed that the susceptibility of different races to yellow fever was derived from some innate propensity that could be revealed and elucidated by dissection. On the contrary, what evidence we have suggests that belief in the flexibility of human constitutions was still the norm. But while traditional notions of predisposition and seasoning continued to be popular, few seemed prepared to embrace the more extreme versions of climatic determinism that attributed colour and other

[99] M'Lean, *Enquiry*, 13.
[100] Ibid., 13–14.
[101] e.g. Statement by Dr E. Negré, Guadeloupe, 31 December 1817, f. 31, Certified copies and original documents relating to Yellow Fever in Guadeloupe and the West Indies, from the collection of Nicolas Chervin (1783–1843), WL.
[102] Statement by Dr John T. Thurston, St Christopher, 20 March 1820, ff. 61–2, Chervin Collection, WL.

markers of race to the direct action of climate. George Pinckard, for example, was prepared to entertain the notion that a change of climate could induce changes in character and that, in time, travellers from cooler regions could take on the predominant characteristics of the locals. Such a belief was entirely in keeping with his cautiously Brunonian beliefs, which saw heat as one of the factors that powerfully influenced the body's nervous tone: 'had the great Bruno visited the tropical regions', he speculated, 'he might have found many facts in support of his plausible and very ingenious doctrine'.[103]

According to Pinckard, heat initially stimulated the bodies of newcomers to the Caribbean, the typical 'Creole inertness' occurring only as the result of several years' residence, in which their nervous energy had been dissipated.[104] Yet he emphatically did not believe that the climate was capable of producing the outward appearances that were the usual markers of race. He noted that many white Europeans who had been resident in Barbados for generations were 'as fair as the fairest Europeans'. 'These facts', he insisted, 'stand in direct opposition to the speculative doctrines of those who derive the various colours of the human race from climate or locality of residence, together with the concomitant circumstances of diet, and mode of life.' 'The opinions of the gentlemen of the island', he claimed, also seemed to be 'all against the idea of such a conversion of the human body.' Indeed, there was evidence that 'multitudes of families . . . now live in Barbadoes, who in progressive descent, through successive generations, for nearly two hundred years, have resided in the island, without the slightest change perceptible in their offspring of the present day'.[105]

The extent to which medical opinions about race and disease rested on evidence from morbid anatomy is unclear, but some practitioners in the West Indies did pursue similar lines of investigation to the likes of Johnson and Twining. One such was James Thomson, whose *Treatise on the Diseases of Negroes* (1820) is grounded extensively on evidence gleaned from post-mortem dissections. Thomson was very interested in the physical differences between blacks and whites, and claimed to have found evidence from the dissection of slave cadavers that disproved notions about there being a distinct membrane in Africans causing blackness of the skin.[106] Evidence from dissections also appeared to show that blacks and whites exhibited different signs post-mortem that matched the symptoms that appeared in patients. Dysentery in Africans, he claimed, 'was extremely different in its nature from the dysentery of Europeans'. In the former, the liver was seldom diseased, quite unlike Europeans, leading Thomson to conclude that different modes of treatment were necessary.[107]

103 Pinckard, *Notes*, vol. 1, 56.
104 Ibid.
105 Pinckard, *Notes*, vol. 2, 135–8.
106 Thomson, *A Treatise on the Diseases of Negroes*, 3.
107 Ibid., 34–5.

Some other British writers on the diseases of the West Indies echoed Thomson's beliefs about the different courses of disease among Europeans and Africans, even though they did not always ground their assertions so explicitly in pathological anatomy. Writing on yellow fever, Colin Chisholm asserted that, 'The influence of colour, or more properly speaking of idiosyncrasy in the negro constitution was so great at Grenada, that, in my practice, at least, only 4 had the fever, of those exposed to it, and only 1 in 83 died of it.' He added that, 'In negroes the manner in which this disease came on was, in some respects, different from that in whites.' The former showed the same early symptoms of fever – quickened pulse, clammy skin, sweating, and so forth – but these quickly subsided and the disease yielded far more easily to simple medication.[108]

Like those who wrote on matters of race and pathology in India, Thomson rejected the possibility that human bodies could be altered fundamentally by external stimuli, believing skin colour, for example, to be a deep-seated, hereditary phenomenon. 'There are facts to shew that three hundred years have little alteration in the complexion, where intercourse with the natives has been avoided', he observed.[109] There was no evidence that Europeans had become blacker or that they had 'degenerated' from black ancestors, as some earlier theorists had claimed.

Thomson's remarks would thus seem to affirm the observations of historians such as Nancy Stepan and Seymour Drescher, who have suggested that the demise of the slave trade and debates over abolition actually sharpened supposed racial differences.[110] However, it is clear that those who located differences in anatomy and physiology did not necessarily see Africans as inferior. For example, Thomson's opposition to climatic determinism led him to disagree with the common belief that Africans were made indolent, weak, and slothful by long exposure to hot climates. In fact, he had a fairly high opinion of Africans and believed them to be 'capable of the most acute sensibility'.[111] This opinion contrasted markedly with opinion in the South of the United States, where it was generally assumed that Africans were far less sensitive to pain and other stimuli than Europeans.[112] Some Continental authors also attributed the susceptibility of Europeans to yellow fever to their supposedly higher sensibilities. The French writer Victor Bally, for instance, claimed that 'exalted sensibility and cerebral activity' were the two characteristics that most predisposed whites to contract yellow fever. 'The whites', he opined, 'differ from blacks by virtue of a more exquisite sensibility'; 'Everyone knows that negroes have a sensibility that is less developed.'[113] Though he differed in his beliefs about the sensibility of

[108] Chisholm, *Manual*, 174, 183.
[109] Thomson, *Treatise*, 4.
[110] Drescher, 'The Ending of the Slave Trade and the Evolution of European Racism'; Stepan, *The Idea of Race in Science*; Stepan, 'Biology and Degeneration'.
[111] Chisholm, *Manual*, 2–3, 7.
[112] See Pernick, *A Calculus of Suffering*.
[113] Bally, *Du typhus d'Amerique*, 303–4.

Africans, Bally shared Thomson's view that racial predispositions to disease were deep-seated: the result of differences in their vascular and lymphatic systems.[114]

Since Thomson believed that racial characteristics were fixed, he had little hope of the acclimatization of white Europeans in the tropics. 'Every region on this earth has its own climate, men, morals, and religion', he concluded, 'In vain would the ambitious self-love of some persuade us that one system should be common to all. The history of our species might read them a melancholy lesson regarding the millions that have been sacrificed in the prosecution of that fatal delusion.'[115] In the 1830s and 1840s, such opinions were expressed more frequently. For example, Robert Armstrong, Deputy Inspector of Hospital and Fleets in the West Indies, and formerly in charge of the naval hospital in Jamaica, criticized notions of seasoning as vague and superstitious, and emphasized instead the fundamental differences between races, as revealed by comparative anatomy, for instance.[116] Reviewing the various explanations given to account for variations in skin colour, Armstrong dismissed notions of climatic determinism, including those of Buffon and (by implication) Hunter, as 'loose and fallacious', and gave short shrift to the views of authors such as Stanhope Smith.[117]

According to Armstrong, climatic determinism was 'opposed by the evidence of our own senses'; echoing Blumenbach's classification, he saw five different varieties of men – Caucasian, Mongolian, Ethiopian, American, and Malay – which had shown no evident change over 4,000 years. He therefore concluded that climate played no part in permanent change in skin colour, although he accepted that it might produce certain modifications to human physiology that could be beneficial to newcomers to a tropical climate. 'The influence of warm climates is apparent after a few years residence within the tropics', he claimed, 'Europeans lose their sanguineous complexions and acquire the power of resisting the heat better than the newcomer.' Likewise, those who came to the West Indies early in life were able to enjoy an exemption from the fevers of the region, at least in their most severe forms.[118] These observations received some support from contemporary physiologists, he claimed, notably Dr W. F. Edwards, whose experiments on animals had afforded proof that adaptation to life in different climates was possible.[119]

[114] Bally, *Du typhus d'Amerique*, 305.

[115] Thomson, *Treatise*, 16.

[116] Armstrong, *The Influence of Climate and other Agents on the Human Constitution*, viii–ix.

[117] Ibid., 5.

[118] Ibid., 8–9.

[119] Ibid., 19. See Edwards, *De l'influence des agens physiques sur la vie*. Edwards was among the second wave of Paris-based physiologists; Lesch, *Science and Medicine in France*, chap. 4.

CONCLUSION

This part of the book has traced the evolution of ideas about disease in hot climates from the seventeenth century to the nineteenth. We have seen how medical practitioners in the colonies asserted their independence from traditional sources of authority in Britain and claimed expertise in important and controversial subjects such as fevers. Their reformist outlook in medicine was often bound up with other forms of radicalism, and many were Dissenters or closely linked with Dissenting figures and organizations in Britain. Their desire to reform medicine was a natural expression of their social and professional marginality but, by the end of the eighteenth century, the authority of colonial practitioners on subjects such as fever was widely acknowledged. Military, naval, and East India Company surgeons were making important and influential contributions to debates over the causation of these diseases and were increasingly cited in the work of practitioners who had never ventured beyond Britain.

The writings of medical practitioners who spent any length of time in the colonies tended to reflect the belief that fevers were the product of local conditions and that they were intimately connected with climate, in particular. This gave rise to a relatively distinctive branch of medicine, which might be termed the medicine of hot or warm climates. But such distinctions did not prevent colonial practitioners from making interventions in debates over the causation and prevention of fevers in Britain. Those who remained professionally active after their return from the colonies often used the experience they gained overseas to inform their practice at home or to champion such measures as the construction of fever hospitals.

Although the natural-historical and empirical orientation of colonial medical writings remained consistent throughout the period examined, the ways in which disease was understood underwent a profound change. Humoral conceptions of disease were adapted in the light of chemical and mechanical philosophy and eventually gave way to concepts derived from nervous physiology. By the early years of the nineteenth century, British medical practitioners had become accustomed to thinking of the human body as a mass of interconnected tissues and nerves, existing in a dynamic relationship with its environment. The humoral system permitted similar interactions, but there was a qualitative difference between bodies that were viewed in Hippocratic terms and the 'nervous' bodies of the early nineteenth century. A body composed of humours was thought capable of being moulded to its environment to an extent that was seldom deemed possible by the early nineteenth century. Hitherto, it was thought that the constitution of the humours, skin colour, and sometimes other aspects of outward appearance, might be altered by long residence in a different climate. In other words, both internal and external features were regarded as amenable to change. After 1800, such views were uncommon: an individual's physiological responses might adapt to new surroundings, it was said, but not their outward characteristics. For the same reasons, the body's response to disease appeared to differ according to racial type, suggesting fixed anatomical differences and the need for different courses of treatment.

These peculiarities owed little to the influence of environment and much to the laws of heredity. But nervous physiology to some degree compensated for distinctions based on racial pathology. While complete acclimatization was generally seen as impossible, it was thought that alien races might adapt to a limited extent if they assisted physiological processes by choosing appropriate modes of diet, lifestyle, and clothing.[120] It also appeared possible to predict the likely responses of different races when subjected to stimuli such as heat. While researchers such as William Edwards were conducting experiments in their laboratories in Europe, colonial practitioners were providing further empirical evidence which correlated the distribution of various diseases with different climatic conditions. In the seventeenth century, the primary identity of a disease had been local in the Hippocratean sense: it possessed a unique character depending on place and time, as exemplified by Sydenham's constitutions of the atmosphere. During the eighteenth century, writers on disease began to generalize to a greater extent and place diseases within classificatory schemes or nosographies. While these were often challenged by medical practitioners in the colonies, their pathological investigations provided some basis for generalization across warm climates, the biliary theory of disease being a case in point. But the shift to a nervous theory of disease enabled such generalizations to be taken a step further. It now seemed possible to predict how human beings would respond if placed in a particular climate, which made it easier to draw parallels between the diseases of similar climatic regions. It was this insight that led James Johnson to depart from established views about the prevalence of hepatitis, for example. Hepatitis was no longer just an 'Indian' disease, or more particularly a disease of India's south-eastern coast, but a malady characteristic of all countries in which human bodies were exposed to extreme heat. Although differences between places such as India and the West Indies continued to be acknowledged, they mattered less than their similarities. A geographical map of disease now seemed possible for the first time, for much the same reasons that Alexander von Humboldt was able to plot the distribution of plant species globally according to latitude and altitude.[121] Underlying von Humboldt's work was a deep conviction in the unity of nature: a conviction that was shared by many natural historians and physicians during the Romantic era.[122]

[120] Harrison, *Climates*; idem, '"Tender Frame"'; Collingham, *Imperial Bodies*.

[121] Dettlebach, 'The Stimulations of Travel'. On 'Humboldtian' disease mapping, see Rupke and Wonders, 'Humboldtian Representations in Medical Cartography'.

[122] Stepan, *Picturing Tropical Nature*, 35–43; Nicholson, 'Alexander von Humboldt and the Geography of Vegetation'; Lawrence, 'The Power and the Glory'.

Belief in the unity of nature was matched by the belief in a unity of sensibility. For much of the eighteenth century, sensitivity to nature had been a mark of refinement, but by the early nineteenth century, this capacity had been democratized. Some writers continued to see working people and 'inferior' races as lacking sensitivity, but there was a growing tendency to believe that human beings responded in broadly similar ways to environmental stimuli. Although some racial characteristics such as skin colour were no longer regarded as amenable to change, all humans appeared to live in a finely balanced relationship with their environment, which, if disrupted in any way, could damage their health. The democratization of sensibility also encouraged a more generous notion of 'sympathy' than that which had existed in the past,[123] embracing all the inhabitants of Britain, if not always of the Empire more generally. This was to become particularly evident among writers who had experience in caring for sick and wounded servicemen during the French Wars. While demonstrating sensitivity to their distress, they also had much to say about the state of the nation to which soldiers and sailors returned. It appeared to be a very different place than the country they had left; and not merely because of protracted conflict. There was a sense that Britons had lost their economic independence and thus much of their dignity; that they were subject to the impersonal forces of the market and financial speculation. And, while commerce with the colonies had brought unparalleled wealth, a deluge of luxury goods and a fast-changing pace of life had left Britons over-stimulated and subject to a host of new diseases. Luxury, sensuality, and volatility were characteristics more usually associated with tropical peoples than with the formerly hardy peoples of a North Atlantic island. As if this were not enough, thousands of Britons were returning from the colonies in a state of moral and physical decay. These 'tropical invalids' were neither fish nor fowl: because their acclimatization to the tropics had been incomplete, they had fallen prey to the ills peculiar to those climates but their partially 'Indianized' or tropicalized constitutions were also ill adapted to life in the cooler climate of their homeland. Like the self-indulgent and 'effeminate' population that had remained at home, these invalids were generally incapable of performing any useful function in society. Some feared that the nation was becoming so denatured by its colonial enterprise that it risked becoming weaker and more degenerate than the peoples over whom it ruled.

[123] Lawrence, 'The Nervous System and Society'.

PART II

TROPICAL THERAPEUTICS

Introduction to Part II

In 1782, the British physician Francis Milman wrote that, 'although the history of diseases has of late years been considerably improved, the Science of Physick (if I may be allowed the expression) has made very little progress'.[1] Milman was reflecting critically on the putrid theory of disease and the methods of treatment based upon it, but his comments betray a sense of frustration that therapeutic practices had not kept pace with advances in the investigation of disease. Indeed, historians have since commented that therapeutics tended to change more slowly than anatomical and physiological knowledge;[2] partly because patients disliked change and partly because of the weight of tradition upon practitioners themselves.[3] We might therefore expect there to be a less considerable difference between therapeutic practices in Britain and its tropical settlements than existed in the realm of medical theory, in pathology and aetiology, for example. And yet, there is ample evidence to show a marked divergence in therapeutic practices between the colonies and the mother country from at least the middle of the eighteenth century. The existence of wide disparities in the normally conservative domain of therapeutics provides compelling evidence that a relatively distinct branch of medicine – a medicine of hot or warm climates – had emerged.

Part II of this book argues that the hospitals of the East India Company, and their military and naval equivalents in the West Indies, were important sources of innovation in therapeutics. Much the same can be said, too, of private establishments such as those on plantations. As is well known, the colonies provided access to medicinal substances that were not commonly available in Europe, but this was not the only or the most important reason why new practices emerged there. More important was the liberty afforded to practitioners in the settings just described and the opportunities they presented for systematic observation and trials. The imperatives of medical practice were also radically different from those in Britain. The medicine of warm climates developed substantially within the medical services of the armed forces and its overriding concern was to find cheap and effective mass remedies, rather than the more

[1] Milman, *Enquiry*, v.
[2] Warner, *The Therapeutic Perspective*, 3.
[3] Risse, 'The History of Therapeutics', 5.

individualized requirements typical of civilian practice.[4] The no-nonsense, practical ethos of the military and naval services was disposed towards such treatment and reinforced an empirical sensibility which had diverse roots in British and colonial medical cultures.

4 Cook, 'Practical Medicine and the British Armed Forces'.

1

Inflamed bodies

In the mid-seventeenth century, the most important objective in the treatment of fevers was the reduction of inflammation. Not all fevers were classed as 'inflammatory' by any means, but some degree of inflammation was common and treatment consisted largely in measures to reduce it: the antiphlogistic regimen, as it was known. Of these treatments, bleeding was probably the most common, followed by other evacuative or depletive therapies such as purging, vomiting, and sweating. It was also common to treat fevers through a dietary regimen comprised of mild and easily digested foods. This 'low diet' was, ideally, modified to the needs of each patient and adapted according to the course of the illness. When the patient reached the stage of convalescence, for example, physicians typically sought to boost recovery through a range of tonics and mild stimulants. As might be expected, recommendations on how to treat fever varied enormously according to its type, the patient's constitution, and the whims of the presiding physician. Fashions came and went, and at any one time there might be several contending 'schools', some preferring warming regimens, others cooling; some aiding natural processes with botanical and chemical remedies, others relying on bleeding or bathing. The permutations were endless, especially if one takes into account what was offered by the diverse array of surgeons, apothecaries, empirics, and, of course, those who resorted to self-medication.

Most practitioners, especially physicians and surgeons, agreed on the importance of letting blood, particularly at the beginning of fevers and in their hot or inflammatory stages. This old Galenic practice persisted through the seventeenth century,[1] despite the challenges posed to orthodoxy by William Harvey and a diverse array of iatrochemical and mechanical practitioners. Although its rationale in Galenic physiology and pathology had been undermined by the discovery of blood's circulation, bleeding could be justified in terms of the New Philosophy, as the practice of Richard Morton (1637–98) illustrates. As the foremost authority on fever of his day, Morton's use of bloodletting alongside newer botanical and chemical remedies maintained its respectability.[2] Patients continued to be bled in a variety of ways, the most common being the use of leeches (the most gentle method), cupping, and venesection (opening the vein), which allowed blood to be

[1] Brain, *Galen on Bloodletting.*
[2] Morton, *Pyretologia.*

taken more rapidly and in larger quantities. Many practitioners were accustomed to doing this, and their patients normally expected them to do so. Just as some Europeans sought to adjust to hot climates by letting blood, many people in rural areas of Europe still came forward in spring and autumn to be bled, in the belief that it would reduce their likelihood of contracting seasonal fevers.[3]

At first, British practitioners in the East and West Indies varied little in the way in which they approached the treatment of fevers, and the majority resorted to bloodletting. Bontius, who came to be regarded as the great authority on the diseases of the East Indies, recommended bleeding in combination with other remedies in the treatment of fevers and liver obstructions.[4] His counterparts in the West Indies also advocated bleeding in fevers, together with purges and emetics. Henry Stubbe explained that:

> The bloud [sic] of the English, which consists of parts more gross, and is extracted from a more substantial food, *viz.* that of Flesh, than in other Countries, did attenuate, and the pulses in some became very lofty and full than before. In some there was a sense of pricking in their flesh, in some a great dulness [sic] and oppression of spirits and heaviness: after which, they pass into a condition of sweating, which pursues them afterwards for so long a time. . . . From this agitation of the humours it is easie to shew the reason why our Ancestors fell sick, and how necessary it is to bleed, when any feels those symptoms in him: for, immediately upon bleeding, the pores are open'd, and they fall to sweat; and by this course, those numbers of people we carried over with us to Jamaica arrived safe.[5]

In Jamaica itself, Thomas Trapham also made frequent use of the lancet when commencing the treatment of fevers and fluxes, before purging his patients with preparations made from local roots. Like Stubbe, his aim was to reduce the sanguinary 'thickness' that was characteristic of European bodies,[6] yet others suggested that the problem was not plethora (fullness of the blood vessels) but the tendency of extreme heat to 'ferment' the blood, an explanation reminiscent of the writings of Thomas Willis.[7]

During the seventeenth century, European practitioners in the tropics differed largely over how bleeding might be combined with other methods and over how much blood to let. Trapham was typical of most English physicians in advising caution and adhering to the Hippocratic dictum that the physician ought to assist nature rather than intervene drastically.[8] The Portuguese, by contrast, tended to let copious amounts of blood, and their practices at the Goa hospital

[3] Porter, 'The Eighteenth Century', 417.

[4] Bontius, *Account*, 32, 62.

[5] Stubbes, 'An Enlargement of the Observations', 708.

[6] Trapham, *Discourse*, 74, 79–80.

[7] A letter from Mr John Clayton, Rector of Crofton at Wakefield in Yorkshire, to the Royal Society, 12 May 1688, giving an 'An Account of several Observables in Virginia, and in his Voyage thither, more particularly concerning the Air', *Phil. Trans.*, 17 (1693), 781–95.

[8] Trapham, *Discourse*, 78–9, 87.

were notorious for this reason.[9] In some respects, this is surprising, as Portuguese doctors were required to work with Indians before they practised at the hospital, and bloodletting seems to have been resorted to less frequently in Indian medicine. The Neapolitan traveller Dr J. F. G. Caveri recalled that 'that the physicians that go out of Portugal into those parts, must at first keep company with the Indian surgeons [sic] to be fit to practice; otherwise if they go about to cure these distempers, so far different from ours after the European manner, they may chance to kill more than they cure'.[10] In fact, most European observers remarked on the tendency of Indians to use methods other than bleeding to treat fevers. Jan Huyghen van Linschoten wrote of the seasonal fever at Goa that, 'This sicknesse is common and very dangerous and hath no remedy for the Portugals [sic] but letting blood: but the Indians and Heathens doe cure themselves with herbes, as Sanders, and other such like ointments.'[11] The French physician Bernier went so far as to claim of Indian practitioners that:

> their practice differs essentially from ours, and is . . . grounded on the following acknowledged principles: a patient with a fever requires no great nourishment; the sovereign remedy for sickness is abstinence; nothing is worse for a sick body than meat broth, for it soon corrupts in the stomach of one afflicted with fever; a patient should be bled only on extraordinary occasions . . . as when an inflammation of the chest, liver, or kidneys, has taken place.[12]

Bernier insisted that Muslim and Hindu practitioners were united in their disdain of bleeding and added that their practices seemed to work in India, however different they might be from those of Europeans.

Most European accounts support the observation that bleeding was used less often by Indians, but some authors claimed the contrary. The French physician Delon, for example, maintained that 'Letting of blood is much used by the Indians, and that with good Success; the Pandites, being by long Experience, convinc'd of the usefulness of this Remedy, will sometimes let Blood twenty times one after another.'[13] Delon was employed as a physician by the Raja of Daman and claimed to have treated 'all the best families', so his remarks are worthy of note, as is his advice that foreign physicians should follow in their footsteps if they expected to succeed in India's climate.[14] This rather confusing picture is probably due to the failure of European observers to distinguish between different types of Indian practitioner. As Dominick Wujastyk has argued, few Europeans at this time managed to penetrate the culture of Sanskritic medicine and did not appreciate either the diversity of practitioners or the

[9] *Les Six Voyages de Jean Baptiste Tavernier*, 160.
[10] 'A Voyage around the World by Dr John Francis Gernelli Caveri', 194.
[11] van Linschoten, 'Observations of the East Indies', 193–4.
[12] Bernier, *Travels in the Mogul Empire*, 338.
[13] Delon, *A Voyage to the East Indies*, 234–5.
[14] Ibid., 233.

philosophical ideas that underlay learned medical traditions.[15] Bloodletting was employed by some (most likely *Unani*) practitioners in Mughal courts,[16] and by some learned men who were not specialized practitioners, but was seldom advocated by traditional *Ayurvedic* practitioners, or *vaidyas*.

At the end of the seventeenth century, then, bleeding remained firmly entrenched in Western medicine, and the diversity of attitudes towards it among Indians gave Europeans there little reason to question its efficacy. Indeed, the practice of bloodletting had recently been revived by Sydenham, who argued that bleeding in fever cases could assist the body's tendency to heal naturally, provided that it was done with caution.[17] Bleeding was advocated even more forcefully by mechanistic physicians such as Lorenzo Bellini, who, in the 1650s, had given a detailed geometrical account of the motions of the heart, bile, and blood in the human body, which he dedicated to his fellow mechanist Archibald Pitcairne, then a Professor at Leiden.[18] One British writer influenced by Bellini was the naval physician William Cockburn, who believed that the profession was deeply indebted to Bellini for his powerful arguments in favour of bleeding in cases of fever, which, he claimed, warranted 'chief consideration among other evacuations'.[19] Most other medicines were of doubtful efficacy and were inclined to be dangerous, he insisted.[20] Cockburn laid down several rules of practice regarding bleeding (derived from Bellini), including that blood could be let safely in any quantity until the patient fainted or became too weak.[21]

Bellini was a controversial figure and his rigorously quantitative approach was criticized and even ridiculed by some other practitioners, such as the Cambridge-educated physician Edward Strotter. While he acknowledged that mathematics had a place in physic, Strotter protested that it had been taken to absurd lengths by Bellini, who claimed to have found in every fluid 'gravitational and lateral pressure, which was perpendicular to the tangent of a circle'. He was similarly critical of British mechanists such as Cheyne and Pitcairne, although Strotter's own theory of fevers was quasi-mechanical and he valued bleeding among other evacuative therapies.[22] Later champions of bloodletting tended to draw on less controversial authorities such as Boerhaave, many having been taught by the great Dutch physician or introduced to his works through the heavily Boerhaavian curriculum of the Edinburgh medical faculty. The Leiden-educated physician John Huxham, whose works on fever enjoyed considerable popularity in the middle of the century, is an excellent example. Huxham gave a Boerhaavian

[15] Wujastyk, 'Change and Creativity in Early Modern Indian Medical Thought'.
[16] *Shah Jahan Nama*, 305.
[17] See Anon., *Medicina Vindicata*, 9–11.
[18] See Bellini, *Opuscula aliquot*, especially the final part – his essay on blood.
[19] Cockburn, *Sea Diseases*, 252.
[20] Ibid., 253.
[21] Ibid.
[22] Strotter, *Criticon Febrium*. See also Oliver, *Practical Essay on Fevers*, xxv.

account of fevers and their causes in his *Essay on Fevers* (1750) and provided a rationale for bleeding in typically mechanical terms:

The Method of Cure is very obvious, which is by lessening the Velocity, Quantity, and Acrimony of the Blood as soon as possible. But nothing so soon abates the too rapid Motion, Quantity, and Heat of the Blood as Bleeding; for by this Means the red Globules of the Blood and *Vis motrix* [its motive force] are lessened.[23]

The quantity of blood to be taken was determined by the size and strength of the patient, his pulse, and the intensity of the fever. After depletion by bleeding, which could be aided by gentle sweating, the patient was given laxative clysters to discharge any acrid bilious matter from the intestines, followed by restorative treatment.[24] Huxham was also prepared to advocate the use of Peruvian bark and other astringents in petechial (spotted) fevers, which he again explained in Boerhaavian terms, as acidic antidotes to the alkalinity of putrefaction.[25] Thus, while strongly in favour of bleeding, Huxham did not advocate it exclusively or indiscriminately, and he stressed the dangers of bleeding carried to excess.[26]

Boerhaave was also the guiding light for those who advocated bleeding in the treatment of fevers in the Indies. The Barbadian physician Richard Towne, for example, insisted that:

The first thing incumbent upon the Physician in these Fevers, is to order the Patient to be blooded as soon as he is called to his Assistance, and the Quantity is to be determined by the Force of the Distemper and the strength of the Person, though it will be rarely be found that any ill Event is to be charged upon performing this Duty with too liberal a hand.[27]

According to Towne, the advantages of bleeding were five-fold: it reduced heat; allowed secretions to become easier; relieved tension in the head; eased the action of the heart; and enabled free passage of blood through the lungs. These were all classically Boerhaavian explanations.[28] Henry Warren was enamoured of bleeding for similar reasons and argued that it was especially important in tropical climates:

'Tis true . . . that common Fevers, in these hot and Sun-burned Parts of the Globe, do generally make a much quicker Progress than in colder Climates, and consequently require large and speedy Evacuations at the Beginning; for which Reason Recourse is had here to Venesection almost upon every little Heat that exceeds the Natural, and often both idly and ignorantly: Nay, the vogue for it is so great, and the Custom is so common, that every raw inexperienced Practitioner . . . immediately use the Lancet, when he does not know the disorder.[29]

[23] Huxham, *Essay on Fevers*, 5.
[24] Ibid., 6–12.
[25] Ibid., 54.
[26] Ibid., 25.
[27] Towne, *Treatise*, 25. Towne cited Boerhaave, *Aphorisms*, 689 in support.
[28] Ibid., 26–7.
[29] Warren, *Malignant Fever in Barbados*, 31.

But, again, Warren urged caution, emphasizing the danger of bleeding in large quantities after the first day.[30]

The picture painted by Warren of an instinctive resort to bleeding is borne out by other authors, not least the Jamaica-based physician William Hillary, who had been taught by Boerhaave at Leiden.[31] Hillary's recommendations appear to have been warmly received in the West Indies, albeit with some caveats, and early venesection was recommended by other practitioners in the treatment of fevers, including yellow fever, as well as in cases of dysentery.[32] The surgeon Mr Ballantyne, who had been stationed in Jamaica with the Guards for some fourteen years, felt strongly that bleeding was the best treatment for yellow fever and, if called on the first day, he took away twelve or fourteen ounces. If the pulse could bear it, he took another ten or twelve ounces at a second bleeding. After this had been completed, he kept the body 'open' with infusions of senna and Glaubers' salts, giving bark on the fourth day if the stomach could hold it.[33] Yet Ballantyne's enthusiasm exceeded that of some surgeons in the tropics. Capt. Forbes, who had recently returned from Senegal, told Sir John Pringle (who generally recommended bleeding in fevers) that, 'The French use repeated bleedings in the cure [of yellow fever], whereas our people only bled once in the very beginning.'[34]

During the 1760s, however, we see the first signs of a shift away from bloodletting in a range of diseases encountered in the Indies, providing one of several indications that practitioners overseas were making a decisive break with European authorities. In the past, any sense of distinctiveness in the realm of therapeutics had manifested itself in the use of exotic remedies or, in some cases, in taking traditional practices like bleeding to extremes. From the 1760s, however, practitioners in the Indies were questioning the efficacy and safety of bleeding on the most fundamental of grounds: that it was unsuited to Europeans who had spent any length of time in a hot climate. This shift seems to have begun in India, where, according to James Lind, Company practitioners like the Calcutta-based surgeon Mr Bogue abandoned bleeding during the rainy season and confined its use only to inflammatory fevers in the dry season. As we shall see in a moment, this move away from bleeding tallied with the growing popularity of chemical remedies such as calomel.[35] However, according to Lind, the dangers of bloodletting in hot climates had also become apparent to practitioners on the

30 Warren, *Malignant Fever*, 30.

31 Hillary, *Observations*, vii.

32 Comments of Dr Fuller, Jamaica, c. 1755, Pringle Papers, Medical Annotations, vol. 1, f. 11; comments of Mr Blair, Guadeloupe, February 1761, vol. 9, ff. 222–3; comments of Dr Macnamara, Barbados, April 1765, vol. 7, f. 272, RCPE.

33 Comments from Mr Ballantyne, 28 July 1765, Pringle Papers, vol. 7, f. 358, RCPE.

34 Capt. Forbes to Pringle, Pringle Papers, vol. 6, f. 221, RCPE.

35 Lind, *Essay on Diseases Incidental to Europeans*, 1808 edn., 107.

West African stations. There, diseases seldom appeared to be inflammatory, making bleeding unnecessary:

> Indeed, so much harm has been done there by the lancet, in the hands of such as have read only Sydenham's works, or authors who treat of inflammatory fevers only, that it is most advisable for the inexperienced in such climates to abstain altogether from its use, and to trust the safety of their patients, in such cases, to vomits and the early application of blisters, together with tartar emeticum, in small doses, or of antimonial medicines of gentle operation, during the fever, and of the bark upon its first remission.[36]

Thus, while bleeding might be suitable for fevers in Britain, it was not so in hot climates, where there was a marked tendency to putrefaction. Lind cautioned that Sydenham's experience was confined to a healthy part of London, not the foetid swamps of Bengal or Bencoolen.[37]

The move away from bleeding over the next few years was most evident in India, where there is little evidence of its being advocated, except occasionally for newcomers. Writing of the differences between medical practices at home and in the Indies, the East India Company surgeon John Clark noted that bloodletting was still generally recommended in Britain for remittent fevers but, on reaching India, he found that his patients were unable to bear it. By 1773, he had become very cautious about bleeding and generally pursued other courses of treatment, such as purging with antimonial drugs followed by the administration of bark.[38] Nor was bleeding of much use in the treatment of other complaints: in liver diseases – which were very common in India – mercurial preparations had entirely supplanted bloodletting, whereas 'plentiful bleeding', according to Clark, was still the norm in other climates.[39] Even after returning to Britain, where he gained employment as a surgeon to the Newcastle Infirmary and Dispensary, Clark remained cautious about bleeding in the majority of cases.[40] The injunction against bleeding in hot climates was widely accepted outside the medical profession, too. In 1799, for example, the Army officer Maj. John Taylor warned that bleeding ought never to be resorted to in cases of fever because of the delicacy of European constitutions in hot climates. Like Clark, his preference was for bark and antimonial preparations.[41]

The rapid and almost complete abandonment of bloodletting in the East Indies reflected the dominance of putrefactive notions of illness, and in particular, of the bilious theory of fevers described in the previous section. The move from bloodletting to purging rested on the belief that diseases originated in

36 Ibid., 78–9.
37 Ibid., 79, 91.
38 Clark, *Observations on the Diseases in Long Voyages to Hot Countries*, 137.
39 Ibid., 269.
40 Clark, *Observations*, 3rd edn., 120–1.
41 Taylor, *Travels from England to India*, vol. 2, 80.

derangements of the liver and other viscera. They were not inflammatory diseases, it was argued, but were characterized by their tendency to rapid putrefaction. As in other 'putrid' diseases like plague, bleeding was increasingly regarded as redundant, but unlike plague, drastic purging was considered vital to the removal of the corrupted bile, which was said to be the immediate cause of most disorders suffered by Europeans in the East Indies.[42] At the same time, the vulnerability of Europeans in hot climates led practitioners to believe that their constitutions were unable to bear bleeding unless they had recently arrived in the tropics, whereas it might still be an appropriate treatment at home. These changes were quite revolutionary, since early and plentiful bleeding had long been the norm, in the tropics as well as in Britain.

In the West Indies, though, the contours of therapeutic practice were not so sharply defined. Between 1760 and 1790, there was a considerable array of treatments which evince a variety of attitudes towards bleeding. Writing of the yellow fever of Jamaica, Charles Blicke advocated a course of treatment that included bleeding for those who recently arrived on the island from northern climates, in order to reduce plethora. 'Bleeding will naturally lessen the degree of heat, and abate the *crasis* of particles of the blood.' This was to be followed by purges and other treatments calculated to carry off corrupted matter and to restore the body's acid/alkaline balance. This was a typically Boerhaavian method and the term '*crasis*' (from the Greek, meaning 'blending') was often used by Boerhaave and his disciples, such as Huxham. Blicke's method therefore shows continuity with the past, even though he appears to have bought into the bilious theory of fevers to some degree.[43] Blicke's text was published in 1772, but in the coming years it appears that West Indian practitioners were beginning to import East Indian methods of treatment, which placed more emphasis on expelling 'redundant' and 'acrimonious' bile from the intestines.[44] Indeed, by the American War of Independence, it seems as if there had been a marked shift away from bleeding. This tendency was regretted by Benjamin Moseley, who complained of 'prejudices . . . in favour of vomits, and against bleeding, that ought to be eradicated' from practice in the West Indies. Furthermore, practitioners who did practise bloodletting tended not to extend it sufficiently beyond the beginning of inflammatory diseases.[45] On balance, though, Moseley reckoned most practitioners in the West Indies were men of 'more science, and of better education' than they were in the time of Towne and Hillary.[46] The rigid doctrines of mechanistic physicians and the 'strange innovations' of Paracelsus

42 On plague treatment, see Dr Timoni, 'An Account of the Plague at Constantinople', 69.

43 Blicke, *An Essay on the Bilious or Yellow Fever or Jamaica*, 67–70. Blicke's text was a revised version of a manuscript given to him by an older acquaintance, yet the practices described in it were ones to which Blicke gave his assent.

44 e.g. Gibson, *A Treatise on Bilious Diseases.*

45 Moseley, *Treatise*, 1789 edn., 113.

46 Ibid.

and van Helmont had given way to a more discriminating practice based on observation and experience.[47] Bleeding also lingered on to some extent in lay beliefs,[48] but there is evidence to suggest that travellers to the West Indies were beginning to place more faith in various chemical and botanical preparations by the end of the century.

[47] Ibid., v–viii.

[48] e.g. Mr Abraham Mason of Barbados mentions the prophylactic and therapeutic use of bloodletting during epidemics of yellow fever. See 'Extract of a Letter to the Reverend Thomas Birch, D.D., Secretary to the Royal Society, from Mr Abraham Mason of Barbadoes, relating to an extraordinary agitation of the Sea there, 31st of March 1761, and an epidemical Disorder in that Island', *Phil. Trans.*, 52 (1762), 477–8.

2

Exotics and antiseptics

The decline of bleeding in the Indies went hand in hand with the increasing use of substances employed to counteract putrefaction. In some cases, practitioners applied remedies that had been known in Europe for centuries, only to a greater degree or in a wider range of diseases. In other cases, they made use of remedies that originated in the tropics and which were only just coming to the attention of practitioners in Europe. The list of substances used and forms of treatment is long, but the following examples reveal something of the nature of tropical therapeutics during the eighteenth century.

Perhaps the most obvious case to begin with is the bark of the cinchona tree, or 'Peruvian bark', which had been known to practitioners in Britain for many years and was highly regarded for its qualities as a febrifuge. In the seventeenth century, the bark was still rather controversial; at a time of religious strife, its origins in the colony of a hostile Roman Catholic power made it suspect, as did the fact that it was generally regarded as a 'specific', which meant that traditionally minded physicians were inclined to dismiss it as a medicine of quacks and empirics.[1] Although Sydenham claimed to have used the bark to good effect,[2] it took some years for practitioners in Britain to openly follow his example. Even those, like the naval physician William Cockburn, who advocated bark in cases of ague, warned that it was not effective in all cases and that it could be detrimental if applied indiscriminately.[3] A series of largely favourable trials conducted in Britain and other European countries meant that bark came to be more widely used in the treatment of fevers.[4] But it was in the colonies that bark first came to be used extensively and the testimonies of practitioners there may have contributed to its growing reputation at home. Although bark had long been used in the Indies in the later stages of treating fevers, usually after the patient had been bled and any offensive matter cleared from the stomach and intestines by vomits and purges, it did not come into vogue until confidence in bloodletting had diminished, and for much the same reason. It was not simply that practitioners were searching for an alternative to bleeding, but that the therapeutic powers of bark

[1] Ackerknecht, *Therapeutics*, 71–3; Honigsbaum, *The Fever Trail*, 40.
[2] Wear, *Knowledge and Practice in English Medicine*, 460–3.
[3] Cockburn, *The Present Uncertainty in the Knowledge of Medicines*, 3–5.
[4] Maehle, *Drugs on Trial*, 223–310; Risse, *Hospital Life*, 190–1.

were increasingly attributed to its qualities as an 'antiseptic', in the sense used by Pringle and his associates, who ascribed to bark certain qualities that prevented or stalled putrefaction.[5] Bark thus became popular for much the same reason as substances touted as preventives or cures for scurvy, ranging from citrus juices, as advocated by Lind, to numerous acidic or fermented products such as MacBride's wort.[6]

In the East Indies, the connection between the rise of bark and the demise of bloodletting is amply illustrated by the writings of John Clark. Clark credited the growing use of the drug to Cleghorn and Lind (at Haslar), who were among the first to use it as part of what he termed a 'rational system of practice in the fevers of hot climates'.[7] Both practitioners did indeed strongly advocate the use of bark, while exercising considerable caution about bleeding. Cleghorn used a wide range of treatments for fevers and, at the beginning of his career, relied heavily on evacuative remedies such as bleeding and purging; however, he declared,

> when Experience had convinced me that the Bark was both a safe and effectual Remedy in these Circumstances, then I plainly perceived that such profuse Evacuations were unnecessary if not prejudicial; and of late Years, as I seldom omitted to bleed or purge once or twice, I rarely repeated either Operation oftener.[8]

Instead, he relied increasingly on the bark to invigorate the body, to prevent and remove dangerous symptoms, and to bring about a crisis sooner. In short, he argued, 'it proves an excellent Assistant to Nature, in what the Antients called the "Concoction and Maturation of the morbid Matter", and (I must add) in the expulsion of it.'[9] It appears to have been partly through Cleghorn's influence that Alexander Russell came to employ bark in the treatment of the endemic fevers he encountered in Aleppo.[10] Their mutual friend, John Fothergill, also came to use bark freely, despite the persistence of some prejudice against its use in England, as did his younger friend and biographer, John Coakley Lettsom.[11]

Although Lind never practised in hot climates, his decision to employ bark in the treatment of tropical invalids at Haslar was informed by the opinions of his many correspondents in the East and West Indies. He learnt from Mr Bogue in Calcutta that the antiseptic properties of bark made it suitable for use against the putrid intermitting fevers of the rainy season.[12] At about the same time, it appears that remedies made from local barks were also being employed in

[5] See Part I, chap. 3.
[6] Carpenter, *History of Scurvy*, 43–74.
[7] Clark, *Observations*, viii.
[8] Cleghorn, *Observations*, 186.
[9] Ibid., 189–90.
[10] Russell, *Natural History of Aleppo*, 141.
[11] Hingston Fox, *Dr. John Fothergill*, 102, 122.
[12] Lind, *Essay*, 1st edn., 90.

India, information about their properties being obtained from Indian practitioners.[13] Lind and Cleghorn did not recommend the use of bark if fevers became continual in nature but they had greatly extended its use, according to Clark. 'Since the days of the judicious Dr Morton', he explained, 'the use of the bark has been greatly limited; but it must give every one a sensible pleasure that in opposition to prejudice, the exhibition of this valuable medicine is becoming every day more general. Physicians now prescribe it liberally in every species of remitting and intermitting fever.'[14] Clark himself prescribed bark, alongside antimonials, in greater quantities and earlier in the course of fevers than most previous writers. 'The bark being antiseptic, cordial, and never suppressing any critical secretion, is well adapted for the cure of fevers in hot climates', he insisted.[15]

When preparing the third edition of his work, which was published in 1809, Clark was given leave by the East India Company to examine the medical journals of its ships from 1770 to 1785 in order to ascertain how and to what extent the practice of treating fevers had changed. He and a fellow physician searched through these journals over a period of six months, finding 189 cases in which both the treatment and the results could be ascertained. Of these, 105 recovered and eighty-four died. In all the successful cases, he claimed, bark had been prescribed, and in those which terminated fatally, the use of bark had been long delayed by the continued use of antimonials or bleeding.[16] These findings supported Clark's views on bark, but he expressed disappointment that his strictures on its early and liberal use had not been generally adopted. Yet he was heartened by the fact that some eminent physicians had followed a similar course, including Dr Francis Balfour in Bengal and the naval surgeon Robert Robertson.[17] Robertson made several voyages to Africa and the West Indies in the late 1760s and 1770s, as well as to the east coast of America. He made use of these voyages to investigate the relationship between weather and disease, making detailed examinations of the kind made by Huxham and Cleghorn. The voyages also afforded an opportunity to test the efficacy of certain well-known remedies. Robertson's experiences led him to reject bleeding as inappropriate in the treatment of tropical fevers. One rationale for bleeding was that it afforded relief from the pain and tension produced during febrile paroxysm, but the tropical heat seemed to render this unnecessary. Humidity opened the pores of the skin

[13] The naval surgeon Pigot, for instance, recalled that: 'In the neighbouring country of Tellicherry there grows a Tree, the Bark of which is recommended by an Eminent Physician, as a very good Medicine in Fluxes, but as it is a very powerful astringent, it is proper only in such Cases where the Disorder arises from Indigestion; or a relaxed State of the Bowels, it is known to the Inhabitants by the name of Coca Palla.' See Pigot, 'Journal of a Passage from Bengal to England', MS 3906, WL.

[14] Clark, *Observations*, 1st edn., ix.

[15] Ibid., 145–6.

[16] Clark, *Observations*, 3rd edn., 315–18.

[17] Robertson, *Essay on Fevers*; Balfour, *Influence of the Moon*.

and loosened the fibres of the body, he observed.[18] Robertson preferred to treat cases of fever with emetics in the first instance, followed by gentle purges, and then to administer bark. The latter was crucial, he insisted, for 'without bark there was no cure'. He arrived at his preferred course of treatment, as well as his preferred dosage (an ounce of bark powder in twelve ounces of water, given every eight hours) after subjecting the remedies to what he referred to as a 'trial', or a kind of systematic evaluation.[19] Robertson's mode of administering bark also changed after a subsequent trial among patients at Greenwich Hospital, in which he confirmed an idea that bark might be easier to swallow and digest if it were given in a fermented liquour.[20] It is not clear exactly how these trials were conducted or if Roberstson employed quantitative methods, although it would have been consistent with his observations on disease if he had.

Many other practitioners also made use of bark in fevers, particularly those of the intermittent variety. Sir Paul Jodrell (1746–1803), personal physician to the Nawab of Arcot, administered bark to good effect in the treatment of the nawab's youngest son.[21] The respected physician William Wright, Surgeon-General with the Army in Jamaica, also claimed to have had excellent results with a native species of cinchona, which was effective both as an antiseptic and as a tonic in cases of remittent fever.[22] By the 1770s, bark was even being used in this capacity without medical advice. Writing to William Fitzherbert, who was about to take up a position in Martinique, a friend long resident there and in Grenada recommended a daily decoction of bark as a means of warding off yellow fever and 'other putrid diseases of the Tropical Climate'. Since he had begun taking a small quantity of bark in a glass of wine every morning, he claimed never to have fallen sick. He also reported that others had benefited from this course of action, including on the deadly west coast of Africa. However, he cautioned that the efficacy of the tonic depended on having the best-quality bark and arranged to send Fitzherbert a pound of it.[23]

Despite this, John Clark's hope that bark would be used more extensively was dashed by the rising popularity of chemical preparations, as we shall see in a moment. Some tropical practitioners also regarded bark as potentially dangerous. Benjamin Moseley warned that giving bark in bilious diseases was an error and that even in intermittent fevers, where it was most commonly employed, it was a 'precarious remedy' in inexperienced hands, and ought 'never be long persisted in, without evidently good effects, and then not without the frequent intervention

[18] Robertson, *Observations on Fevers*, 140–1.
[19] Ibid., 142–4.
[20] Robertson, *Directions for Administering Peruvian Bark*, 6, 7.
[21] e.g. 'The Journal of Sir Paul Jodrell', 1 November 1792, Jodrell Papers, MSS Eur. 136/1, APAC, BL.
[22] Wright, 'Description of the Jesuit's Bark Tree of Jamaica'.
[23] L. MacLean to William Fitzherbert, 7 November 1770, D 239 M/F 8269, Fitzherbert of Tissington Papers, DRO.

of rhubarb and calomel'.[24] Bark, he explained, could not be given with advantage while the patient's viscera were full of acidic and glutinous matter, and the blood and lymphatic vessels clogged with 'sizy blood and lymph'. Furthermore, where inflammation was present, bark tended to increase it. He even claimed that bark had induced madness in some soldiers who had received it.[25]

Peruvian bark was one of the best-known and most widely employed exotic medicines in Europe, though never so extensively used there as in warm climates. Other substances from the East and West Indies also began to enter the Western pharmacopoeia, but their popularity tended to be ephemeral or they were used by a comparatively small number of practitioners.[26] A good example of a medicine that remained essentially local was the so-called Tanjore pill, one of many Indian preparations reputed to be a cure for snakebite. Like much other valuable scientific and commercial information, the British came to hear of the Tanjore remedy through a Danish intermediary – Christian Schwartz (1726–98), the 'Southern Oracle' – who had witnessed the pill being used to good effect. Although some British practitioners were prepared to take Schwartz at his word, the Medical Board of Madras decreed that the remedy should be subjected to testing before it could be employed in its hospitals. An unnamed Indian practitioner was brought into the Madras hospital and his methods of working were observed as he administered the pills to patients suffering from snakebite. The effects on the patients were noted over time and the pills subjected to further trials, with apparently favourable results.[27] This led to the pills being declared fit for use in the Company's hospitals throughout the Madras Presidency, although, in the 1780s, following less favourable trials in Vizagapatam by Patrick Russell, they fell largely, though not entirely, into disuse.[28]

Trials of indigenous drugs continued in the Company's hospitals well into the nineteenth century, in parallel with similar experiments in other European colonies, such as Spanish America.[29] In the 1830s, however, these trials were complemented and to some extent replaced by chemical analysis, which aimed to determine the active properties of medicinal plants and compound medicines.[30]

[24] Moseley, *Treatise*, 1789 edn., 162.
[25] Ibid., 159, 162, 163, 174.
[26] Styles, 'Product Innovation in Early Modern London'.
[27] Chakrabarti, '"Neither meete nor drinke"'.
[28] Russell to Banks, 22 November 1788, MSS 1788, RCPE.
[29] See, for example, the account given by Martin de Sesse y Lacosta, director of a botanical expedition to New Spain (Mexico). In this case, the Hospital General de San Andrés was used to carry out clinical trials of drugs found by the expedition between 1800 and 1804. See 'Experiences clínicas y terapeuticas de la Real Expedición Botánica a la Nueva España', 1804; 'Expediente sobre los efectos de plantas medicinales en los enfermos del Hospital de San Andrés', WMS Amer. 43–4, WL. See also papers of M. J. de Herrarte, WMS Amer. 40, WL.
[30] e.g. O'Shaughnessy et al., 'First Report of the Committee for the Preparation of a Pharmacopoeia for Bengal'.

The increasing subjection of local remedies to clinical and chemical trials shows that, while indigenous information was sought after, word of mouth was seldom sufficient for it to gain broad acceptance by Western practitioners. This is indicative not only of the growing reliance in European medicine on trials and scientific procedures to evaluate the efficacy of drugs,[31] but also, perhaps, of a growing disinclination to trust indigenous sources of information. Such procedures mirror, and to some extent prefigure, other new forms of knowledge collection described by C. A. Bayly, in that they aimed to produce objective knowledge that was not mediated by indigenous informants.[32] As the physician and orientalist John Tytler was later to put it, 'our method of proceeding must be to make ourselves masters of their systems of sciences and distinguish clearly and impartially what in them is truth and . . . distinctly point out what is erroneous'.[33]

The curious episode of the Tanjore pill also serves to illustrate the importance to British medical practitioners in India of their relationship with members of the Danish settlement at Tranquebar. War and imperial rivalry with France meant that intellectual connections with its *savants* were limited, but the religious affinity between the British and the Protestant missionaries at Tranquebar, together with Denmark's benevolent neutrality, served to foster close and important connections between the British and the Danes.[34] In addition to acting as intermediaries between the British and Indian informants, the missionaries played a crucial role in communicating British medical and natural-historical work to a wider European audience.

The importance of the Tranquebar connection is clearly evident in the career of William Roxburgh (1751–1815), who was among the most eminent of the Company's botanists.[35] Roxburgh studied medicine in Edinburgh before joining the Company as a surgeon. He began his botanical research after encountering J. G. Koenig (1728–85), a Baltic German who had been a student of Linnaeus. Koenig was initially employed as a naturalist by the Nawab of Arcot but transferred to the Company in 1778. He and Roxburgh went on several botanical expeditions together in the Carnatic, while the latter held the post of surgeon at the garrison station of Samalkot, in the Northern Circars.[36] In 1793, Roxburgh

[31] Maehle, *Drugs on Trial.*

[32] Bayly, *Empire and Information.*

[33] Tytler to H. H. Wilson, Calcutta, 26 January 1835, ff. 105–6, H. H. Wilson Collection, MSS Eur. 301/2, APAC, BL.

[34] The small Danish settlement at Tranquebar, on India's Coromandel Coast, was established in 1620 as a trading station but later became the location of a Protestant mission, founded by Frederick IV of Denmark to counteract Catholic influence in the region. It was run by the Danes in conjunction with the Moravian mission based at the University of Halle in Saxony. On the scientific interests of the missionaries, see Mohanavelu, *German Tamilology.*

[35] For more on Roxburgh and on scientific relations between the British and the Royal Danish missionaries, see Grove, *Green Imperialism,* chaps 7 and 8.

[36] Roxburgh, *Plants of the Coast of Coromandel,* vol. 1, i–iv.

left Samalkot, where he had created a botanical garden, to become superintendent of the garden at Calcutta; a post he held until 1813.[37] Like most colonial botanists, Roxburgh corresponded with Sir Joseph Banks and was eager to impress him with his drawings and descriptions of Indian plants. Recognition from Banks undoubtedly meant a good deal to Roxburgh, and it was probably through the latter's influence that he secured the position at Calcutta.

Among the subjects of their correspondence is the bark of an Indian tree – *Swietenia febrifuga* – that was supposedly an effective treatment for fevers. Roxburgh devoted a great deal of time to testing the bark, which he believed might be of great benefit to humanity; Banks was also interested in it as it had enormous commercial potential as an alternative to the bark of the cinchona tree of South America.[38] But Roxburgh did not rely on Banks alone. Like many others in the Company's medical establishment, he maintained strong links with Edinburgh and sent the *Swietenia* bark to the city's Royal College of Physicians, in the hope that its members would subject it to clinical trials.[39] Of even greater importance was Roxburgh's connection with the Tranquebar missionaries and, in particular, with Father Christopher Samuel John (1747–1813), who became a close friend. John looked after Roxburgh's eldest son (a rather difficult child) while the latter botanized in the Carnatic. Roxburgh also wrote regularly to John, who shared his interest in natural history and their correspondence shows a strong commitment to human betterment as the principal motive for prospecting medicinal plants. John depicts Roxburgh as a devoted public servant with little regard for his own welfare or profit,[40] while both men had an Edenic view of Indian forests. John, for example, contrasted the natural beauty of the Northern Circars, and the innocence of forest-dwellers, with the 'sinfulness, misery and confusion' of life at Tranquebar.[41]

As well as providing moral support for Roxburgh's endeavours, John was of great practical use, transcribing articles in European medical and philosophical journals and sending them to Roxburgh in the Carnatic. He also arranged for clinical trials of *Swietenia* to be conducted by Drs Klein and Folly at the Danish hospital in Tranquebar, and, in answer to Roxburgh's queries, compiled lists of other medicinal plants with the help of a local assistant, a 'black Natural Philosopher'.[42] In one letter, John wrote to Roxburgh: 'You have made me almost a Malabar Doctor by your Inquiries'.[43] But the most important assistance

[37] Desmond, *Discovery*, 39–51.
[38] e.g. Roxburgh to Banks, 10 December 1791, Banks Correspondence, 1790–4, 116–17, Add. MSS 33979, BL; Banks to Roxburgh, 29 May 1796, Banks Correspondence, 1795–1801, p. 65, Add.MSS 33980, BL.
[39] Roxburgh, 'Observations and Cases Relative to the Swietenia febrifuga', MS 1792, RCPE.
[40] John to Roxburgh, Tranquebar, 7 April 1793, Roxburgh Papers, MSS Eur. D.809, APAC, BL.
[41] John to Roxburgh, 18 August 1784.
[42] John to Roxburgh, 7 April 1793.
[43] John to Roxburgh, 9 September 1790.

provided by John was that he arranged for Roxburgh's specimens to be dispatched to natural historians in Europe. After getting a favourable report from the doctors at Tranquebar, bark and seeds from the *Swietenia* were sent to Professor Jade at the University of Copenhagen, and to other individuals at the universities of Halle (the centre of Protestant missionary activity), Berlin, and Strasbourg, so that trials could be conducted as extensively as possible.[44] Due to Denmark's outward neutrality in wars between Britain and France, Roxburgh was able to continue to send botanical specimens on Danish vessels during periods of hostility with France. Danish shipping thus became nearly as important to the British in the arena of natural knowledge as it was in the field of commerce.[45]

Independent verification was clearly important to Roxburgh, but it would be a mistake to conclude from this that he was dependent upon European authorities to substantiate his claims.[46] Roxburgh conducted his own exhaustive trials with *Swietenia* and other plants, experimenting with all kinds of infusions and concentrations in the clinic and in the laboratory, but he believed that it was 'only by the concurring testimony of others, that the real virtues of a medicine are to be ascertained'.[47] For Roxburgh, this meant testing the remedy in as many contexts as possible; not just in India, or in Europe, but in the Levant and other parts of the world that were regularly afflicted by fevers.[48] What we see here is not evidence of subservience, as is sometimes claimed, but the recognition that experimental work could be flawed or affected by a variety of local circumstances; that what might work in Calcutta might not necessarily work in Copenhagen or Constantinople. In fact, the need for verification in a variety of contexts was stressed by most of those engaged in scientific work in India, being integral to the experimental approach to medicine for which the Company's surgeons become renowned.

Neither the bark of the *Swietenia* nor the Tanjore pill made the transition from what were generally known as 'country' or 'bazaar' medicines to become an established part of the European pharmacopeia. But some remedies widely used in the East did make an impact upon practice in Britain. One such was the fabled 'bezoar stone' of India. Also known as the 'snake stone' or 'Goa stone', this alleged antidote to poison did not become a permanent feature of British medicine, but it was extremely popular in the late seventeenth and early eighteenth centuries. The first mention of the stone in a European text is probably

[44] John to Roxburgh, 26 July 1792; 17 August 1792; 26 November 1792.
[45] Feldbaek, *India Trade under the Danish Flag.*
[46] Kumar, *Science and the Raj*, 65.
[47] Roxburgh, 'A Botanical Description of a new Species of Swietenia (Mahogany) with Experiments and Observations on the Powers of its Bark comparing them with those of Peruvian Bark for which it is proposed as a Succedaneum', MS 1792, RCPE.
[48] Ross to John Forbes, 6 November, Madras, MSS Rox, 1793, Botany Library, Natural History Museum, London.

that in da Orta's *Coloquios*, in which he claimed that three grains of the bezoar stone 'miraculously' dilated the heart, giving patients renewed vigour.[49] He found it especially useful in diseases which resulted in rapid loss of vitality. The Persians also understood the stone as an antidote to poison and it appears to have been favoured, not only in Goa, but in the courts of Mughal India. It is mentioned, for example, in the *Shah Jahan Nama* as an antidote to plague, the rationale being again that it had the power to restore vitality when disease had brought about debility.[50]

But what appears to have interested European observers at this time was the fact that these stones were supposedly effective in cases of snake bite, hence the terms 'snake' and 'cobra' stones. The Huguenot traveller J. B. Tavernier told his readers that 'the Indians say it grows on the heads of certain snakes, but I should rather believe that it is the priests of the idolators who make them think so, and that this stone is a composition which is made of certain drugs.' Whatever its true composition, he thought that it had 'an excellent virtue in extracting all the poison when one has been bitten by a poisonous reptile'.[51] Another French traveller, de Thevenot, shed some light on the nature of the mysterious stones, having seen them being made at the Portuguese settlement of Diu in Gujarat. 'In this town . . . ', he recorded, 'the so much famed stones of cobra are made, they are composed of the ashes of burnt roots, mingled with a kind of earth, which afterwards is made up into a paste, of which these stones are formed. They are used against the stingings of serpents and other venomous creatures, or when one is wounded with a poisonous weapon.'[52] The stones are also mentioned by the English clergyman John Ovington who again claimed to have seen them at Diu. His description is in many respects similar to Thevenot's and one is tempted to suggest that it is derivative; however, some additional details are added concerning the administration of the stones. 'This stone cures by the application of it to the part envenomed, he observed, 'to which it immediately sticks fast, and by its powerful attraction sucks back the infused venom, till its pores are full. Then, like a glutted horse leech, it falls off.'[53] But a rather different account of the stone was given in 1698 by one Dr Manuchi, who witnessed similar stones at Fort St George, Madras. Referring to stones known as 'bezoar', he claimed they were found in female goats in the province of Panzar in southern India. Manuchi had been a physician to the Mughal Emperor for between twenty and thirty years and can be supposed to have had reliable informants. However, some of the English physicians and surgeons in Madras doubted that the stones came from only one breed of goat and suspected that they were also produced in the

[49] Da Orta, *Coloquios*, 155–9.
[50] *Shah Jahan Nama*, 500.
[51] Tavernier, *Les Six Voyages de Jean Baptiste Tavernier*, vol. 2, 120–1.
[52] 'The Third Part of the Travels of Mr. de Thevenot', 56.
[53] Ovington, 'Voyage to Suratt', 115–16.

stomachs of other ruminants. Nevertheless, all seem to have agreed that the stones had great therapeutic power.[54]

Through the works of Thevenot and Ovington, and presumably on the basis of personal recommendation, bezoar stones came to be used by many practitioners in England at the turn of the century. William Oliver describes their use in what was known as the 'warm regimen' in the treatment of fevers, together with other substances including mithradite, snake root, and cochineal. The aim of this treatment was to 'exalt' the blood and to ferment the humours with a view to removing obstructions by creating free perspiration. Oliver states that the warm regimen was fashionable in London, but he thought the practice dangerous because it could over-stimulate the patient, possibly fatally.[55] Another eminent physician, Frederick Slare (like Oliver, a Fellow of both the Royal College of Physicians and the Royal Society), was also critical of the use of bezoar stones. However, Slare attacked claims about the stones' efficacy rather their safety. He acknowledged that 'The Authors that write of it, both Ancient and Modern, give extravagant Encomiums of its Vertue [sic], and of its Power to cure Diseases; and the Price it bears at this time in London, being Three Pound and Ten Shillings, the finest Four Pound, equals it with Gold, and shews what value we have of it here.'[56] Yet he and some other physicians had conducted experiments with the stone that showed no grounds for its reputation. Rather, he hoped to 'have the Satisfaction of seeing it neglected, if not blotted out of Materials that belong to Medicine'.[57] It appears that Slare was granted his wish, for in the coming decades fewer claims were made about the miraculous properties of the stone and it seems seldom to have been used by British practitioners either in India or at home. Only rarely did it again come to the attention of the profession in Britain, cropping up occasionally in travellers' tales and other non-medical accounts.[58] It is not clear whether its fall into disuse can be attributed at all to the criticisms made by Slare and Oliver, but it is likely that bezoar was a victim of medical fashions, and that it was eclipsed by growing interest in other drugs such as antimonials. It did, however, make a brief reappearance as a treatment for cholera in the early 1820s and continued to be used as a treatment in *Unani Tibb*.[59]

Another medicine originating in Asia but which enjoyed a measure of support in Britain was 'camphire'; a febrifuge used quite extensively in traditional medicine in the East Indies and which was employed by Bontius in the treatment of a range of diseases, including fevers.[60] References to camphire in the seventeenth and

[54] Slare, *Experiments and Observations upon Oriental and other Bezoar Stones*, 26–8.
[55] Oliver, *Practical Essay*, 10–13.
[56] Slare, *Experiments*, iii.
[57] Ibid., viii.
[58] Vernati, 'Of the Nature of a Certain Stone'.
[59] Ainslie, *Observations*, 83; Dalrymple, *The Last Mughal*, 78.
[60] Bontius, *Account*, 6.

eighteenth centuries can be misleading, however. Practitioners do not appear to be referring to the substance translated as 'camphire' in the Bible (a form of henna, which grew in the Middle East and North India) but to a preparation of camphor; indeed, the terms 'camphor' and 'camphire' were used interchangeably. Most references to 'camphire' in medical texts at this time describe an aromatic resin closely resembling that obtained from the camphor plant, the *Laurus* tree, particularly *Cinnamomum camphora.* 'Camphire' was collected from the roots, leaves, and bark of the tree, cut into pieces and boiled in water, whereupon the oil rose as vapour to be collected in cakes at the top of conical vessels placed over the pots. The brownish-white cakes were then purified by a second evaporation, producing a white, aromatic resin. Camphire was seldom employed in European medicine until early in the eighteenth century, when Hoffman endeavoured to bring it into more general use. He reckoned camphire to be chief of all the alexipharmic drugs; that is, those which worked as antidotes to poisons. The first person strongly to advocate its use in Britain was probably Robert Whytt, who rated it as a remedy for nervous complaints. Unlike previous authors, he believed that the substance acted directly on the nervous system, rather than by mixing with the blood. Also, whereas Hoffman had attributed the powers of camphire to its cooling properties, Whytt thought that it acted generally by heating the body, but acknowledged that it could act differently depending on how it was administered. Despite these weighty endorsements, camphire does not seem to have been popular with practitioners in Europe in the middle of the century, perhaps because of continuing uncertainty over how it worked and its often powerful side-effects. As Whytt acknowledged, large doses of camphire could produce madness, vomiting, purging, epileptic convulsions, and even death.[61]

In 1771, in an essay on the uses of camphire and calomel, Dr Daniel Lyssons invited the profession to reconsider the drug. A physician in the fashionable spa resort of Bath and a Fellow of All Souls College, Oxford, Lyssons did not travel to any of Britain's tropical colonies, but he was well acquainted with practices there. He began his essay by noting that camphire was used extensively by practitioners in the East Indies, along the coast of Guinea and, indeed, in all hot countries to treat the fevers which typically afflicted Europeans on their arrival.[62] Lind and other writers on the diseases of hot climates had mentioned the use of the drug to treat continual fevers in the tropics, but Lyssons thought that they might have done even better if they had administered the drug in larger quantities.[63] Lyssons had experimented with larger doses in treating patients during an epidemic of fever in Gloucestershire and some of the adjacent counties.

[61] Whytt, 'Observations on the Nature, Causes, and Cure of those Disorders which are commonly called Nervous, Hypochondriac, or Hysteric', 646–7.

[62] Lyssons, *An Essay upon the Effects of Camphire and Calomel in Continual Fevers,* v–vi.

[63] Ibid., 44–5.

He began with evacuations if necessary and then administered twenty grains of camphire, together with ten grains of nitre, bound with a glutinous substance into a pill. He described five cases, all of which appeared to respond favourably to this treatment. His practice resembled that of Hoffman, except the latter used only twelve grains of camphire.[64]

According to Lyssons the drug worked because it pervaded even the smallest vessels of the body, where it rapidly dissolved any stagnant humours, animated relaxed fibres, and forced the humours back into circulation. Camphire also appeared to remove the symptoms of fever, including perspiration.[65] Lyssons was pleased that his recommendations received support independently from the experiments of Dr William Alexander at Edinburgh,[66] who found that camphire had warming properties that were beneficial in the way that Lyssons had described. According to Lyssons, nitre was the ideal companion for the drug, because of its widely recognized cooling properties.[67] The simultaneous interest in camphire exhibited by Lyssons and Alexander perhaps reflected a growing interest in exotic remedies as described in the works of Lind and other writers, but Lyssons' *Essay* also indicates that ideas about the relationship between heat and disease, which had been elaborated by practitioners in the colonies, were beginning to take root in Britain.

Lyssons could see similarities between the action of heat upon the body in Britain and its more extreme consequences in India and the West Indies. In principle, the relationship was the same, though the degree of heat was substantially different. What Lyssons found most compelling in the works of colonial practitioners was their observation that the seat of most fevers lay in the stomach and the intestines. He cited Bontius's conclusion that bad air affected the stomach and numerous similar observations by Lind; these also happened to accord with the observations of Hoffman, for whom Lyssons clearly had a great deal of respect.[68] One of the effects of heat and miasma upon the viscera, according to Lyssons, was the production of excessive bile; a belief which was fundamental to therapeutics in the topics. Thus the bilious nature of the fever he encountered in Gloucestershire could be explained by the action of heat (it was a summer epidemic) and the beneficial action of camphire was attributed to its ability to prevent the bile from stagnating and corrupting. In particular, he argued, it was important to get the bile moving before it irritated the duodenum where it caused many febrile diseases. In support of these views, he cited Hippocrates, alongside modern authorities, who maintained that bile was generated by the heat of the weather and that it was the cause of additional heat in human bodies and, hence, sometimes, of fever.[69]

Camphire never caught on to the extent that Lyssons had hoped, at least in mainstream practice, although it continued to be widely used in the East

[64] Ibid., 6–14. [65] Ibid., 24–5. [66] Alexander, *Experimental Essays*.
[67] Lyssons, *Essay*, 81. [68] Ibid., 72, 76–8. [69] Ibid., 55–6.

Indies.[70] In this sense, it points more to the distinctiveness of tropical therapeutics than to the export of ideas from the colonies to Britain. The difference between British and colonial therapeutics was also evident in the use of antimonial medicines. Unlike camphire, antimony was already widely known amongst European practitioners. During the eighteenth century, it was thought that its origins lay in ancient Egypt, where it had been used for ceremonial magic as well as in medicine. From there, it was said to have found its way into Arabic medicine, being imported into Europe by pilgrims and Crusaders returning from the Holy Land. The mineral itself was subsequently mined in a number of European countries, the highest quality being found in the centre and east of the continent; British antimony was of the poorest quality, usually being mixed with lead. In the relatively recent past, practitioners in Europe had come to know of the drug largely through the writings of Paracelsus, who recommended it – like Glauber and other modern writers – as an external application in the treatment of cancers and all so-called 'corroding diseases'. Paracelsus, however, strictly forbade its internal use unprepared and warned of the harmful effects caused by the mineral in its crude form; his interest in antimony was also as much alchemical as medical.[71]

By the eighteenth century, however, and probably as a result of Helmontian advocates, antimony was being widely used in powdered form as a remedy for various diseases including fevers. Despite protests against 'Enthusiastic Chymists' and their secret preparations,[72] numerous patent medicines containing antimony were available by the middle of the century, and were eagerly employed by many surgeons and apothecaries, as well as some physicians. One such was the fever powder which was apparently used with great success by German surgeons during the War of Austrian Succession. This powder began to be used by the British military surgeons, much to the chagrin of John Pringle, then the Inspector-General of British Hospitals in Flanders, who ordered their preparations to be destroyed. But this did not stop the reputation of such powders from spreading and one of these, Dr James's fever powders, came to enjoy tremendous popularity in Britain and its colonies.[73] Indeed, it was to become one of the most frequently used treatments in the fevers of hot climates through to the nineteenth century.

Dr Robert James (c. 1703–76) was a physician who advocated forceful intervention in fevers to assist the course of nature, citing Sydenham (disingenuously) in his support.[74] He was particularly critical of the contemporary fashion

[70] It was, however, recommended by Buchan as both an antidote to poison and a cure for melancholy, so it may have been used fairly widely in self- or family medication. See Buchan, *Domestic Medicine*, chaps 43 and 46.

[71] Anon., *Paracelsus his Aurora*, chap. 14.

[72] Anon., *Medicina Vindicata*, 5–6.

[73] This account is based largely on John Millar's *Observations on Antimony*, 4–5, 16–17, 39–40.

[74] James, *A Dissertation on Fevers and Inflammatory Distempers*, 2–3.

for treating fever by sweating the patient, in the hope of removing the 'poisons' causing the disease. Those who used sudorific drugs in cases of fever, he argued, were 'guilty of an Error equal to that of a Housewife, who should endeavour to anticipate the Term of Incubation, by boiling her Eggs with a view of producing Chickens more expeditiously'.[75] The best course of action, according to James, was to give the patient large doses of his secret preparation to purge the patient of all poisonous matter. In support of his claims, James adduced thirty-seven case histories in which he and others had used his powders with success and it is noteworthy that he claimed it had been used with profit in cases of yellow fever. 'I have just receiv'd an agreeable, and very material Account of the Efficacy of these Powders, in the Yellow Fever', he claimed, 'a Distemper much dreaded in the West-Indies, and generally fatal'.[76] Indeed, James targeted those who were bound for foreign lands, and who might often find themselves beyond the services of a physician:

> Those who make Voyages by Sea and those who travel by Land, either on account of Commerce, War, or any other Business, will find their particular Accounts in being provided with this Medicine, as it will be some security for their Lives, under those unavoidable Accidents, which daily happen, in warm Climates especially, where proper Assistance is not always to be procured. And I hope I may without Arrogance esteem myself a Benefactor of Society, if I am an Instrument of preserving many in the Army and Navy, for the Services of their King and Country.[77]

Such inflated claims were regarded as preposterous by many physicians. Writing in the early 1770s, Dr John Millar noted that there was a variety of antimonial drugs currently available. The mildest and probably the most useful were those containing calx of antimony, which was often mixed with sea salt and had been employed effectively as an emetic by Morton in fevers and by the Viennese physician, van Swieten as a deobstructant. Crocus of antimony – an equal mix of antimony and nitre – by contrast was a violent emetic and generally to be avoided, while antimonial wine – also a strong emetic – was said to be useful in cases of ague and other fevers. The most common form, however, was tartar emetic, prepared by boiling equal quantities of washed crocus of antimony and crystals of tartar in water. This was generally effective and safe, according to Millar, but if given in high quantities could be fatal. On balance, he concluded, 'the evidence in favour of antimony and its preparations is too slight to justify the extravagant encomiums with which it has been extolled'.[78] But Millar reserved his sternest condemnation for 'secret' antimonial preparations such as James's, which, on some occasions, he claimed, had caused 'fainting, convulsions, and other violent symptoms, which terrified those who gave it'. Furthermore, in all

[75] Ibid., 3, 5. [76] Ibid., 57. [77] Ibid., 50.
[78] Ibid., 50–1, 53, 56–7, 57–8, 68.

cases he had seen treated by it, it had proved unsuccessful and the cure had afterwards been accomplished by other means.[79]

But James knew his customers well. By the early 1760s, antimonial vomits were apparently the 'chief means of cure' employed in cases of yellow fever by military surgeons in the West Indies and were said to be the best remedy for bilious fevers.[80] Some Army surgeons in the Caribbean also used antimonials as purgatives in cases of yellow fever, but only after the third or fourth day.[81] James Lind, too, showed a marked preference for antimonial drugs in the treatment of fevers, prior to administration of Peruvian bark.[82] He singled out tartar emetic and Dr James's Powders as being particularly useful, claiming that the latter was a powerful febrifuge. Indeed, he noted that the Admiralty had ordered supplies of James's powder to be sent to all naval hospitals and ships, with instructions to observe and report on its effects.[83] It has not been possible to obtain these reports, although Lind's experiences with the powder at Haslar were obviously favourable. Other sources also indicate that antimonials were used extensively in the Indies. Clark's comments on the journals of the Company's Marine surgeons, for instance, communicate his displeasure at the fact that antimonials were often employed to the exclusion of other remedies and sometimes to the detriment of patients. Yet, despite these warnings, he made use of antimonial medicines together with bark at different stages in the treatment of remitting fevers and other putrid diseases.[84]

In fact, James's powder and other antimonial preparations remained very popular in India and the West Indies through to the nineteenth century. As James had intended, his powders were considered indispensable for travellers to tropical climates. In 1783, for example, one J. Stuart, who had lived in the West Indies, offered the following advice to Sir William Fitzherbert who was about to travel there:

> Permit me to recommend to you to provide a little assortment of the following articles – viz.: The very best bark, and its tincture – Dr James's powder – magnesia – rhubarb – Tartar Emetic – Cream of Tartar – Laudanum – and chamomile flowers. The best means of preserving health in hot countries, are, to keep the bowels always soluble, occasionally to fortify the stomach with bark, or chamomile tea, immediately to remove any accidental obstructions in the perspirations, and to live generously, but avoid any excess in eating. The few medicines I have mentioned are sufficient for all these purposes – and Lewis's

[79] James, *Dissertation*, 93.

[80] Communication from Mr Rupel, Master Surgeon, British Expeditionary Force in the West Indies, 20 December 1763, Pringle Papers, vol. 7, f. 271, RCPE.

[81] Communication from Mr Ballantyne, Jamaica, August 1771, Pringle Papers, vol. 9, f. 296, RCPE.

[82] Lind, *Essay*, 1808 edn., 78–9, 267.

[83] Ibid., 270–1.

[84] Clark, *Observations*, ix.

Dispensary would shew you the proper doses of them. I earnestly hope, however, that you may not have occasion to use them otherwise than as mere preservatives.[85]

Lay conceptions of disease thus tended to reflect medical ideas about the origins of disease in tropical climates, with attention being directed towards keeping the body free from morbid material such as 'redundant' bile. The popularity of James's powder, together with other antimonials such as tartar emetic, was a direct consequence of this belief and provides further evidence that hot climates were thought to require distinct methods of treatment and preservation.

The fact that most practitioners in the Indies were military or naval surgeons may have inclined them towards relatively inexpensive mass remedies,[86] but it seems to have been the peculiar demands of tropical practice that led them to favour antimonials in particular. There was also a much stronger interest in the therapeutic uses of chemistry and, as we shall see in the next two chapters, chemical medicines eclipsed both bleeding and bark in the treatment of diseases in the Indies. In developing these therapies, the surgeons of the Army, Navy, and East India Company moved consciously away from metropolitan orthodoxy and clashed openly with Britain's elite physicians. By the end of the century, however, some of the chemical therapies pioneered in the Indies were finding their way into Britain, where they had a major impact on medical practice. We shall therefore find evidence not only of divergence and distinctiveness, but of the growing reputation and authority of practitioners with colonial experience.

85 J. Stuart to Sir William Herbert, 28 December 1783, D 239/M/F 8316, DRO.
86 Cook, 'Practical Medicine'.

3

Empire of experiment

MERCURY: 'A SAFE AND TRACTABLE MEDICINE'

Of the chemical remedies which came to dominate tropical practice, mercury, in the form of calomel or mercurous chloride, was king. The transformation of mercury from a treatment of venereal disorders into a panacea for tropical ailments owed much to the putrefactive theory of fevers, which came to dominate Anglo-Indian and then West Indian medicine in the last decades of the eighteenth century. Mercury seemed to cleanse the system of corrupted humours by acting as a powerful purgative; it was also reckoned to have a cleansing effect upon organs such as the liver. But the growing reliance on mercurial remedies placed colonial practitioners at odds with their colleagues in Britain. There, mercurial drugs were used predominantly for the treatment of syphilis and, in some circles, were still considered disreputable because of their Paracelsian connotations. Although Boerhaave and some other writers had recommended mercurial drugs in the treatment of flux and plague, the idea had yet to catch on.[1] The widespread and liberal use of mercury in the tropics was therefore a wholly new phenomenon in British medicine and one which proved highly controversial. Yet, by the end of the eighteenth century, variants of the practices developed in India were being employed, not only in other tropical colonies but in Britain itself. Mercurial therapy for non-venereal complaints thus represents a clear case of a therapy making the transition from the colonies to affect British medicine as a whole.

In the middle of the eighteenth century, Company surgeons began to administer mercury in the form of calomel pills to patients suffering from inflammatory diseases of the liver. In these pills, calomel was generally mixed with gum arabic and ipecacuanha, which was already an established medicine for dysentery. These were generally given every three to four hours, until the patient's urine turned pale,[2] or sometimes in sufficient quantities to make the patient salivate. This practice began in the Company's hospital in Madras in the 1750s, under the

[1] See Maehle, *Drugs on Trial*, 15–17; Bynum, 'Treating the Wages of Sin'; Risse, *Hospital Life*, 199–200; Goldwater, *Mercury*, 239–48; Anon., *Traité de la Peste*; Laitner, *De Febrius et Morbis Acutis*.

[2] Goodeve, 'Sketch', 145.

direction of two surgeons, John Wilson and Gilbert Pasley.[3] Acute and chronic hepatitis had long afflicted European troops on the Coromandel Coast and had recently assumed epidemic proportions. The unusually severe nature of the disease affecting European troops prompted immediate dissection of those who had died, revealing livers full of white pus. This damage was attributed to a combination of intemperance and great heat, which had apparently stimulated copious secretions of bile which could not be absorbed through the process of digestion. Finding that traditional antiphlogistic treatments made no impact on the disease, the two men turned to calomel as their primary remedy, seemingly in an attempt to clear the system of redundant bile.[4]

Wilson and Pasley may have known that Boerhaave endorsed the use of calomel for non-venereal complaints, but the drug was then seldom used in this in way. It seems more likely that they drew their inspiration from the bazaar located near to the Madras hospital, in which Indian practitioners regularly sold mercurial remedies. Mercurial drugs entered *Ayurvedic* medicine in the fourteenth century, partly through the influence of tantrism and partly through *Unani Tibb*. In south India, the local medical tradition, *Siddha*, which was more directly influenced by tantrism, made extensive use of chemical remedies including mercury and itinerant salesmen-practitioners moved from town to town selling and using mercurial remedies.[5] In view of the fact that the latter were likely to be practising medicine without much reference to classic texts, we cannot be sure of the ways in which they employed mercury. But in *Siddha* medicine it was common to use mineral remedies including mercury (*rasam*) to relieve 'obstructions' of the humours and cure fevers, which is similar to the manner in which calomel was employed by Pasley and Wilson. Both men had a contract to supply their hospital with bazaar medicines and would have been familiar with local practices;[6] they would have also regularly purchased mercury, which was already extensively used to treat venereal complaints. Separate rooms appear to have been constructed in the Madras hospital exclusively for the salivation of patients with mercury.[7] The hospital also possessed a laboratory so as to

[3] Pasley's name is spelled in at least three ways in contemporary sources, *viz.*, 'Pasly', 'Paisley', and 'Pasley'.

[4] *Medical Museum*, 2 (1764), 611–12.

[5] T. L. Folly, 'The Preparation or Sublimation of Mercury by the Malabars of which three compositions are made', Tranquebar, 1798, cited and discussed in Thode Jensen, 'The Medical Skills of the Malabar Doctors'.

[6] No. 192, 3 May 1763, No. 143, 12 April 1763, P/240/21, Madras Public Consultations, APAC, BL.

[7] Letter from Robert Twining and James Wilson detailing repairs and additions needed to make the hospital larger and fit for the purpose, No. 462, 1757, P/240/14, Madras Public Consultations, APAC, BL.

enable the manufacture of medicines from local ingredients and Indian practitioners were engaged to work in the laboratory as compounders.[8]

In the coming decade, the fame of Wilson and Pasley spread throughout India and practitioners in other stations corresponded with them. Patients in need of treatment for liver diseases also travelled to Madras to seek their assistance, and, by the early 1770s, mercurial remedies were being taken by many who wished to relieve themselves of tropical ailments. In 1771, for example, Gustavus Ducarel, an officer in the Bengal Army, requested his uncle to send him Kyser's Pills, not 'for a certain Disorder' (syphilis) but because 'they will always be of great value either for myself or my Friends, as the mild preparation of the Mercury renders them the fittest Medicine for this Country'.[9] But as news of mercurial treatment filtered back to Britain, it was greeted with scepticism and dismay by some eminent physicians. Dr Silvester of London wrote to Sir George Colebrooke, at the East India Company's Court of Directors, claiming that 'Your People have not always the best Physical Assistance' and recommended that castor oil be used instead of calomel to treat liver diseases. Pasley replied to the Court of Directors in a long letter dismissing the suggestion. 'There are Bilious Disorders in India which sometimes end in general obstruction of the Viscera' he explained, 'where the Liver and every other glandular part contained in the Belly enlarge considerably and form together a production of the Bowels, which becomes a Chronick Case of difficult Cure. Castor Oil under such Circumstances would be trifling with the health of the Patient.'[10]

Pasley seems to have been supported by both the Governor of Madras and the Court of Directors, for the practice of using mercury continued at the hospital in Madras and, indeed, quickly spread elsewhere in India. The fact that the Company was prepared to protect its surgeons against interference from physicians at home is significant because it demonstrates that the opinions of the former carried greater weight. Claims made by Company surgeons about the peculiar dangers of the Indian disease environment, and of the need for remedies more powerful than those used in Britain, were therefore accepted. Indeed, in the same decade, some Company surgeons were committing their observations to print with the sanction of the Company. The first to do so was the Company marine surgeon John Clark, who had spent several years in Madras. Like Pasley and Wilson, Clark recommended calomel in cases of inflamed and obstructed liver:

[8] Madras Public Consultations: No. 177, 26 February 1762, P/240/20; No. 155, 9 March 1762, P/240/20; No. 491, 18 October 1765, Letter from Mr Gilbert Pasley to Robert Palk, President and Governor Fort St George, 14 October 1765, No. 494, P/240/23, APAC, BL.

[9] Gustavus Ducarel, Purnea, to James C. Ducarel, St Germaine, France, 4 January 1771, Records of Ducarel Family, D.2091, F/7/5, GCRO.

[10] Letter from Gilbert Pasley to Governor of Madras in Council, Nos. 167–72, 29 March 1771, P/240/31, Madras Public Consultations, APAC, BL.

In cold climates, the cure, as in all other inflammations, depends on plentiful bleeding, antiphlogistic purges, and the application of a blister to the part affected. But in the East Indies, this method being found unsuccessful, and the disorder in general proving soon fatal, the most experienced practitioners in that part of the world prescribe mercury as a specific. They apply it externally upon the part, and give it internally in such doses as excite a general salivation.[11]

However, Clark was uncertain about the efficacy of mercurial preparations in cases of fever and warned that the profuse sweating caused by large doses of mercury could actually prove injurious in the putrid fevers of hot climates.[12]

But it was not long before calomel and other mercurial remedies came to be recommended for a much wider range of diseases. As the efficacy of mercury lay in its effects on the liver and in its ability to clear large quantities of putrescent matter rapidly, it seemed logical to use it in complaints which were also supposed to arise from excessive bile. By the 1780s, this included most of the ailments common among Europeans in India, including nearly all fevers and fluxes. The first British-Indian writer to recommend mercury for the treatment of fevers was the Calcutta-based physician Dr Francis Balfour. Balfour was one of a number of practitioners in British India who wrote on sol-lunar influences on fever and, for this reason, he attempted to devise a therapeutic regimen in accord with the lunar cycle.[13] His first monograph – a *Treatise on the Influence of the Moon in Fevers* (1784) – advocated a mixture of treatments, in which mercurial therapies did not figure largely.[14] But mercury was far more in evidence in his later *Treatise on Putrid Intestinal Remitting Fevers* (1790), in which Balfour's favoured method of treatment was to expel putrid matter with a mixture of emetics and purgatives. Of the latter, he believed calomel to be especially valuable.[15]

By the late 1780s, mercury in the form of calomel pills had come to dominate British medical practice in India, where it was used in high doses to treat many common ailments, including dysentery and fevers. In Britain, by contrast, mercury was still used largely for venereal complaints and most physicians regarded its liberal use in cases of hepatitis and fevers as dangerous and unsophisticated, preferring less drastic and more individualized remedies.[16] But the

[11] Clark, *Observations*, 269.
[12] Ibid., 139.
[13] Harrison, 'Medical Astrology'.
[14] At this point, Francis Balfour believed that the so-called 'Pucca Fever' of Bengal could not be cured with anything but bark, which checked the process of putrefaction; see *Treatise*, 17–20. Balfour was in correspondence with Pringle and was aware of the latter's experiments which appeared to show that bark had an antiseptic quality. However, Balfour allowed that purely bilious fevers could be cured simply through evacuation (ibid., 21).
[15] Editorial, *India Journal of Medical Science*, n.s. 2 (1837), 306; Balfour, *Treatise*, 111–12, 129–30. See also Balfour, *Treatise on Sol-Lunar Influence*; idem, 'Observations'.
[16] *Medical Museum*, 3 (1764), 611–12; Gilbert Pasly to Hon. Court of Directors, 29 March 1771, Madras Public Proceedings, P/240/3, APAC, BL; Gustavus Ducarel to James Ducarel, 4 January 1771, Ducarel Papers, D.2091, GCRO; James Lind, 'An Account of the Efficacy of

Company's surgeons paid little heed to criticism from doctors in Britain. Like their counterparts in the Army and Navy, the vast majority did not possess medical degrees; at most, they had attended a course of lectures at one of the Scottish universities – usually Edinburgh – or one of the new surgical schools established in London. The ethos of these institutions was empirical and experimental, and was compatible with the robust practicalities of military life. Although physicians were perhaps more inclined to experiment than we have been led to believe, the Company's surgeons saw the medical elite of London – the Oxbridge-educated MDs of the Royal College of Physicians – as effete and irrelevant. Until the end of the eighteenth century, there was a good deal of suspicion and ill feeling on both sides. Sir Paul Jodrell, personal physician to the Nawab of Arcot, noticed that 'it is not the custom here to practice Physic as we do in England, the Company's Servants being all Surgeons'.[17]

Mercury was now 'lord paramount' of the remedies administered in the hospitals of British India,[18] its dominance being clearly indicated in the writings of the prominent surgeon and orientalist, John Wade.[19] Wade wrote at length on its use in the treatment of fevers in an essay on the *Nature and Effects of Emetics, Purgatives, Mercurials, and Low Diet, in Disorders of Bengal and similar Latitudes* (1792) and in his *Paper on the Prevention and Treatment of the Disorders of Seamen and Soldiers in Bengal* (1793). In common with many other British practitioners in India, he believed that vitiated bile was the cause of intermittent fevers and many other 'tropical conditions'. This seemed to be confirmed by Wade's post-mortem examinations of patients who had died of fever and which usually showed that the liver was more damaged than other organs.[20] Since it was now normal to treat hepatic disorders with mercurial preparations, he argued, it seemed reasonable to apply them in all cases of fevers linked to some derangement of the liver. In his first publication, which was addressed to his brother Charles Wade, a physician in Lisbon, he claimed that calomel generally worked where the bark did not, such as in the deadly 'pukka' and jungle fevers of Bengal.[21] Indeed, Wade had found on many occasions that 'the medicines chiefly in use in Europe' had been employed in vain and that calomel was often the only remedy that was effective.[22]

Wade had been converted to the bilious theory of fever and mercurial treatment by Pasley, who recommended an initial purge with castor oil, followed

Mercury in the Cure of Inflammatory Diseases, and the Dysentery', *London Medical Journal*, 8 (1787), 53–4; Wade, *Paper*, 150–62.

[17] Jodrell to Earl of Salisbury, f. 4065, undated, Letters from Sir Paul Jodrell, 9/35/177, Wiltshire and Swindon Record Office.

[18] Wade, *Paper*, 145.

[19] S. K. Bhuyan, 'More about John Peter Wade', MSS Eur. D.501, APAC, BL; Wade, *Select Evidences*.

[20] Wade, *Paper*, 116–17, 129.

[21] Wade, *Nature and Effects of Emetics*, 57.

[22] Ibid., 297.

by the gradual administration of mercury pills.[23] In a letter to a 'young surgeon on the Bengal establishment' – which was probably Wade – Pasley had declared that 'Mercury, in judicious hands, is a safe and tractable medicine, and it is the only safe and powerful deobstructant in glandular obstructions'.[24] Wade was convinced of the efficacy of Pasley's remedies and believed that his knowledge of liver complaints was unparalleled. The successful treatment of liver disorders, he claimed, 'has long been understood in the honourable company's settlements in the East Indies, and perhaps there only'.[25] Wade thought that the use of calomel and other purgatives to treat fevers amounted to a 'therapeutic revolution'. Certainly, from the 1780s to the 1820s, scarcely anyone in India doubted the 'absolute necessity of mercurializing every patient affected with fever, dysentery or hepatic affections'.[26]

The sovereignty of mercury in British India was due in large part to widely held assumptions about the climate and its effects on the human body, but its dominance can also be attributed to the harsh manner in which the medical establishment dealt with contrary viewpoints. Although most advocates of mercury were wary of excessive salivation, and seldom relied on mercury alone, they took pains to denounce rival systems of treatment. Wade argued that hitherto common therapies such as Peruvian bark were of little use in India. He could accept that bark was 'a medicine occasionally applicable to the various modifications of fever . . . as they occur in Europe' but maintained that such occasions were 'very infrequent in warm climates', even in the case of intermittent fevers which were generally thought to respond well to this treatment.[27] Stimulants such as wine were also of little use in the tropics, he claimed, and in some cases had been positively detrimental because they had been given in enormous quantities. Those who advocated such practices, he argued, had usually little experience of fevers in India.[28] Wade therefore insisted that surgeons arriving in India dispense with any 'prejudices acquired at the university or at the shop', and warned that 'the diseases of warmer latitudes differ very materially from such as afflict the inhabitants of cold climates, and the methods of treating them should consequently vary'.[29]

A new orthodoxy had emerged in British-Indian medical practice; grounded in the bilious theory of fevers, and manifest in the overriding emphasis on mercury as a therapy. Although the military context provided many of the conditions necessary for innovation in medical practice, and though military surgeons prided themselves on their empiricism, it also enabled senior medical officers to impose their views upon juniors. This could be done to some extent through the exercise of patronage, without which the aspiring surgeon had no

[23] Wade, *Paper*, 155. [24] Pasley quoted ibid., 162. [25] Ibid., 112.
[26] Goodeve, 'Sketch', 147.
[27] Wade, *Paper*, 59.
[28] Ibid., 62–3. [29] Ibid., 48.

chance of appointment to the Company or the armed forces medical services, or of advancement through the ranks. Once in the service, surgeons or physicians in charge of hospitals were in complete control of the purchase of medicines and were in a position to regulate their use. Above these surgeons came the inspectors and deputy inspectors-general of hospitals and the medical boards (in India, there was one for each presidency) that had the power to enforce certain practices on pain of disciplinary action. Some viewed the powers wielded by these individuals as tyrannical,[30] and there is one well-documented case of a surgeon falling foul of the Indian medical authorities for pursuing practices at variance with the official line. The British Army surgeon Thomas Clark was arrested and threatened with a court-martial on the grounds that his assistants were no longer keeping a log of treatments. It seems likely that the charge was merely a pretext to remove Clark who preferred to administer drugs other than mercury for the treatment of dysentery and other diseases. Clark was kept under lock and key for three months, after which he was released without trial.[31]

Although mercurial therapy did not entirely eclipse other forms of treatment in British India, therapeutic practices began to display a certain amount of rigidity. But it is likely that enormous doses of calomel were indicative of desperation as much as doctrinal attachment. In one of his first letters home, the Company surgeon Francis Maxwell told his father (who seems to have possessed some knowledge of medicine) that:

> You would be surprised, and, I'll venture to say, so would every Medical man in Glasgow, at the quantity of Mercury we give in Feveres [sic], Fluxes, etc., for diseases here are such that if we do not stop them soon by vigorous remedies, they will save us trouble by killing the patients. As you are a bit of a doctor, you may form some idea of your practice when I inform you I frequently give a man 70 or 80 grains of Calomel in 24 hours, and perhaps continue the same for some days.[32]

However, patients often took some convincing that mercurial therapy was in their best interests, as George Cormack, a cornet in the Bengal Army, recalled when recovering from an attack of bilious fever:

> The fatigue I underwent brought on a Bilious Fever and this is the first letter I have written since my recovery. The Fever did not annoy me above five days, but the Doctor, a cabbage headed West Country Medicine Pounder, crammed me with such a quantity of Calomel as salivated me completely for 25 days. I had no use of either gums or teeth.[33]

[30] Maclean, *An Analytical View*, 90.

[31] See Clark, *Observations*; Harrison, 'Disease and Medicine in the Armies of British India'.

[32] Maxwell to his father, undated c. August 1798, Letters from Dr Francis Maxwell, MSS Eur. C.101, APAC, BL.

[33] Letter from George Cormack, 17 November 1804, in Alexander Allan Cormack (ed.), *The Mahratta Wars 1792–1805: Letters from the Front by Three Brothers – Nicholas, George and Thomas Carnegie of Charleton, Montrose*, RAMC 715/6, CMAC, WL.

The unpleasant side-effects of mercury and its failure, in many cases, to arrest the progress of disease, later induced many practitioners in India to turn against it. But in the 1790s, mercurial remedies were being employed as a matter of course, not only in India but in the West Indies, too. The Jamaican physician William Wright had heard of the method used at the Madras hospital as early as 1760 and, four years later, he began to use mercury in the treatment of visceral obstructions. After encouraging results, he began to use the drug more freely, not only in hepatic disorders, but in all acute diseases he encountered. At about the same time, according to Wright, one Dr Drummond, also of Jamaica, began to use calomel to treat fevers and pleurisies, but at that time the two practitioners had no knowledge of each other. Rather, Wright had learned of Drummond's method from a Dr Smith of Savannah, Georgia, who gave calomel in doses of twenty grains in acute diseases.[34]

However, mercurial treatment for non-venereal complaints does not appear to have been common in the West Indies until the 1790s, when its rising popularity owed much to the desperation many felt in the face of the fever epidemic that claimed so many lives in St Domingue. One of its chief advocates was Colin Chisholm, author of *An Essay on the Malignant and Pestilential Fever* (1795).[35] Commonly known as yellow fever, this disease was generally thought to be a putrid bilious fever – like many of the fevers in India – even though the symptoms, most notably yellow staining of the skin, marked it out as different to some degree.[36] The black vomit that was characteristic of the later stages of the disease seemed to suggest that the victim's bile had putrefied; hence the apparent utility of treatment with mercury. Chisholm's argument appealed to a number of other surgeons working in the West Indies. One such was James Bryce, formerly a surgeon on the East-Indiaman, the *Busbridge*; his own experience in using calomel in the treatment of yellow fever rested on a conviction 'that the greatest part, if not all the acute diseases of those regions, proceed, either immediately or remotely, from accumulations of offending matter in the bowels'.[37] The powers of mercury also excited the Army surgeon James Clark, who like many other British surgeons employed it in the treatment of the disease on St Domingue. Of the different treatments for yellow fever used on the island, mercury stood out as being by far the most effective. Its main rivals, including bloodletting, which was still used extensively by the French, were considered dangerous by Clark and most other British surgeons.[38] The British method of treatment consisted in

[34] William, 'Practical Observations', 23–4. Wright learned of the regime at Madras from Lind of Haslar.

[35] Chisholm, *An Essay on the Malignant Pestilential Fever*, 163. The treatment was also developed by others simultaneously, e.g. Maclarty, 'History of a Case of the Epidemic Fever'.

[36] See also Blicke, *Essay on the Bilious Fever of Jamaica*; Priestley, *A Few Interesting Remarks on Bilious Disorders*; Gibson, *Treatise on Bilious Diseases*, 1–2; Dancer, *The Medical Assistant*, 85; Fisher, *Tentamen medicum inaugurale*, 10–11.

[37] Bryce, *An Account of the Yellow Fever*, 52.

[38] Clark, *Treatise on the Yellow Fever*, 24–5.

moderate purging with jalap followed by between six and eight mercurial pills given as quickly as possible, followed by two or three more every hour until they began to take effect. If this course of treatment did not arrest the symptoms, the dose of calomel was increased to ten grains. Calomel pills continued to be administered throughout the febrile stage and often for several days afterwards, but, according to Clark, this method 'seldom failed to remove the fever in twenty-four or thirty-six hours'. He was aware that some would consider the amount of calomel used too large and even dangerous, but, he explained, in 'this most desperate of all diseases, it is necessary to oppose, very speedily, the most powerful, and seemingly desperate remedies'. Like Bryce and Chisholm, he believed that it worked by expelling and correcting 'a vitiated and superabundant secretion of bile'.[39]

By the 1800s, the treatment of yellow fever with mercury was well established among British Army surgeons in the West Indies,[40] and, in 1812, when Robert Jackson took charge of the medical department of the British Army there, the practice generally adopted in fever was still to 'saturate the system with mercury'.[41] The same was true of naval outposts in the West Indies, according to Leonard Gillespie. In 1799, he recorded in his journal that the method employed by most surgeons on that station was to bleed, if necessary, on the first attack of fever and then to administer a calomel purge: about five grains every hour until the mouth became affected. He added that a concoction of ginger was sometimes necessary to allow such large quantities to remain in the stomach until the point of salivation was reached.[42] Calomel was also used to treat dysentery on naval vessels in the West Indies, one surgeon noting that a combination of calomel and ipecacuanha worked particularly well, notwithstanding the opinion of some British authorities such as Dr Robertson. The same surgeon noted that he and his naval colleagues in the West Indies had learned of the practice from 'the writings of East India Practitioners'.[43]

Some, like the plantation doctor John Quier, believed that the propensity of mercury to produce salivation was greater in tropical climates, but the quantities used in the East and West Indies suggest that this did little to moderate its use.[44]

39 Clark, *Treatise on the Yellow Fever*, 30, 37–8.

40 Mabit, *Essai sur les Maladies de l'Armée de St.-Domingue*, 17.

41 M'Cabe, *Military Medical Reports*, 13.

42 Leonard Gillespie, 'Medical Journal of His Majesty's Ship, Arab, from the 27th day of March 1799 to the 27th day of March 1800', ADM 101/85/4, The National Archives.

43 Alexander Meline, 'A Journal of Physical and Surgical Cases that occurred on Board of His Majesty's Ship L'Amiable between the 5th day of September 1797 and the 4th day of September 1798; during which time the said ship was employed in the West Indies and on her passage for England', 15–23, 36–7, ADM 101/81/4, The National Archives.

44 Quier, 'An Account of the Success of Inoculation for the Small-Pox at Jamaica,' in idem et al., *Letters*, 22. Quier was a physician on a major plantation, where he fathered several children with the slaves among whom he practised medicine. See Carton, 'Dr John Quier'; Hamilton, *Scotland, the Caribbean and the Atlantic World*, 118–19.

Salivation had become the touchstone of mercurial treatment, being recommended by some of the principal authorities on yellow fever such as Clark and Benjamin Rush of Philadelphia, who most likely learned of the treatment from West Indian practitioners.[45] It is therefore misleading to view the heroic doses of mercurial drugs given in the West Indies at this time as 'malpractice'.[46] It may seem so when viewed with the hindsight of centuries, but, as we have seen, there was a clear rationale for such practices. Indeed, medical men in the West Indies were so confident in using calomel that they cared little about criticism at home. An anonymous correspondent to a London-based surgeon, Mr Chamberlain, claimed that:

> I am astonished to hear that some of the practitioners in England have written to their friends here [Jamaica] of the 'madness of our practice'. I shall not call them mad; but I think them blameably presumptive in writing of what they know nothing at all. For, if they are eminent, their opinions may poison the minds of such unfortunate strangers as may be taken ill, so as to make them object to the only treatment that has a chance of saving them from the most fatal of all diseases yet known, scarcely the plague itself excepted.

He added, 'whenever you may have an opportunity of giving advice to adventurers coming this way, never neglect to recommend having the salivary glands slightly affected before they embark, or immediately on their arrival on the spots of infection'.[47]

By the end of the century, those who had first encountered the use of calomel to treat fevers in the tropics were beginning to use it elsewhere. We find numerous references to the use of calomel to treat plague in James McGrigor's account of the military expedition to Egypt in 1801, for example. He noted that the drug had never been used for this purpose before, regretting that 'no traveller, acquainted with the modern practice with mercury and analogous remedies, ever resided in the countries where this disease is endemic'. However, during the campaign in Egypt, several military surgeons made extensive use of it, purportedly to good effect. They employed calomel not simply as a purgative but used it with the intention of inducing salivation, as an indication that the patient had been sufficiently oxygenated. In other words, the rationale for the use of mercury among these practitioners was a chemical one, the beneficial effects of calomel being attributed to the fact that it was supposed to contain large quantities of vital air.[48] This provides further indication of the extent to which pneumatic

[45] 'Medical and Physical Intelligence', *Medical and Physical Journal*, 1 (1799), 79. It remains to be seen whether the popularity of calomel in American medicine – particularly in the warmer, southern states – owed anything to the practices that had developed in the British Caribbean. See Warner, *Therapeutic Perspective*.

[46] Hamilton, *Scotland, the Caribbean and the Atlantic World*, 118–19.

[47] Letter to Mr Chamberlain, Kingston, Jamaica, 15 September 1800, 'Miscellaneous Intelligence, Observations and Hints', *Medical and Physical Journal*, 4 (1800), 568.

[48] M'Gregor, *Medical Sketches*, 110–11, 119, 138.

ideas were flourishing in the medical establishments of the Company and the Army, particularly among practitioners with experience of hot climates.

The early and liberal use of calomel in hot climates was justified on the grounds that tropical diseases required more drastic treatments than those in Britain, but it was beginning to catch on there, too. Practitioners in Britain came to hear of the way in which mercury was used in India as early as the 1760s, with an account given of its use in the treatment of dysentery in the journal, the *Medical Museum.*[49] Favourable reports of its use had also been communicated by Lind in his *Essay on the Diseases of Hot Climates*,[50] and it was used with apparent success by Clark after his return from India to treat cases of hepatitis and other 'obstinate distempers' encountered in his practice in Newcastle.[51] When venesection and other commonly used cures had failed to alleviate such complaints, Clark had no hesitation in giving mercury, 'in nearly the same manner as recommended in the East Indies'.[52] Mercurial drugs were also strongly advocated by Lyssons, together with camphire, in the treatment of epidemic fevers.[53] But it was not really until the late 1770s that publications on the subject appeared with sufficient frequency to make much of an impact in Britain.[54] One of those who advocated its use then was Dr Robert Hamilton, a physician in the Norfolk town of King's Lynn, who had employed mercury in the treatment of inflammatory diseases for some eighteen years. He had discussed the treatment with Pringle who had given him encouragement and expressed the hope that it would be given trial in some of the public hospitals. But 'so little was it consonant to common practice', he claimed, 'and so difficult is it to overcome prejudices, that I apprehended it never was tried'.[55] Hamilton had learned of the practice from a 'worthy surgeon of the navy' who had worked at a hospital on the Coromandel Coast for eight years, before his return to England in 1764. It was he who had suggested that the same practice might work in England, particularly in the low-lying country around Lynn which in several respects resembled India. 'Our diseases are nearly the same with those of similar situations in India', Hamilton wrote, 'particularly the bilious autumnal remittent and intermittent fevers, an allowance being made for their difference in violence and magnitude.' Like

[49] 'Inflammation of the Liver', *Medical Museum*, 3 (1764), 611.

[50] Lind, *Essay*, 1808 edn., 104, 107.

[51] Clark, *A Collection of Papers*, 177. Clark also urged that special mercury wards be included in the fever hospital which he was attempting to establish in the city.

[52] Clark, 'Observations on the Hepatitis', 423.

[53] Lyssons, *Effects of Camphire and Calomel*; Bryce, *Account*, 54–5. Bryce refers to the use of calomel by Dr Carmichael Smyth of London to treat victims of an outbreak of jail fever at Winchester.

[54] e.g. Falck, *A Treatise on the Medical Qualities of Mercury*; Letter from Dr Robert Hamilton, to Dr Duncan, giving 'An Account of a successful Method of treating Inflammatory Diseases, by Mercury and Opium', *Medical Commentaries*, 9 (1783–4), 204.

[55] Ibid., 191–2.

the south-east coast of India, the fens also suffered from 'a most dangerous hepatitis'.[56]

A few years later, the physician James Lind (of Windsor) extolled the virtues of mercury in the treatment of inflammatory diseases and dysentery. In 1787, he was already able to report that it was used in such cases by a number of distinguished practitioners on Britain, although he warned that British physicians ought to be more moderate in the quantity they administered and guard against salivation.[57] The naval physician Gilbert Blane, who had served as personal physician to Lord Rodney in the West Indies during the American War of Independence, also employed mercury in his civilian practice, which included a number of aristocratic patients. In 1801, Blane was using calomel to treat James Harris, the 1st Earl of Malmesbury for a range of maladies including digestive disorders, constipation, and gout. But the dosage was more moderate than that given in tropical fevers. He recommended the earl to take half a pill every other night and to keep this up despite some unease on the part of his patient, who had complained of chills which he attributed to the drug. Blane insisted that calomel was 'certainly of all the medicines you take, the most calculated for producing a radical and permanent effect'.[58]

By the early 1800s, many doctors in Britain were recommending purgation with mercury for non-venereal complaints, all having accepted the biliary theory of fevers. These included the fever expert Sir William Fordyce,[59] the liver expert Dr William Saunders, and a host of other practitioners who believed it useful in everything from chronic hepatitis to the diseases of children.[60] But there were still, of course, many sceptics. The military surgeon, Colin Chisholm, declared that there was a 'powerful prejudice' against the practice in the medical department of the Navy,[61] for example, although this was by no means true of all naval surgeons. To the extent that it was true, resistance to mercury may be partly ascribed to the nervous theory of fevers popularized by such eminent naval practitioners as Thomas Trotter (1760–1832), which formed the basis of an entirely different therapeutic regime which will be considered later.[62] There were also many practitioners who remained suspicious of calomel on pragmatic grounds, fearing its toxicity and its associations with quackery.

[56] Ibid., 194.
[57] Lind, 'An Account of the Efficacy of Mercury', 43–4.
[58] Blane to Malmesbury, undated, 9M73 183/78; see also letters of 25 July, 29 August, and undated, 183/77, 80, 85, Hampshire County Record Office.
[59] See Wade, *Paper*, 52–3.
[60] See, for example: Houlston, *Observations on Poisons*; Saunders, *Treatise on the Structure, Economy, and Diseases of the Liver*, 4th edn.; Letter from 'A Medical Practitioner', Gloucester, 13 November 1801, *Medical and Physical Journal*, 7 (1807), 38–9; Currie, *Examination of the Prejudices commonly entertained against Mercury*.
[61] Chisholm, *Essay*, 163.
[62] Trotter, *Medicina Nautica*, 334–6.

HELENUS SCOTT AND PNEUMATIC MEDICINE

Mercurial therapy stands out as being one of the most successful therapeutic exports from Britain's colonies in terms of the extent to which it altered the complexion of medical practice in Britain and its Empire. Another chemical therapy which for a time made a huge impact on British medicine was the nitric acid treatment first developed in India by Dr Helenus Scott (c. 1757–1821).[63] Raised near Dundee, the son of a clergyman, Scott took science courses at Aberdeen University after being educated in the classics at the Dundee Grammar School. He then studied medicine in Edinburgh and appears to have taken the degree of MD. His greatest inspiration at Edinburgh was the chemist Joseph Black (1728–99), famous for his work on pneumatic chemistry and especially on what was then known as 'fixed air' (carbon dioxide). After finishing his studies, the Scott family's modest means were exhausted and Helenus was forced to earn a living. Although his initial impulse was to go to America to fight with George Washington (Scott was a professed lover of liberty), his more sober friends induced him to take up a position as a cadet in the service of the Company. After two unsuccessful attempts to reach India, Scott arrived there in 1782, with his new wife, Anna, aged twenty-four or twenty-five.[64]

One of his first appointments in India was as an apothecary in the Company's hospital in Bombay. In this capacity, he would have had close contact with indigenous practitioners and traders. He argued that the Board had not taken sufficient advantage of materials available locally, from which most of the medicines normally sent from Europe could be constructed.[65] A few years later he was writing to the Governor of Bombay with much the same purpose, describing various minerals and their use in the making of soap, glass, dyeing, and bleaching, as well as in a number of unspecified local 'manufactures'. On a number of occasions, Scott urged the Governor to use his influence with the Company's Court of Directors, so that they might consider exporting these minerals to Britain, thereby reducing its dependence on potentially hostile nations at a time of war.[66] The Governor dutifully passed the letter to the Court of Directors but nothing came of it.[67] In 1792, when Scott again wrote to the Hospital Board, he had not yet received any reply from the Directors.[68]

63 Like many other surnames during this period, one encounters different spellings of Scott's surname, which is sometimes, as in the foreword to his novel, spelled with a single 't'.

64 Biographical details from Scott, *The Adventures of a Rupee*, i–x.

65 Letter from 'Helenus Scott, Apothecary' to the Hospital Board, 3 October 1787, Bombay, Hospital Board Diary, 1787–9, vol. 289, 40–2, MSA.

66 Scott to Governor of Bombay, 2 April 1790, Bombay, Public Department Diary 1790, no. 96, Part II, 228–9, MSA.

67 Ibid., 229, 233.

68 Scott to Hospital Board, 9 February 1792, Public Department Diary, 1792, no. 100, Part II, 222–5, MSA.

The failure of Scott's earnest representations may help to explain why he was so eager to enlist the help of Banks, whom he may have thought sympathetic on account of the latter's enthusiasm for science and statecraft. In January 1790, he wrote the first of several letters to Banks, in which he described the various techniques used in cleaning and dyeing cotton cloths, and about local antiquities such as the Elephanta Caves. He offered to send Banks further remarks on the sciences and manufactures of India, adding that 'I often think that their arts improved by the practice of so many years might afford matter of Enlightenment and Instruction to the most enlightened philosopher of Europe.'[69] Scott was evidently encouraged at finding a receptive ear and in a letter of March 1792 wrote: 'I had the favour of your letter of the 17 March 1791 by the Essex, the last ship that arrived here from Europe. I was greatly flattered to find that what I had done was acceptable to you and that gave me encouragement to prosecute the subject I proposed to you.' Scott began with an account of the state of Indian medicine and surgery, which, like even the most ardent orientalists, he assumed had degenerated under centuries of despotism and war. Yet, like Sir William Jones, he acknowledged that Indians were the equal of Europeans in certain areas of therapeutics, including surgical operations such as the removal of cataract and lithotomy. The letter went on to give further details about Indian dyeing techniques and the manufacture of goods using local minerals. He ended with a promise to send some objects of scientific interest to Banks and expressed a desire to publish his findings in England.[70]

Most of the other letters from Scott to Banks convey similar information about vegetables and minerals useful in manufacturing and the sciences, continually stressing their utility to Britain at a time of war with France.[71] In 1796, however, the subject matter of the letters changed and Scott began to relate what he believed to be the extraordinary effects of nitric acid 'procured from a Mixture of three parts of Alum and one of Nitre'. He believed that 'such a remedy would be highly useful to mankind if judiciously employed, especially in Warm Climates where a tendency to Animalization gives a particular character to all our diseases'.[72] This notion may have been prompted by the work conducted by Joseph Priestley, who was awarded the Royal Society's prestigious Copley medical by its then president, John Pringle, for the discovery of 'nitrous air', among other things. This discovery had aroused expectations that air impregnated with nitrogen could be used to fumigate ships and other confined spaces to combat infectious and contagious atmospheres.[73] During the 1780s, a number of medical practitioners in British prisons and

[69] Scott to Banks, 7 January 1790, Add. MSS 33979, Banks Correspondence, 1765–1821, vol. III, ff. 1–13, BL.

[70] Scott to Banks, 14 March 1792, ff. 127–30, BL.

[71] e.g. Scott to Banks, 7 February 1792, f. 135, 8 January 1794, ff. 233–5, BL.

[72] Scott to Banks, 6 May 1796, Add. MSS 33979, Banks Correspondence, vol. IV, ff. 16–17, BL.

[73] Lawrence, 'Priestley in Tahiti'.

in the Royal Navy had subsequently experimented with the substance and their efforts were subsequently popularized by the radical physician Thomas Beddoes.[74] It is highly likely that Scott would have been aware of these experiments, but his application of nitric acid in a therapeutic capacity was wholly novel. Practitioners in other colonies had been experimenting with therapies incorporating 'fixed air', but none with nitrous airs or acids given internally.[75] It was with some excitement, then, that Scott sent Banks a copy of the article detailing his experiments with nitric acid, which appeared in the *Bombay Courier* in April 1796. Dedicated to his senior officer Dr James Anderson, the article began with an account of Scott's laboratory experiments on bile, which was then widely thought to be the causative agent in many of India's most deadly diseases. Scott concluded that mercurial drugs worked to dissolve bile because they contained a vital principle – oxygen. He explained that his belief in the therapeutic power of oxygen had led him to experiment with nitric acid, which he also believed to contain about 'four parts of Vital Air, united to one of Azote [nitrogen], with a certain proportion of water.' Scott had reason to believe that nitric acid was preferable to mercury because it dissolved even more completely 'the resinous Base of the Bile'.[76]

Before Scott embarked on his intended course of experimentation, he read as much as possible on nitric acid and concluded that it had been seldom used in medicine, except occasionally in very small quantities as a diuretic. In view of this, Scott did not think it right to experiment on others in the first instance and resolved to take the acid himself. 'I was particularly qualified to determine its effects', he wrote, 'as I had reason for a long time before to complain of my Liver.' He began to take the substance in September 1793, mixing about a drachm of the strongest acid he could procure with a quantity of water. He observed that he was 'happy to find, that I could finish that quantity in the course of a few hours, without any disagreeable effects from it'. From that day, Scott kept a journal, briefly recording the effects of the acid on his own body:

11th September, 1st day. Took at different times about a dram of strong nitric acid, diluted with water. Soon after drinking it, I feel a sense of warmth in my stomach and chest; but I find no disagreeable sensation from it, nor any other material effect.

2d. I have taken to-day a considerable quantity of acid, diluted with water, as much as I could easily drink during the forenoon.

3d. I have continued the acid. I feel my gums affected from it, and they are somewhat red, and enlarged between the teeth. I slept ill; but could lie for a length of time on my left side, which, from some disease in my liver, had not been the case for many months before. I perceive a pain in the back of my head, resembling what I have commonly felt when taking mercury.

[74] See *Report from the Committee on Dr C. Smyth's Petition*; Trotter, 'On the Means of Destroying Contagion'; Review of Blane's *Observations*.

[75] e.g. Curtin, *De febre flava Indae Occidentalis*, 40.

[76] Scott to Banks, 6 May 1796, Add. MSS 33979, Banks Correspondence, vol. IV, ff. 18–19, BL.

4th. My gums are a little tender. I continue the acid as before. I still find a pain in the head, and about my jaws, like what arises from mercury. I perceive no symptoms of my liver-complaint.

5th. I have taken the acid; and always feel an agreeable sense of heat after drinking it. I spit more than usual.

6th. I continue the acid. I observe my mouth sorer to-day, and spit more.

7th. I think I am now sufficiently oxygenated. I feel my mouth so troublesome that I shall take no more acid.

From this time my mouth got gradually well, and I found my health considerably improved.

Scott now supposed that he had found a remedy for the chronic liver complaints that afflicted hundreds of his countrymen in India and after their return to Britain. Moreover, it was a remedy that had fewer unpleasant side-effects than mercury; although it should be noted in this regard that Scott may have been using what we now know as nitrous acid rather than nitric acid, which is far more corrosive. Both terms were used by those who emulated Scott's trials, which makes it difficult to be certain. Whichever acid he used, Scott was sufficiently emboldened by his results to try it on some of his patients who were suffering from hepatic diseases: not all were cured, but many improved markedly. He moved next to the treatment of those suffering from 'tedious intermittents': fevers often connected with diseases of the liver and spleen. He claimed that those who had been given nitric acid had 'recovered their natural colour from a leaden or bilious hue' and that they had regained their strength after a 'long continued weakness'. Indeed, he concluded that the acid might be used instead of mercury, which had hitherto been regarded as a specific to cure bilious, putrid, or nervous fevers.

Having perceived similar effects to those of mercury – though with less serious side-effects – Scott began to wonder if nitric acid could be used to remove the various symptoms of syphilis. In September 1793, he persuaded his friend Dr Anderson to administer nitric acid in the treatment of syphilitic cases from the 77th Regiment in Bombay. The trial was encouraging and Scott achieved similar success with some cases that he treated himself. He concluded that nitric acid was at least as good as mercury in treating syphilis and in some cases better. 'We appear to be able to carry the degree of oxygenation of the body to a greater length by means of the nitric acid', he believed, 'and to continue it longer than we can do by mercury.' But Scott was still cautious about claiming too much for nitric acid. He was well aware that some medicines that had acquired a reputation as specific cures had turned out to be disappointing. He was aware, too, that results could vary depending on the strength of the acid and he relied on taste to determine its potency. His method of administering it was to fill half or three-quarters of a Madeira wine glass with the acid and to mix it with two pints of water; a quantity sufficient for one day, taking a glassful at one time. Using this method, he claimed that he had removed syphilitic symptoms within a fortnight and sometimes in as few as five days. He confessed that he had sometimes failed, but his failures happened to be intractable cases that had not responded to mercury either.[77]

Scott was adamant that nitric acid should be judged on the basis of rigorous trials. He had little time for theory and speculation and satirized the tendency of physicians to produce elaborate systems in his picaresque novel, *The Adventures of a Rupee* (1782):

> Ye theorists (a powerful band!) who corrupt all true philosophy and genuine induction by not attending to the never erring operations of nature with sufficient accuracy; who mistake your own disordered notions for eternal truths; who jumble effects with efficients, and causes with their consequences; it is not for you gentlemen to judge of my production.[78]

It was with some modesty, then, that Scott offered his opinion to Banks and he could hardly have imagined that his paper would excite so much controversy. Indeed, until now, Banks had been no more than quietly encouraging of Scott's endeavours, but he found the experiments with nitric acid sufficiently interesting to secure the publication of Scott's *Bombay Courier* article in the new London-based medical journal, *Annals of Medicine.* The article was published in full in the 'Medical News' section of the journal in 1796, with a copy of the forwarding letter to Banks and a short comment from the editor. The initial of Scott's first name was mistakenly printed as 'W' rather than 'H', but otherwise the letter and article are exact copies of those sent to Banks from Bombay. The editor was clearly excited by the prospect of a new remedy for one of the most common diseases afflicting the British Army and the Royal Navy, and one which had few of the disadvantages of mercury. If Scott's claims were correct, the implications were tremendous.[79]

The reaction to the publication of Scott's letter and article was almost immediate. A number of practitioners began trials with nitric acid straight away, the most prominent of the early attempts being the trials begun at the Royal Naval Hospital at Plymouth, which regularly treated patients with syphilis. These trials were conducted by one Mr Hammick under the inspection of Mr Geach, the hospital's senior surgeon. Hammick selected the worst cases of syphilis that had been admitted to the hospital and administered nitric acid in fifty cases, with what he claimed was great success. The acid appeared to cure the disease in a short period regardless of dietary regimen, and with none of the harmful side-effects of mercury. He found no instances of it having affected the gums of his patients, nor of vomiting or diarrhoea, unless patients were given too much at any one time. Excited by these discoveries, Hammick wrote to

[77] Scott to Banks, 6 May 1796, Add. MSS 33979, vol. IV, f. 19.
[78] Scott, *Adventures of a Rupee*, xi–xii.
[79] *Annals of Medicine*, 1 (1796), 373–86.

Beddoes, who was about to found a Pneumatic Institute in Bristol, with the aim of furthering medical reform. Beddoes and his supporters – which included members of the Lunar Society such as James Watt junior – hoped that oxygen and other gases could be used therapeutically to treat a wide range of diseases and that it would revolutionize the practice of medicine.[80] Beddoes responded enthusiastically to Hammick's first letter of 22 July 1797, sending him numerous pamphlets on the subject and encouraging further trials. In return, Beddoes secured publication of Hammick's letter together with details of twelve cases involved in the trials, as a *Report, principally concerning the Effects of the Nitrous Acid in the Venereal Disease, by the Surgeons of the Royal Hospital at Plymouth, and other practitioners*, which appeared in 1797.[81]

Unfortunately, there is no account of these trials in the records of the Plymouth naval hospital, but the latter do contain some relevant information. A Mr Stephen Hammick is listed in 1796 as the hospital's dispenser rather than as a surgeon, which places him in much the same position as Scott, who developed his interest in chemical therapies while an apothecary at the Bombay hospital. Both would have been experienced in handling chemicals and would have been in a position to obtain them more readily than most practitioners. With this in mind, it is interesting to note that in October 1796, Hammick issued an order for the supply of concentrated vitriolic acid of nitre to be used on four naval vessels due for overseas service. It is likely that the ships were supplied with the acid to be used as a fumigant in the event of an outbreak of fever, but Hammick may have obtained sufficient acid from these supplies to conduct his own experiments. By January 1797, Hammick had been promoted to the post of Surgeon at the hospital and was now in a position to conduct trials with the acid under the supervision of his superior, Francis Geach.[82]

Hammick and Geach later wrote to Beddoes expressing their gratitude, adding, in September 1797, that 'Since we have had the Honor [sic] of writing to you, we have found it effectual in the Gonnorhoea, after the discharge began to thicken, and then we have successfully injected four times a day, the nitrous acid about five drops to eight ounces of water.'[83] Beddoes sent this letter and details of the experiments carried out in Bombay and Plymouth to some of his friends, including the Jacobin sympathizer James Watt junior, who had a keen interest in the application of pneumatic chemistry to medicine.[84] Among the enclosures was

[80] Porter, *Doctor of Society*, 17. On Beddoes and the Lunar Society, see Levere, 'Dr Thomas Beddoes'.

[81] Beddoes (ed.), *Reports*.

[82] Private minutes and memoranda of Capt. Richard Creyke, Governor of the Royal Naval Hospital, Stonehouse, Plymouth, 1795–9: list of staff, 1796; entries of 6 October 1796 and 21 January 1797, Plymouth and West Devon Record Office.

[83] Mr Hammick, Royal Naval Hospital, Plymouth, to Dr Beddoes, 29 September 1797, Papers of James Watt, JWP W/9 (reel 22), BCA.

[84] On Watt's and Beddoes's other radical associates, see Levere, 'Dr Thomas Beddoes'.

a circular letter which Beddoes later published in a number of medical journals as an inducement to other practitioners to emulate the work of Scott and Hammick. He added that some other surgeons had already done so, and that there were now – by September 1797 – some 100 cases that had been cured 'beyond all reasonable doubt' by the acid. He went on: 'By the co-operation of practitioners, a thousand cases might soon be collected. And it is hoped that you will not refuse your assistance. If profits accrue they shall be divided among charitable establishments for venereal patients.' Beddoes requested that any such reports should be sent to his publisher, Mr Johnson, a bookseller of St Paul's, Bristol.[85]

In view of the large number of venereal patients treated in naval and military hospitals, practitioners in those services responded enthusiastically to the call. No less a figure than Thomas Trotter, who had until recently been Physician to the Channel Fleet, began trials on several vessels of the fleet, including his own. In November 1797, he claimed that:

> A number of successful Trials of the Nitric Acid in the Treatment of old and obstinate Venereal Complaints . . . have been made through my Directions; many under my own eye. . . . [T]his Medicine promises to be one of the greatest Blessings which the Science of Physic has ever conferred on Mankind, and particularly a Sea Life; this Discovery we owe to a Physician in the East Indies.[86]

Army surgeons were quick to follow their counterparts in the Navy. One such was William Cruikshank, who was both a chemist at the Royal Ordnance and a surgeon with the Royal Artillery. Cruikshank was eager to satisfy himself of the veracity of Scott's claims about nitric acid and the extent to which its therapeutic efficacy was due to its containing oxygen. He administered nitric acid to four patients suffering from syphilis, and other substances thought to contain large amounts of oxygen to two other groups of patients, one group of four being treated with oxygenated muriate of potash, the other group of three, with citric acid. The patients in all three groups were discharged as cured, leading Cruickshank to the conclusion that nitric acid and all other oxygenated substances might be usefully employed in cases of syphilis.[87]

But it was not long before those who experimented with nitric acid began to report less favourable results; indeed, some practitioners denounced the practice. As the *Annals of Medicine* put in 1798, 'The use of nitric acid for the cure of the venereal complaints, has of late attracted more notice than any other new practice. While some men of distinguished eminence are strenuous advocates in support of it, others, of no less high reputation, have no scruple in representing

[85] Beddoes to Watt, February 1798, enclosing circular letter on nitric acid, 5 September 1797, JWP W/9 (reel 22), BCA.

[86] Letter from Trotter, 4 November 1797, cited in *Report from the Committee on Dr C. Smyth's Petition, respecting his Discovery of Nitrous Fumigation* (1802), House of Commons Parliamentary Papers Online, 86.

[87] Cruickshank, *The Results of the Trials of various Acids.*

it as inefficacious, and even as pernicious.'[88] Some of the hostility came from practitioners – predominantly physicians – who had doubts about any new remedy touted as a 'specific', almost as a matter of principle. Others came to doubt the efficacy of nitric acid after subjecting it to systematic trials. William Blair, surgeon of the Lock Hospital and Asylum at Finsbury in north London had mixed results when he tried the acid on his syphilitic patients. Although some cases appeared to be cured by the acid, others were not, or relapsed after an initial disappearance of symptoms. He was led to conclude that nitric acid probably counteracted the venereal poison to some degree, but that it was usually necessary to supplement it with mercury. Indeed, in some cases, the acid seemed to have no effect at all.[89]

James Currie, an Edinburgh-trained physician and a correspondent of the former Company surgeon John Clark, also had mixed results when he attempted to use nitric acid at the Liverpool Infirmary. Induced to try the nitric acid by Scott's apparent success, Currie concluded that the efficacy of the remedy had been 'exaggerated by a warm imagination', as the *Annals of Medicine* put it in a review of Currie's 1797 work on fevers.[90] The review, however, was selective in what it gleaned from Currie's book. Currie had, in fact been quite pleased at the way in which syphilitic patients responded to nitric acid, but had less success when he attempted to use it as a substitute for mercury in the treatment of cases of yellow fever among soldiers returning from the West Indies.[91] Scott may have taken solace from Currie's success with venereal patients, but he was clearly shaken by the increasing volume of negative reports. In 1799, he wrote to Banks informing him that he had 'no great inclination to appear to the world in the light of a mistaken enthusiast' but insisted that 'I still believe I shall be able for the benefit of mankind to establish what I have asserted.' He continued, 'I think I can now assert from more experience in the nitric acid that the failures that have occurred in venereal cases have arisen from the remedy being administered in an insufficient quantity.' As an alternative, he recommended introducing the acid into the body via the skin, by means of a bath, which enabled the quantity of acid to be increased above the dose that could be safely taken internally.[92] After this letter, Scott does not appear to have to written to Banks again on the subject of nitric acid, confining himself to other topics, such as his praise for Edward Jenner's vaccination against smallpox and his belief that the older practice of variolation had caused many deaths in India.[93]

[88] *Annals of Medicine*, 3 (1798), 91.
[89] Blair, *Essays on the Venereal Disease*, chap. 4.
[90] *Annals of Medicine*, 3 (1798), 3.
[91] Currie, *Medical Reports on the Effects of Water*, v–vi; Dr James Currie to Sir Joseph Banks, 25 January 1797, HILL 39/9, Papers collected by Sir Francis Hill, Lincolnshire Archives.
[92] Scott to Banks, 20 January 1799, ff. 20–1, Banks Correspondence, BL.
[93] Scott to Banks, 12 October 1800, f. 22, Banks Correspondence, BL.

Scott's treatment with nitric acid might have continued to inspire many more trials in Britain had it not been for what proved to be a decisive intervention by John Pearson, Senior Surgeon of the Lock Hospital and Asylum at the Public Dispensary in London. Pearson subjected a wide range of substances touted as cures for venereal disease to trials among his patients. He began his trial of nitric acid at the Lock Hospital at the beginning of 1797, following the publication of Scott's letter to Banks. In 1800, he provided details of fifteen cases treated with acid at his Lock Hospital and of trials conducted by Dr Mathew Baillie, Physician at St George's Hospital, by Dr Marcet, Physician at the London Dispensatory, and by a Dr Ramsbottam of Wakefield, Surrey. These results indicated that 'nitrous acid', as he termed it, did not cure venereal disease permanently, even though it may have temporarily removed some of its symptoms; nor did it assist the action of mercury. Its sole benefit, as far as he could see, was that it promoted the appetite and reduced salivation when mercury was administered.[94] Other critics, such as Blair, also acknowledged that the acid could offset some of the unpleasant side-effects of mercury, including allaying salivation. On this basis, a number of practitioners, including Thomas Dancer of Jamaica, began to try it alongside mercury in the treatment of certain fevers.[95] It was used in this way by military surgeons during the Egyptian expedition, for example, being given to plague patients internally and externally in the form of a bath, apparently to good effect.[96]

Pearson's *Observations on the Effects of Various Articles of the Materia Medica, in the Cure of Lues Venerea* was well received in the medical press. A reviewer in the *Medical and Physical Journal* declared that:

> This work is extremely well calculated to calm the agitation in the minds of those, whose opinions have been unsettled on the treatment of the Venereal Disease, since the introduction of the new remedies. The situation the respectable author has long held, gives him full claim to the confidence of the public; and the work evidently shews that it is the production of a mind well adapted for careful observation and sound judgement.[97]

The implication was that both judgement and observation had been lacking in previous trials of nitric acid and other modish therapies.

Beddoes nevertheless continued publicly to support Scott's contention that nitric acid was a cure for venereal disease. It was natural that there should be an affinity between the two men. Both had radical sympathies and had been pupils of Joseph Black at Edinburgh; moreover, Scott's support added greatly to the respectability of the pneumatic enterprise in Bristol. In 1799 and 1800, Beddoes thus published further collections of reports on nitric acid, which in his view

94 Pearson, *Observations on the Effects of Various Articles of the Materia Medica in the Cure of Lues Venerea*, 154–83.

95 Dancer, *The Medical Assistant*, 82.

96 M'Gregor, *Medical Sketches*, 136–7, 139.

97 *Medical and Physical Journal*, 3 (April 1800), 380.

provided substantial evidence in its favour. These included letters from Scott, praising Beddoes for having induced others to follow his example. Scott had apparently been experiencing difficulties in obtaining sufficient supplies of nitre of late and was pleased that practitioners in Britain had taken the initiative. Scott also made it known that he had been applying the nitric acid in venereal cases in the form of a compress and as a bath. His letters make it clear that the effective principle in these treatments was oxygen; a view confirmed by Beddoes' associate Humphry Davy. He had thus experimented with other means of 'oxygenating the body' such as giving black calx of manganese in a drink containing acids of vitriol or nitre, although apparently with little success.[98]

In a letter to the *Medical and Physical Journal*, in May 1800, Beddoes thus felt able to state that trials conducted at the Pneumatic Institution had proved nitric acid to be 'strikingly efficacious'.[99] As to the issue of relapses, he later admitted that these sometimes occurred, but less frequently than was the case with mercury.[100] By the late summer of 1801, Beddoes was evidently frustrated that the nitric acid cure upon which he had staked his reputation – and that of his Institute – was running out of steam. In another letter to the *Medical and Physical Journal*, he bitterly attacked Pearson and declared that he was 'impatient that it should be known to the public, whether careless management, with foul play and an insufficient range of powers, occasioned the loss of many lives, and the destruction of many constitutions, which acids would have saved'.[101] He appended a plan for 'Public Scrutiny of certain Medicines, lately proposed as antivenereal, at the Pneumatic Institution near Bristol'. Through this, he hoped to open trials of various acids to public scrutiny. 'It remains that the Inquiry be unexceptionably conducted', he added, 'so that Europe may be no longer defrauded of that benefit from acids which India is unanimously attested to enjoy. All doubt as to the nature of the cases must be obviated.' Beddoes suggested that each case should be verified by no fewer than three physicians before the trials took place and that 'the public must be satisfied that the medicines alleged are administered, and no others' and that 'A person worthy of confidence, must . . . be engaged to superintend the treatment'.[102]

Beddoes appears to have received little support for the scheme as references to it in medical journals soon disappeared. Still, a few practitioners continued to speak up for nitric acid, though mostly with less enthusiasm than before. Dr T. Vage informed the *Medical and Physical Journal* that: 'Among what are

[98] Stansfield, *Thomas Beddoes*, 178–9.

[99] Beddoes to Dr Bradley, editor of the *Medical and Physical Journal*, 'Medical Intelligence', 3 (May 1800), 486.

[100] Beddoes to editors of the *Medical and Physical Journal*, 12 December 1800, 4 (January 1801), 71–2.

[101] Beddoes to the editors of the *Medical and Physical Journal*, 18 July 1801, 4 (August 1801), 164–5.

[102] Ibid., 167.

termed new discoveries, the nitric acid seems to claim the chief regard; for although it is not adequate to a perfect cure in confirmed cases, yet if given at proper intervals it very much prevents some of the ill effects of mercury, particularly upon the teeth and gums, and the debility of the digestive viscera.' He therefore concluded that nitric acid was best given alongside mercury, where it could be used to cure not only venereal complaints but cases of scrofula and cancer.[103] The most enthusiastic reports came from outside Britain. A correspondent from India confirmed that Scott had recently cured one of his servants of venereal disease using a bath containing nitric acid. He had heard of two other such cases, in which Scott had apparently cured Indian servants. The fame of nitric acid had spread outside the British Empire, too. Professor Wurzer of Bonn claimed to have cured cases of venereal disease with nitric acid after mercury had failed. But another German physician, Professor Huseland, was more measured, insisting that it proved effective only in treating the 'morbid remainders' of venereal disease, rather than the disease proper.[104] After 1802, the British medical press carried fewer reports about nitric acid. The medical profession in Britain appears to have grown weary of such claims and, though nitric acid was never entirely discredited, the trials by Pearson and distinguished physicians such as Baillie – a royal physician respected for his work in morbid anatomy – ultimately counted for more than the optimistic proclamations of Beddoes.

However, nitric acid continued to be promoted aggressively in the British Army by its Director-General, Sir James McGrigor, with whom Scott had a long-standing friendship. According to his autobiography, McGrigor had met Scott in Bombay and remained in close contact with him until the latter's death. Both were graduates of Aberdeen and it was Scott who introduced McGrigor to the then Col. Arthur Wellesley, who, as the Duke of Wellington, would later play an important part in McGrigor's rise to prominence.[105] McGrigor was intensely interested in the therapeutic and preventive power of chemical substances and, like other practitioners working in the colonies, believed that chemistry had the potential to unlock the secrets of nature, elucidating the mechanisms of contagion and infection for example.[106] Indeed, during the 1790s there was a real vogue for pneumatic medicine in the colonies and many individuals were carrying out eudiometrical investigations of the atmosphere as well as experimenting with chemical drugs.[107] Impressed by Scott's work, McGrigor began his own trial of nitric acid at the Bombay military hospital in 1799. He gave forty-six European dysentery patients in the 88th Regiment nitric acid and other drugs commonly used to treat the condition, including calomel, gum camphor, and

[103] Vage, 'Criticism on the Treatment of the Venereal Disease', 465.

[104] 'Medical and Physical Intelligence', *Medical and Physical Journal*, 4 (August 1800), 183.

[105] McGrigor, *The Scalpel and the Sword*, 82, 88, 104, 109.

[106] M'Gregor [McGrigor], *Medical Sketches*, 68.

[107] e.g. Davidson, 'Experiments'; Chisholm, 'An Account of the Cachexia Africana'; Currie, 'An Enquiry'. On eudiometry generally, see Schaffer, 'Measuring Virtue'.

ipecacuanha. The nitric acid patients seemed to show the best results. McGrigor also used the 'new oxygenated remedies' in the treatment of syphilitic complaints. He was so excited by the response to nitric acid treatments that he wrote to Beddoes, explaining the experiments in detail.[108] McGrigor's enthusiasm for nitric acid and other chemical therapies was matched only by his passion for morbid anatomy, in which, like other British surgeons in India, he hoped to gain indications of how pathological signs related to symptoms. His principal object was to gain some insight into the nature of disease so that the curative properties of medicines could be better understood. McGrigor thus lost no opportunity for dissecting soldiers who died in the Company's hospitals and took detailed notes of both symptoms and post-mortem findings in a range of diseases.[109]

When Scott returned to Britain after twenty-five years' service in India, with 'an ample fortune', he joined McGrigor in London. There they attended lectures on anatomy and chemistry given by Mr Brande at the Windmill Street anatomy school.[110] McGrigor's belief in the efficacy of nitric acid never wavered and in 1817 he wrote to his friend John Thomson, Regius Professor of Surgery at Edinburgh,[111] inquiring whether there had been any trials in that country of Scott's nitro-muriatic baths in the treatment of hepatic disease; a treatment which he claimed was 'much in view here [London] at this time'.[112] He was probably referring to a trial of Scott's bath on twenty venereal patients at the York Hospital, Chelsea, which was an Army establishment.[113] McGrigor also requested Thomson to 'give a full and fair trial to the nitro-muriatic bath of my old and highly respected friend Dr Scott of Bombay and continue the trials for a year in cure of syphilis and venereal disease'.[114] He was quite persistent in these requests and several months later reminded Thomson to encourage military surgeons in Glasgow, Aberdeen, and Stirling to send any cases fit for the nitro-muriatic bath to him so that they could be included in a trial.[115] This suggests that McGrigor was using his influence to promote Scott's treatment among friends and patrons despite the indifference of the profession as a whole.

[108] McGrigor to Beddoes, 1 December 1800, MACS/10/5/6, McGrigor Papers, Medico-Chirurgical Society, University of Aberdeen.

[109] e.g. McGrigor, Case Book XIX, 40, 76.

[110] McGrigor, *The Scalpel and the Sword*, 247.

[111] Thomson had a strong interest in military medicine, and briefly (in 1803) enlisted in the Army as a hospital mate in case it became necessary to establish a military hospital in Edinburgh during the Napoleonic Wars. Afterwards, he continued to lecture on military surgery and diseases. Like McGrigor, he had a strong interest in chemistry, but was politically active in Whig circles rather than the Tory ones in which McGrigor moved. See Power, *rev.* McConnell, 'John Thomson (1765–1846)'; Jacyna, *Philosophic Whigs*.

[112] McGrigor to Dr Thomson, 22 July 1817, MS Cullen, 905, Special Collections, University of Glasgow Library [hereafter, SCUG].

[113] McGrigor to Thomson, 19 September 1817, MS Cullen, 909, SCUG.

[114] McGrigor to Thomson, 31 August 1817, MS Cullen, 906, SCUG.

[115] McGrigor to Thomson, 28 October 1817, MS Cullen, 911, SCUG.

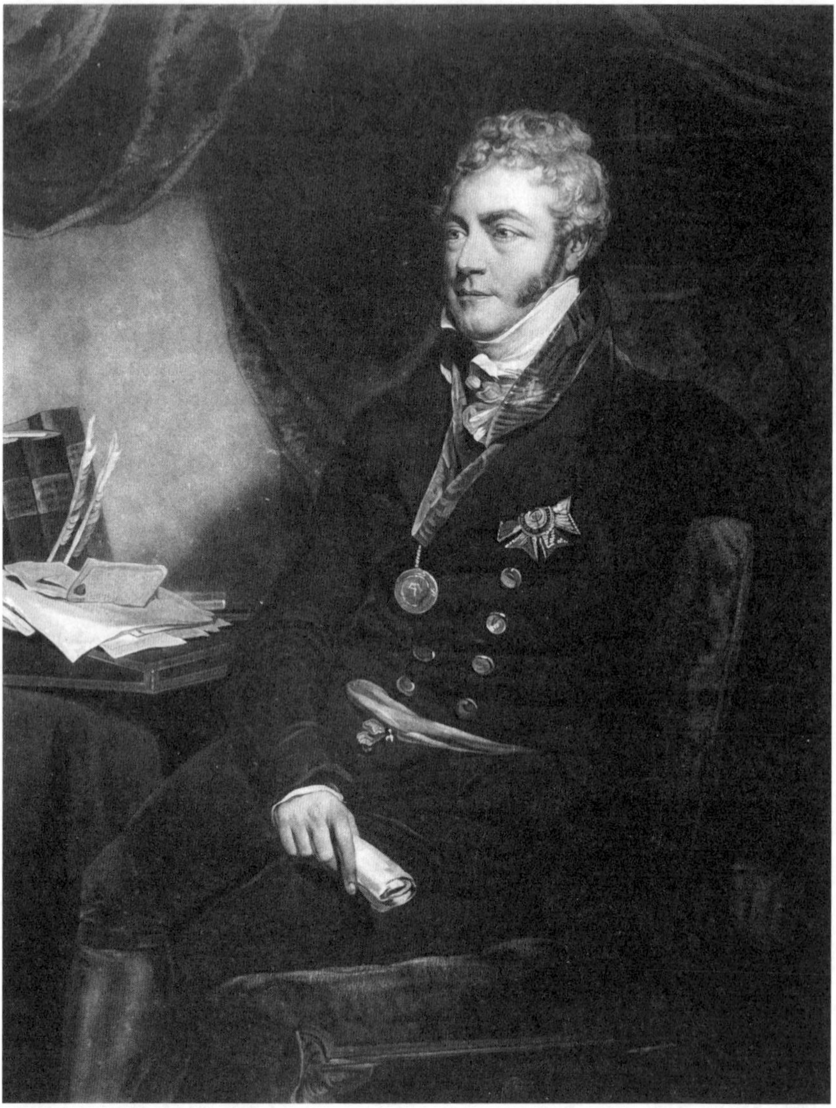

II.1. Sir James McGrigor

In the tropical colonies and among former colonial practitioners, nitric acid treatment in its various forms continued to be advocated for a range of conditions. In the 1820s, no less an authority than Colin Chisholm claimed that 'It is beyond all doubt that oxygenated medicines, particularly the oxy-muriate of potass [sic] and the nitric acid, are possessed of much greater powers in hot than in cold climates – in the East and West Indies than in Great Britain. I can assign no satisfactory cause for this, but the fact is indubitable.' Indeed, Chisholm 'fully confirmed' the claims of Scott during trials conducted at the hospital under his charge in Martinique.[116] He had also begun to experiment with Scott's method of using a nitric acid bath to treat a range of disorders, although he had not yet sufficient evidence to give an opinion of its worth.[117] These hot, medicated air baths, using vapours from nitric and other forms of acid, were popular until at least the 1850s.[118] Chisholm was no crank but one of the most respected writers on the diseases of the West Indies; he had been Inspector-General of Ordnance Hospitals in the West Indies, and was a Fellow of the Royal Society and an honorary member of learned societies in Switzerland and America.

While nitric acid continued to be used by colonial practitioners and by the Army more generally, it failed to take root in British medicine the way that calomel did after its fame had spread to Britain in the 1790s. Nevertheless, the fact that nitric acid was widely evaluated by systematic trials represents something of a larger victory for the practitioners in the military and naval medical establishments, who had long championed such methods. More importantly, perhaps, the case of nitric acid, like that of calomel, serves to demonstrate the importance of informal, 'horizontal' connections between colonial and metropolitan practitioners, in addition to the more hierarchical and centralized ones operating through the offices of the Company and influential patrons such as Banks. It is clear that there was a strong and enduring bond between radical or dissenting practitioners and natural philosophers in Britain and some of the luminaries of medicine in British colonial settlements. These links serve to emphasize the point that the nature of medical and philosophical activity in the colonies was complex and that it cannot be easily squared with conventional depictions of colonial 'scientists' as servile 'fact gatherers'. Rather, it would seem that Britain's settlements in the East and West Indies afforded reformist practitioners with unparalleled opportunities to experiment with new drugs and to develop courses of treatment which were at odds, at least initially, with mainstream opinion at home.

116 Chisholm, *Manual*, 74–5.
117 Ibid., 75–6.
118 Letter from Dr Jackson, Presidency Surgeon, Bengal, to Dr Forsyth, Secretary Medical Board, 22 September 1852; No. 266, Medical Board to Marquis of Dalhousie, 22 October 1852, Bengal Military Consultations, APAC, BL.

4

A therapeutic revolution

Part I of this book argued that the early 1800s marked a turning point in the way in which disease was understood. Until that time, the medicine of warm climates rested largely on theories of putrefaction and particularly that which ascribed most diseases to excessive bile. Despite a few dissentient voices, the theory and its advocates held sway over the medical services of the East India Company and, perhaps less securely, those of the Army and Navy. By the late 1790s, however, nervous theories of the kind articulated by Cullen and his rebellious student John Brown began to take hold, first in the West Indies and then more generally, affecting even the East Indies, where notions of putrefaction were deeply entrenched. The growing dominance of nervous physiology had a marked effect on the way in which people construed their relationship with the environment and particularly the influence of the atmosphere upon their bodies. It also had a profound effect upon the practice of medicine. Those who had understood disease as putrefaction of the humours had tended to rely on purging the body of substances which had become corrupt; hence the popularity of antimonials and calomel. In most cases, such practices rested on empirical observation, with some grounding in morbid anatomy and pneumatic chemistry. By the early 1800s, the dominant rationale for therapeutics was very different. The main principle was not the evacuation of dangerous substances but alleviation of the causes and symptoms of nervous debility. Debility was widely regarded as the proximate cause of fevers or, if not actually a cause, then one of their primary symptoms. Therapeutics was thus turned on its head, and remedies hitherto regarded as unsuited to the tropics came back with a vengeance, particularly bloodletting. In most of these respects, what happened to the medicine of warm climates mirrored and reinforced trends in Britain and other temperate countries, but, as we shall see, the pattern is somewhat different from that in Britain, France, and the United States.

BRUNO TROPICANUS

The new therapeutics emerged in its most extreme form in the guise of Brunonianism. John Brown, who was the originator of this movement, set himself up as a tutor in medicine in Edinburgh, in opposition to the teachings of his former mentor William Cullen. In place of Cullen's subtle teachings, he favoured a doctrine of revolutionary simplicity, which his followers compared to the intellectual advances of Newton a century earlier. According to Brown, all diseases were due to either too much or too little natural energy, or excitability, which in turn depended upon the action of external stimuli. A healthy body required just the right amount of stimuli, but if these were excessive or inadequate then it would quickly lapse into a state of ill health. There was no room in his system for the Hippocratic notion of the healing power of Nature. Rather, the practitioner needed to intervene quickly and often drastically to restore the body's fragile equilibrium. In what he termed *sthenic* diseases (in which energy had been depleted by over-stimulation), weak stimulants were employed in the form of bleeding, vomiting, purging, cold applications, low diets, and so forth. In *asthenic* cases, in which energy was deficient, more powerful stimulants such as camphor, wine, opium, and ether were required, as well as an ample diet and plenty of fresh air. To modern readers it may seem odd to see substances such as wine and opium listed as stimulants, but to Brunonians anything which initially administered a small shock to the system was classed as such, including articles which ultimately had a soporific effect. Most of the drugs used by Brown and his followers were already in common use, but Brunonians classified them differently. They were not seen primarily as emetics, purgatives, and the like, but were employed according to the degree of stimulation which they were capable of producing.[1]

Brown's doctrines enjoyed a fair amount of support in Britain and on the Continent, appealing to different practitioners for different reasons. But in Britain, his ideas appealed most to those who saw themselves as radicals, sometimes in political matters as well as in medicine, and for this reason they were regarded sympathetically by the likes of Darwin and Beddoes and his circle in Bristol. By stripping medicine to its essentials, Brunonians dispensed with the accumulated wisdom of ages, believing they would inspire confidence in a public weary of the elaborate nostrums of physicians. It was this radical simplicity that attracted many practitioners working in the East and West Indies, especially those employed in military or naval establishments. Simplicity was important to them for two reasons. Firstly, once a general principle had been established, it was much easier to organize therapeutics on the scale required for patients in military and naval hospitals. Secondly, and most importantly, any new doctrine that offered clear guidelines was welcome to practitioners who regularly saw scores of patients die through want of effective medical treatment. As Charles Maclean, one of the foremost followers of Brown in India put it, 'In climates and countries where the transition, from health to disease, and from disease to death, is often alarmingly rapid, and health always precarious, the knowledge of a

[1] Brown, *The Works of Dr John Brown*; Risse, 'The Brownian System of Medicine'; idem, 'Brunonian Therapeutics'.

doctrine, which reduces the practice of medicine to a degree of certainty hitherto unknown, cannot but be attended with great and evident advantages.'[2]

Maclean and his colleague William Yates are among the very few practitioners in the East Indies that it is possible to identify with certainty as followers – though not uncritical ones – of Brown. That there were more is clear from the statements of their antagonists, but very few identified themselves as Brunonians in the manner of Yates and Maclean, perhaps because they feared they would be punished or otherwise disadvantaged for departing from orthodoxy. But many at least flirted with Brunonian ideas or, as Michael Barfoot has put it, 'simply absorbed an approach which was . . . widely diffused throughout the culture'.[3] In the late 1790s, Maclean and Yates were both at the Calcutta General Hospital, where they treated mainly European soldiers and mariners employed by the East India Company. Little is known of Yates's background, but Maclean was formerly a surgeon in the Company's Marine,[4] and their jointly authored volume, *A View of the Science of Life* (1798), includes case notes from this part of Maclean's career.[5] Maclean is far better known for what he did after leaving the Company's service than in it, particularly his vehement opposition to the doctrine of contagion in diseases such as plague and to quarantine as a measure to prevent them.[6] Relatively little has been written about either his earlier career or his advocacy of a modified version of Brunonian therapeutics, yet without considering the first part of Maclean's career one cannot fully understand the intellectual basis for his opposition to contagion.[7]

As Maclean makes clear in *A View of the Science of Life*, contagion was a disputed theory that fitted awkwardly in a Brunonian view of disease. To the extent that different 'poisons' could be considered causes of disease, they owed 'their deleterious operation . . . wholly [to] . . . their superior degree of stimulant power'.[8] But most diseases classed as epidemic and pestilential, according to Maclean, were due simply to 'a certain state or vicissitudes of the atmosphere, together with the casual application of other powers, producing indirect debility'.[9] However, the idea of disease to which both authors subscribed was subtly different from that of Brown. Whereas Brown had thought that many diseases were due to excessive excitement, Yates and Maclean believed that there were no diseases that could truly be so called

[2] Maclean in Yates and Maclean, *A View of the Science of Life*, 22.

[3] Michael Barfoot, 'Brunonianism under the Bed: An Alternative to University Medicine in Edinburgh in the 1780s', in Bynum and Porter (eds.), *Brunonianism*, 25.

[4] Maclean is listed as Surgeon on the Indiaman, the *William Pitt*, and received payment of £35 8*s*. for service on that vessel from 1 April 1788 to 3 June 1789. The fact that he was a full surgeon as opposed to a surgeon's mate suggests that he already possessed some experience of the craft. See paybook of the *William Pitt*, 1788–9, L/MAR/B/184S(1), APAC, BL.

[5] Yates and Maclean, *Science of Life*.

[6] e.g. Mullett, 'Politics, Economics and Medicine'.

[7] Brown, 'From Foetid Air to Filth'; Kelly, '"Not From the College"'.

[8] Yates and Maclean, *Science of Life*, 26.

[9] Ibid., 153; Maclean, *Results of an Investigation respecting Epidemic and Pestilential Diseases*.

because all diseases manifested themselves in debility. The main distinction lay between diseases of exhaustion (or indirect debility) at one extreme and 'diseases of accumulation' (or direct debility) at the other. The former were those diseases which occurred when the body's vitality had been exhausted by massive stimulation of the nervous system, and included most of the maladies common in warm climates.[10] The latter were diseases in which there had been a steady erosion of the body's vital powers, perhaps because of prolonged exposure to cold, lack of nutritious food, or even subjection to mental 'stress'. Such diseases included scurvy, pneumonia, and rheumatism.[11] In terms of therapy, the authors believed that Brown's chief error had been his belief that certain substances (especially evacuants) could be debilitating. Yates and Maclean saw them unambiguously as stimulants, causing an increase in pulse or 'general invigoration'.[12]

The drug most favoured by Yates and Maclean in treating the diseases they encountered in India was calomel.[13] Thus, in terms of what they actually administered, the remedies employed by Yates and Maclean differed little from their more orthodox colleagues in the Bengal establishment. This was true, also, of the quantities in which mercurial preparations were given by Maclean and Yates, which were just as generous as those administered by their military colleagues. The difference lay largely in the rationale for their therapy, and in some cases their willingness to use additional 'stimulants' (especially opium) or non-purgative preparations of mercury in addition to calomel.[14] Their sole principle of treatment was to raise the system – gradually, if necessary – to a level of stimulation which compensated for the debility suffered by the patient.

In writing the *Science of Life*, the authors' avowed aim was to 'promulgate the doctrine of Brown, with some modifications, in India' where it seemed to be 'almost wholly unknown'.[15] According to Maclean, knowledge of Brown's system had been difficult to obtain because of the 'strenuous and authoritative manner in which this doctrine has always been opposed'.[16] How far this is true of other colonies is hard to say, but there is some evidence that Maclean may have been correct about India. One of the principal exponents of the biliary theory in Calcutta in the 1790s was John Wade, whose *Paper on the Prevention and Treatment of the Disorders of Seamen and Soldiers in Bengal* (1793) explicitly denounced the way in which Brown had used wine and opium. Rather than being stimulants, these substances had a sedative effect, he claimed; he also noted

10 Yates and Maclean, *Science of Life*, 29–30.
11 Ibid., 26–9.
12 Ibid., 37.
13 Calomel was also used in this way by some practitioners in the West Indies; see Davidson, 'Practical and Diagnostic Observations on Yellow Fever', 249.
14 Yates and Maclean, *Science of Life*, 44–100; see also Maclean, *A Treatise on the Action of Mercury*.
15 Yates and Maclean, *Science of Life*, Preface.
16 Ibid., 103.

that wine had been given indiscriminately by some practitioners in Bengal to native troops, despite the fact that Muslim sepoys opposed it on religious grounds.[17] More fundamentally, he claimed that Brunonian practice was unsuited to the diseases of hot climates:

> Doctor Brown's practice may possibly apply to some circumstances of low fever in Europe; but the occurrence of such fevers will be found very rare in the meridian of Bengal, particularly in the upper provinces, where the most acute disorders have, what would be deemed in Europe, and according to Doctor Moseley in the West Indies, an inflammatory aspect, and are also characterized by larger secretions of bile.[18]

Wade felt the need to caution his readers because several notices had appeared in Calcutta newspapers in 1788 and 1789 recommending Brown's practice; notices which he attributed to 'surgeons of the honourable company's ships'.[19] It is very likely that one of these was Maclean, who was then serving on the *William Pitt*.

It was not the only occasion on which Maclean fell foul of the Company for writing what its senior administrators regarded as inflammatory and seditious articles. Maclean commenced employment with the Company in 1788, in which year he began to use calomel as a stimulant. The following year, on the passage from Bengal to England, he subjected it to a trial, using himself as an experimental subject: he was suffering from fever.[20] Three years later, while visiting his friend Hector M'Lean in Jamaica, he began to use mercury in the treatment of fevers on that island and later claimed (falsely as it happens) that he was the first person there to use it in non-venereal conditions.[21] In 1791, Maclean was re-employed in another of the Company's ships, the *Northumberland*, and in 1794 was appointed surgeon to the *Houghton*, which formed part of a squadron sent to protect Batavia against the French.[22] What happened then is unclear. It has been claimed that Maclean deserted from the Marine, but in 1796 he was working with Yates in the mariners' ward at the Calcutta General Hospital.[23] In the same year, he became the proprietor of a newspaper and magazine and was denounced by the new Governor-General, the Marquis of Wellesley as 'a most audacious and turbulent demagogue'.[24]

Wellesley's invective was fuelled by rumours of a French alliance with the Company's great enemy, Tipu Sultan of Mysore. There were fears that Jacobin agents were active in Calcutta and that Maclean was among them. No evidence has survived to support this, but Maclean was clearly seen by Wellesley as a

[17] Wade, *Paper*, 62, 63, 65.
[18] Ibid., 67.
[19] Ibid., 68.
[20] Maclean, *An Analytical View*, 153–4.
[21] Maclean, *Practical Illustrations*, 1, 9; idem, *Results*, vol. 2, 501.
[22] Maclean, *Illustrations*, 11, 25, 27.
[23] Maclean, *Results*, vol. 2, 504; idem, *The Affairs of Asia*, 2nd edn., 9–10.
[24] Wellesley to Mr Henry Dundas, President of the Board of Control, 21 March 1799, letter 9 in Ingram (ed.), *Two Views of British India*, 235–6.

troublemaker and, when a chance to remove him arose, Wellesley swiftly took advantage. On 28 April 1798, Maclean wrote a letter critical of the magistrate of Ghazipore (Mr Jacob Rider) in the Calcutta newspaper, *The Telegraph*. A friend of his, who also bore the surname Maclean, had been locked up on the magistrate's orders, on what Charles Maclean regarded as false pretences, having allegedly assaulted his business partner, the indigo planter Benjamin d' Aguillar. The magistrate had failed to give Mr Allen Maclean notice that he was to be imprisoned on the grounds that 'he was not a gentleman'. He was later released without charge, with a judgement from a superior court, the Nizamat Adalat, that the magistrate had not been authorized to detain him.[25] But Maclean provided Wellesley with the pretext he needed, for he refused to comply with Wellesley's order that he apologize for insinuating improper conduct on the part of the magistrate.[26]

An attempt had been made to expel Maclean on a previous occasion for desertion but, for reasons which are unclear, the authorities were unable or unwilling to apprehend him.[27] Maclean and his family – he was then married – were ordered to leave India for the second and final time in August, yet he appears to have left India alone. He departed in poor health but had managed to avoid repayment of a substantial debt to an Indian money-lender, although Wellesley was later to claim that the suit of debt against Maclean was fictitious; a desperate attempt to enable him to remain in India.[28] Maclean's creditor, one Bysenaut Mitter, insisted that Maclean had borrowed from him the sum of Rs. 1,332.12, of which he had paid back only Rs. 200. Mitter instituted a suit against Maclean in the Supreme Court as soon as he heard that Maclean was about to return to Europe and took out a warrant for his arrest. However, he found that Maclean was already under confinement in Fort William and petitioned the government to prevent him from being deported before the debt could be settled.

It is doubtful that Wellesley's allegation was true, as Mitter persisted with his demand for compensation after Maclean left India, seemingly unaware of his departure. He sent a petition to Wellesley dated 9 September 1798, despite the fact that Maclean had departed Bengal on the *Busbridge* on 18 August.[29] Mitter's persistence in the matter suggests that his appeal against Maclean's removal had

[25] Proceedings of the Nizamat Adalat, 19 April 1798, Consultation No. 8, 19 April 1798, Judicial (Criminal) Consultations, West Bengal State Archives [hereafter, WBSA].

[26] Maclean, *To the British Inhabitants of India*, 1–2, 20–1.

[27] Governor-General in Council to Hon. Court of Directors, 29 September; answer to same, giving approval, in Gupta (ed.), *Fort William–India House Correspondence and other Contemporary Papers*, 209–10, 529–30.

[28] See petition delivered by Bysenaut Mitter, 9 September 1798, Consultation No. 9, 9 November 1798, Judicial (Criminal) Consultations, WBSA.

[29] Maclean is recorded as a charter party passenger on the *Busbridge*, which left Bengal on 18 August 1798. He disembarked at Portsmouth on 11 July 1799. Journal of the *Busbridge* 1796–9, list of ship's company and passengers, L/MAR/B/413G, APAC, BL.

not been orchestrated, although his claim that non-payment of Maclean's debt would reduce him and his family to poverty may well have been exaggerated. But with Maclean gone, Wellesley had little interest in the matter and noted contemptuously that, 'The Governor-General in Council observes that it does not appear to him necessary to take any notice of the foregoing petition.'[30]

Before leaving India, Maclean collected most of the correspondence connected with the incident, in an attempt at vindication and to illustrate the repression of free speech by the Governor-General, who had attempted to crush all exhibitions of what he referred to as 'Jacobin' sentiments. It is unclear whether Maclean's pamphlet was published shortly before or after his departure from India, but in the coming years he lost no opportunity to criticize Wellesley, comparing him to Bonaparte and blaming him and his kind for the steady erosion of liberties at home as well as in India.[31] However, while Wellesley's imperious leadership was clearly not to Maclean's tastes, he later defended the Company's monopoly of navigation (despite otherwise advocating free trade) and its general record in India, having found occasional employment with the Company as a lecturer on the 'diseases of hot climates'.[32] From this position he continued to espouse the use of calomel as a treatment for diseases of the tropics and he later claimed that the remedies he had pioneered whilst a servant of the Company had been generally accepted. Writing of the progress made in medicine over the last thirty years, Maclean observed that calomel had now 'become domiciliated even in the nurseries'.[33]

There are certainly contradictions, if not tensions, in the positions adopted by Maclean in the course of his career, not to mention a whiff of opportunism and financial impropriety. Nevertheless, he consistently railed against anything that he regarded as tyranny, in public and in professional life. In this sense, there is a clear link between his advocacy of a modified version of Brown's doctrine and his political outlook, both during his time in India and subsequently in Britain, where he was critical of smallpox vaccination, quarantine, the Royal College of Physicians, senior members of the Army Medical Department (which he later joined), the Roman Catholic Church, King William IV, and the repressive administration of Lord Liverpool.[34] His own political position is hard to define, but in the late 1810s and early 1820s, he was aligned with the Benthamites, the Radical MP John Cam Hobhouse, and the Liberal MP John Smith, who championed quarantine reform in Parliament. By the late 1820s, Maclean was

[30] Consultation No. 9, 9 November, Judicial (Criminal) Consultations, WBSA.

[31] Maclean, *Affairs of Asia.*

[32] Maclean, *A View of the Consequences of laying open the Trade to India*; idem, *Remarks on the Evidence delivered before both Houses of Parliament, on the East-India Company's Affairs.*

[33] Maclean, *Evils of Quarantine Laws*, vii–viii.

[34] See Maclean, *On the State of Vaccination in 1810*; idem, *Suggestions for the Prevention and Mitigation of Epidemic and Pestilential Diseases*; idem, *The Triumph of Public Opinion*; idem, *Specimens of Systematic Misrule*; idem, *Remarks on the British Quarantine Laws.*

supporting a proto-Chartist platform of universal suffrage and annual parliaments.[35] Just as in medicine, radical reform was not to be expected from the corridors of power, he argued, but from below, from popular agitation.[36]

THE JACKSONIANS

Most of the followers of John Brown are shadowy figures: the occasional objects of professional venom, or less often, of approbation. In 1818, Maclean mentioned only three practitioners other than himself and William Yates, who were happy to be known as Brunonians: Dr James Robertson of Bengal, Mr Syme, a surgeon on the Indiaman *Dublin*, and Mr Crout, surgeon on another Indiaman, the *Dover Castle*.[37] Apart from these, it is possible to identify a handful of others, among them the military surgeon, George Pinckard, who served in the West Indies. But whatever the number of practitioners who considered themselves Brunonians, in spirit if not in letter, they were certainly less numerous than the followers of the military surgeon Robert Jackson. Like Maclean, Jackson inspired loathing and admiration in equal measure, but with the crucial difference that he rose to a position of power and influence within the military hierarchy. Jackson enjoyed the support of Mr Knight, the surgical member of the Army Medical Board,[38] and was on good terms with Sir James McGrigor, the first Director General of the new Army Medical Department, who referred to Jackson as his 'venerable friend'.[39]

Jackson began his career as a surgeon during the American War, serving in North America and Jamaica, where he noted the practices used to treat fever in different localities. Bark, for instance, was more popular in America than in Jamaica, where purging with various substances was the order of the day. However, Jackson noted that there were some surgeons who recommend bloodletting in fevers when he was on the island, some years before the practice was recommended by Dr Moseley, who was one of the few people to advocate it in print after it had fallen into disuse. Jackson claimed that Dr Spence, 'a practitioner of some eminence at Lucca', in Western Jamaica, had written a pamphlet on the subject before Moseley, in around 1776.[40] It seems to have been Spence rather than Moseley who induced Jackson to try the practice after finding other therapies such as bark and some antimonials wanting.[41] Bark, he argued, was very effective in the treatment of intermittent fevers but tended to be employed

[35] Pelling, *Cholera, Fever, and English Medicine*, 27–8; Maclean, *Specimens*, xiv–xxi.
[36] Maclean, *Specimens*, xxv; idem, *Public Opinion*, 1.
[37] Maclean, *Practical Illustrations*, xvi.
[38] Maclean, *Analytical View*, 91.
[39] McGrigor to Dr Thomson, 20 March 1818, MS Cullen, SCUG.
[40] Jackson, *Treatise on the Fevers of Jamaica*, iv–v.
[41] Ibid., 211–14.

by British practitioners to treat other kinds of fever in which it was not so efficacious; furthermore, it was often rendered effective only by very careful management of the patient.[42] Jackson reckoned bleeding to be far more effective in cases of the endemic fever of Jamaica as well as the more deadly yellow fever.[43] He also came to favour restorative treatment in the form of bathing in warm and cold water, which he claimed excited 'the tone and vigour' of the system'.[44]

At this time, however, Jackson's influence was relatively weak and it was not until after his return to the West Indies in the 1790s that his ideas had much impact on his colleagues in the Army. When Jackson was posted to St Domingue, he had the opportunity to make further observations, both of the island's endemic fevers and the yellow fever, which claimed thousands of lives among British troops. His experiences led him to alter his thinking about the identity of this disease – which he came to see as a type of endemic fever – and to work out a clearer rationale for treatment. Jackson attributed most fevers to exposure to unwholesome influences, including what he termed the 'principle of vegetation', which he deemed to be excessive in tropical countries.[45] The precise cause of fever was obscure, according to Jackson, but he believed that it operated in a way analogous to electricity, accumulating invisibly in the body until it 'exploded',[46] the timing and intensity of the explosion depending upon the state of the body's defences.[47] In such cases, morbid influences acted upon the nervous system, resulting in 'debility and impaired energy'. This depletion of the body's vital power gave rise to a range of febrile symptoms including trembling, chills, sweating, and, in extreme cases, led to death.[48] Superficially, this looks like a version of Brunonian doctrine, but theories of disease and therapeutics that rested on notions of excitability and vitality were part of the *Zeitgeist*, and it is difficult to attribute them to any single authority, be it Cullen, Brown, or Darwin.[49]

The primary intention of treatment was therefore to restore vitality and to alleviate the symptoms caused by nervous debility. In Jackson's view, such treatment ought to comprise two stages: the first to prevent the disease forming properly, and the second to treat fevers that had already taken root. In the treatment of the endemic fever of the West Indies, for example, Jackson recommended bloodletting in the first instance, particularly among patients newly arrived from Europe, with a view to removing upwards of twenty fluid ounces; this was to be followed by a dose of calomel or antimonial medicines. If this was

[42] Jackson, *Treatise on the Fevers of Jamaica*, iv–v, 317–26.
[43] Ibid., 223, 268.
[44] Ibid., 245.
[45] Jackson, *Outline of the History and Cure of Fever*, 107.
[46] Ibid., 247.
[47] Ibid., 252.
[48] Ibid., 253.
[49] Barfoot, 'Brunonianism under the Bed'; Lawrence, 'Cullen, Brown and the Poverty of Essentialism'.

not sufficient to stop the disease, then more blood could be taken, together with bathing the patient alternatively in cold and warm water. If the fever proceeded to a second day, then modification of treatment was required, with further bleeding until the patient's headache was removed or until the pulse was lowered. Cold water was then to be poured over the patient's shaven head and a blister applied to the back of the neck and between the shoulders; afterwards, the patient was to be laid in bed and given cooling, refreshing, and gently stimulating drinks. Jackson also suggested that patients might be taken on an invigorating carriage ride in pure air. This process was to be repeated until a remission of symptoms occurred.[50]

The rationale behind exposure to airs and waters of different temperatures was to stimulate a nervous system that had become debilitated by febrile influences; the rationale for bleeding was that it alleviated some of the symptoms of the fever which resulted from a rapid pulse, produced as the vascular system was forced to work harder as nervous vitality diminished. Underlying exposure to airs and waters was the idea that all parts of the body were intimately connected by the nervous system and that a sensitive organ such as the skin would communicate any stimulation rapidly to other parts of the body, including the vascular system.[51]

Jackson was acutely aware that his recommendations were likely to prove controversial, particularly his advocacy of bloodletting. When he arrived on St Domingue, bleeding had 'no credit' and 'the prejudices of the greater number were against it'.[52] At that time, the majority of the profession, according to Jackson, subscribed to the view that purgatives such as calomel were singularly adapted to treating the fevers of hot climates, which they attributed to an abundance of bile, and saw bleeding as dangerous because it further debilitated the body.[53] Nevertheless, he insisted that it was among the most important therapies in cases of fever, not only because it reduced the pulse but also because it relieved the venous congestion that typically followed debility. The blood of fever patients appeared to stagnate as nervous power was lost and in post-mortem dissections it was revealed to be much darker in colour than healthy blood.[54] Indeed, Jackson proceeded with bleeding only after trials had given him sufficient proof and after he had conducted a number of autopsies to reveal the nature of the disease.[55] Purgatives, by contrast, appeared to have little effect in cutting short fevers and in certain cases could aggravate them.[56] In moving away from purgatives and towards venesection, Jackson was conscious that he was advocating a revolution in therapeutics: a return to the antiphlogistic treatments advocated by Sydenham and Boerhaave a century before.[57]

[50] Jackson, *Outline*, 266–7. [51] Ibid., 270, 287–8. [52] Ibid., 280.
[53] Ibid., 283–4.
[54] Ibid., 273–4, 289.
[55] Ibid., 280.
[56] Ibid., 285–6. [57] Ibid., 263–4.

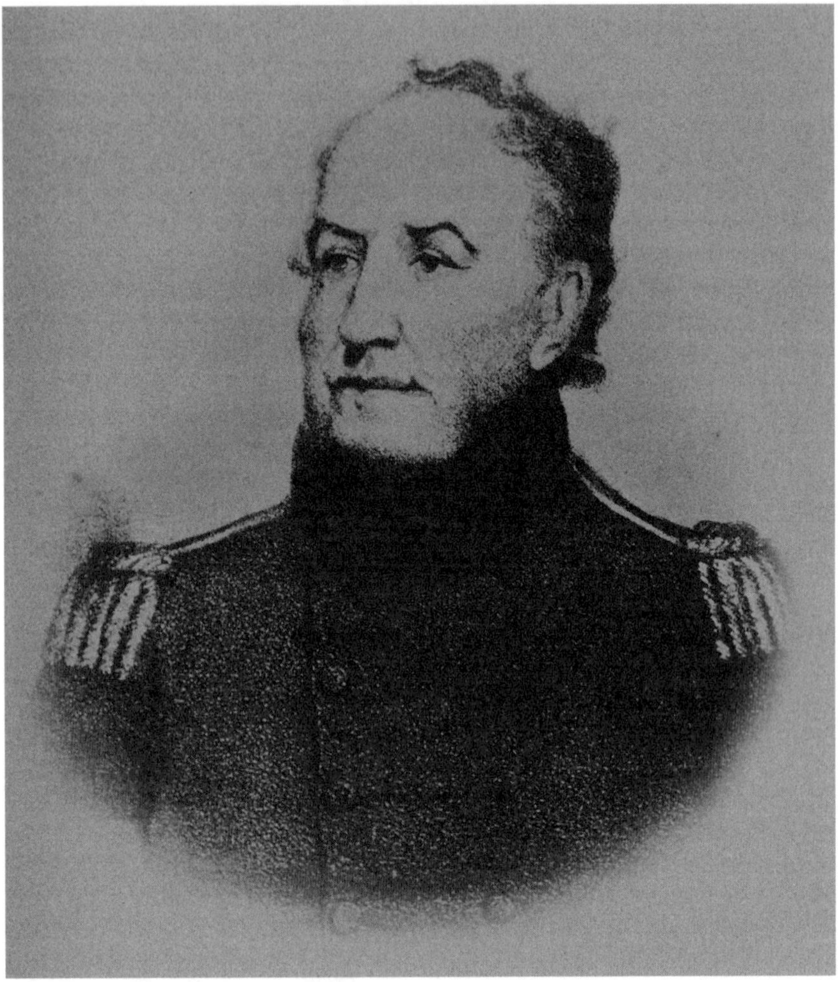

II.2. Robert Jackson

By the time Jackson's second treatise on fever was published, in 1798, he had acquired a number of followers who expressed near-identical views about the nature and treatment of these diseases. All served under Jackson for some time on St Domingue and were clearly impressed by his forceful personality. One of these men was Hector M'Lean, who spent three years as a surgeon at the Army's general hospital at Port-au-Prince. Like Jackson, M'Lean was an enthusiast for cold bathing in the treatment of fevers.[58] Bathing, he argued, increased the

[58] Jackson, *Outline*, 63, 137.

body's 'sensibility' and left it more amenable to other treatments; he defined 'sensibility' as 'the great characteristic of animated matter, it is what chiefly distinguishes it; and forms the great basis on which changes are introduced'.[59] This is almost identical to the explanation of its efficacy given by Jackson in his first and subsequent treatises on fever; however, M'Lean had also seen evidence of the beneficial effects of bathing in the East Indies, before he had met Jackson or read his work. At Diamond Harbour near Calcutta he had witnessed a man recover from a remittent fever after jumping ship in the throes of delirium. Although he had little success when he tried to throw water over his patients at the harbour hospital, he later concluded that this may have been because the water was insufficiently cool. After reading Jackson's book, he had no doubt at all that cold bathing could be useful, for the author had provided ample evidence.[60]

M'Lean also followed Jackson in recommending the more controversial practice of bloodletting. Like most practitioners at the time, he had been led to believe that bleeding was inappropriate for those who had spent any length of time in hot climates and had completely abstained from the practice. It was only after encountering Jackson that he realized that he had been ill-advised, for

> Dr Jackson, whose sagacity and attention are equally conspicuous, was much more successful, after he made more free with the lancet. The 56th regiment had been suffering from the Remittent very severly [sic] . . . but when Dr Jackson took the management of the sick, and bled more freely the mortality diminished considerably. And though the fever described by Rush, differs materially in being highly contagious, yet there are circumstances of great similitude in the symptoms; and I look on Rush's practice as a confirmation of the benefits of blood-letting.[61]

The eminent Philadelphia physician, Benjamin Rush, bled plentifully when treating cases during the city's epidemic in 1793, prompting the journalist William Cobbett to dub him 'Dr Sangrado'. Rush actually took far less blood than was advocated by Jackson and did not regard himself as an apostle of bleeding like his British counterpart. But the fact that a prominent physician like Rush had endorsed bloodletting strengthened Jackson's case, at least with a reforming element in Britain. The two men certainly had a good opinion of one another, although it is unclear whether they ever met.[62]

Some West Indian surgeons also found that Jackson's rationale for bleeding made sense of what they had experienced themselves, emboldening them to go further. Having arrived in Jamaica, the military surgeon Edward Doughty used a range of treatments in cases of yellow fever and had good results with some of them, including mercury. After a while, he was given medical charge of a detachment hospital of the 67th Regiment and was left to his own discretion

[59] M'Lean, *An Enquiry*, 147. [60] Ibid., 150–1. [61] Ibid., 137.
[62] Rush conveyed his greetings to Jackson and Pinckard via a colleague, John Syng Dorsey. See Rush to Dorsey, 23 May 1804, in Butterfield (ed.), *The Letters of Benjamin Rush*, vol. 1, 883.

regarding treatment. It was then that he attempted bloodletting, being guided as he put it, 'by no particular system', and found that he did not lose one man to it in the six weeks he resided in Fort Augusta.[63] By January 1802, he had had time to reflect on his experiences and also to read the opinions of others, including Jackson, which encouraged him to bleed more copiously than before: 'I had recourse in the first instance to the lancet. I bled to the extent frequently of two pounds, as I never ceased to let the blood flow until I observed its effects, by a disposition to syncope.' After bleeding, he administered purgatives, including calomel and Dr James's Powder.[64] Although he did not recommend bleeding in all cases, he found it to be the most important component of his therapeutic regime, as apparently did others, including Dr Harness, the Commissioner of Sick and Wounded Seamen.[65]

In the 1810s, a number of Edinburgh MD dissertations, most of which were written by military and naval surgeons returning from the Caribbean, also advocated the use of bleeding in cases of yellow fever and, indeed, in other forms of fever. Walter Steel, a former Army surgeon, recommended the lancet as first resort in all cases of fever in the islands, followed by a mixture of mild purgatives, emetics, and bark.[66] Other doctoral advocates of bleeding (as well as cold bathing) in Caribbean fevers included William King and Archibald Arnott.[67]

It is not surprising that Jackson's ideas should have taken hold so firmly among military surgeons as, in 1812, he was appointed Inspector-General of Hospitals for the Army of the West Indies. At that time the general practice was still to 'saturate the system with mercury', as his disciple James M'Cabe put it, while surgeons of a Brunonian persuasion attempted to cure yellow fever by giving substances regarded as stimulants, such as wine. Brunonian treatments were superficially attractive because debility was common in the tropics. But those military surgeons who subscribed to these notions made the mistake of thinking that debility was a cause of disease, rather than its consequence, according to M'Cabe. Jackson did his best to stamp out these practices and to replace them with his system of bleeding and bathing, which M'Cabe regarded as having sound foundations in pathology. The post of Inspector-General was one that conferred a great deal of power and, as Charles Maclean lamented a few years earlier, 'The Inspectors and Deputy Inspectors of Hospitals seem invariably to consider themselves as entitled to interfere in the practice of all inferior Officers.'[68] He was referring to those, like Francis Knight and Dr (later Sir) James Borland, who had formerly supported Jackson,[69] but now it was Jackson himself

[63] Doughty, *Observations*, 7–8.
[64] Ibid., 11–12.
[65] Ibid., 15.
[66] Steel, *De febre insularum Indae Occidentalis*, 25–9.
[67] King, *De febre flava*, 24; Arnott, *De febre remittente*, 27–30.
[68] Maclean, *Analytical View*, 90.
[69] Ackroyd et al., *Advancing with the Army*, 29–30.

who enjoyed a similar position of power. Moreover, while Jackson occupied the post for just a few years, his successor Dr William Fergusson, continued the same regime and according to M'Cabe treatment on Jacksonian lines became 'generally established'.[70] M'Cabe reckoned that Jackson's influence now extended well beyond the Army and that he had been responsible for the revival of bloodletting, 'not only in tropical climates, but also in every part of Great Britain and Ireland'. It was now taught in universities and practised in the leading teaching hospitals, such as the Edinburgh Royal Infirmary.[71] But some of Jackson's friends lamented that he had he begun to dabble in things that were not strictly medical. McGrigor for one wished 'he had not mixed Lord Castlereagh and politics with his doctrine of fever'.[72] It is not certain whether Jackson was a supporter or a detractor of Castlereagh, but in view of his reformist tendencies, it is likely that he had become critical of the latter's role in the suppression of radical assemblies or, more likely, his disinclination to alleviate distress in agricultural communities (Jackson was a champion of wholesome rural virtues).

But these forays into politics seem to have made little difference to Jackson's younger supporters. For M'Cabe, a former military surgeon and Edinburgh MD, bloodletting and the principles on which it was established were emblematic of modern, scientifically based medicine. He and other advocates of bloodletting, not least Jackson himself, went to great pains to stress that their practice was based on extensive observation, that it had been subjected to systematic trials against other remedies, and that it had a sound basis in pathological anatomy. In other words, the supposed efficacy of the practice vindicated the methods they had been espousing for years in the face of opposition from physicians involved in the running of the Army Medical Department. In the 1800s, especially following the disastrous landing at Walcheren, the department had been assailed from several directions, with Jackson and other former colonial practitioners in the forefront of the attack. The controversy was a bitter one in which Jackson actually came to blows with one of his antagonists. But, by the late 1810s, these reforming surgeons felt themselves to be on the winning side. They were coming to dominate the faculties of universities such as Edinburgh and to exercise authority within the medical services of the Army and Navy.[73] They revelled in their modernity and declared old practices, including those of their former colleagues in the military and naval services, redundant. They were able to explain many of the pathological appearances of diseases such as yellow fever without having recourse to notions of putrefaction, which leant towards the 'exploded doctrine of the humoral pathology', as M'Cabe put it.

[70] M'Cabe, *Military Medical Reports*, 13–15, 20.
[71] Ibid., 11–12.
[72] McGrigor to Dr Thomson, 23 March 1818, MS Cullen, 914, SCUG.
[73] Ackroyd et al., *Advancing with the Army*.

Most of Jackson's followers, including M'Cabe, attributed the symptoms of yellow fever, for example, and its appearances post-mortem, to a collapse of the nervous system which followed the excitement of the first stage of fever. In the last stages of such a fever, the vital principle was exhausted to such a degree that some parts of the body started to decompose, giving rise to the characteristic 'putrid' symptoms. The pulse also became weaker for the same reason, leading to stagnation and morbid changes in the blood. Bleeding was particularly important at the start of a disease, they argued, because it could lessen the initial excitement of the fever and consequently the subsequent exhaustion.[74]

Bloodletting was back with a vengeance and Jackson's supplementary treatment of fever by bathing was also in vogue. One of its main advocates in Britain was the radical physician James Currie, who appears to have used cold and warm bathing in fevers even before he had heard of Jackson's work.[75] Currie spent his early years in Virginia and had traded in the Caribbean before returning to Britain to attend Edinburgh and then Glasgow universities, graduating MD from the latter in 1780.[76] Although Currie never visited the Caribbean in a medical capacity, his practice in Liverpool brought him into contact with surgeons who worked there and on the coast of Africa; he was also called upon to treat soldiers returning from the Caribbean with fever.[77] Through these contacts, he introduced other practitioners to the benefits of bathing, which was subsequently used on board ships sailing to the tropics. It was only just before the publication of his *Medical Reports on the Effects of Water* (1797) that Currie claimed to have read Jackson's work, but he was pleased to endorse it.[78] Indeed, he was glad that cold water bathing – which he saw as especially useful in the diseases of warm climates – was now being employed in the treatment of yellow fever, which had caused so many deaths on St Domingue. His earnest wish was that the practice would spread more widely among military and naval surgeons and his aim was to interest Joseph Banks in the treatment so that it would receive wider publicity.[79]

It is therefore clear that there was a continual circulation of ideas between practitioners in Britain and the Caribbean, especially in cities such as Liverpool, which were closely linked with the region by trade. The exchange of information is also evident from the correspondence which followed the publication of Currie's *Medical Reports.* Dr James Robertson, who had practised in Barbados, told Currie that he had recently met one Dr George Davidson who had been using cold affusion in the treatment of fevers for a long time. Robertson supplied Currie with extracts from two letters written to him by Davidson, in which the latter mentioned the use of cold bathing in Barbados and Tobago as long ago as

74 McCabe, *Military Medical Reports*, 26–7, 32, 34.
75 Currie, *Medical Reports on the Effects of Water*, iii, 1.
76 DeLacy, 'Currie, James (1756–1805)'.
77 Ibid., v, vii, 8–9.
78 Ibid., 167–8.
79 Ibid., ix.

the 1770s. But, crucially, Robertson added that 'I am inclined to think his practice in the use of this remedy in fevers was a desperate measure taken at a venture and not guided by rational principles.'[80]

There was a great deal of difference between the isolated advocates of bleeding and bathing in the 1770s and 1780s and the likes of Jackson and Currie, who made a strong case for their efficacy on physiological grounds. As Robertson explained when writing of his own use of cold affusion, it worked because of the 'stimulus of sensation' which subdued febrile heat and interrupted all morbid associations and motions. His own preference was for what Currie termed 'cool' rather than 'cold' water, as water that was too frigid could produce a fatal shock to the system. Also, rather than throwing cold water over patients, he dipped their faces in it, rubbing their hands and neck with camphorated vinegar and arranging vine leaves or similar foliage around the temples to keep them cool. These articles, he explained, were mildly cathartic and diaphoretic. The practice was particularly useful in treating cases of fever among merchant seamen and sailors because it could be performed quite easily on board ship without the need to send them to a hospital on the shore.[81]

Other West Indian writers also came to advocate the practice of bathing in fevers on the principles outlined by Jackson and Currie. Thomas Dancer, a private physician of Jamaica, maintained that cold baths were necessary 'whenever there is a general loss of tone and vigour in the system', whereas hot bathing worked in the opposite circumstances, affording relief in cases of inflammation, colic, and other common conditions.[82] He did not, however, follow Jackson in bloodletting, preferring to bleed sparingly, if at all.[83] The naval physician Leonard Gillespie, who had been stationed in the Leeward Islands in the mid-1790s, was also sympathetic to Jackson's practice of bathing in fevers, but had little success with bleeding.[84] In Demerara, too, the physician George Pinckard, who had been introduced to his first case of yellow fever by Jackson, found that his old master's practice of bathing was being used to good effect. He formed a high opinion of one 'Dr E', whom he described as a 'man of talents and observation', who placed very little reliance on bark, mercury, or any of the remedies commonly employed in cases of yellow fever, but 'he thought that he had witnessed the most decided benefit from the Indian method of employing hot and cold bathing'.[85] Pinckard was referring here to the practice of Native Americans who treated a range of diseases using hot or 'vapour' baths;[86] whether

[80] Robertson to Currie, 25 March 1801, Robertson Papers, Amer. MS 137, WL.

[81] Robertson to Currie, 16 March 1801, Robertson Papers, Amer. MS 137, WL.

[82] Dancer, *The Medical Assistant*, 56–8.

[83] Ibid., 50–1, 67, 81–2, 83–6. Others were also sceptical of bleeding, claiming that it killed more often than it cured, but used bathing in the treatment of fevers, e.g. Renny, *History of Jamaica*, 199–200.

[84] Gillespie, *Observations*, 71–2, 78.

[85] Pinckard, *Notes*, vol. 3, 377.

[86] Pinckard, *Notes*, vol. 2, 430.

or not Jackson and other advocates of bathing were aware of these practices is unclear. As in the case of bloodletting, hot and cold bathing also figured in a number of the Edinburgh MD theses of the 1810s and it is notable that many of those who recommended it also favoured bloodletting.[87] Indeed, it would not be going too far to say that Jackson's ideas on the treatment of fever dominated the Edinburgh medical scene in the 1810s and 1820s.

Foreign writers on fever – especially yellow fever – also came to recommend cold bathing, for precisely the same reasons as Jackson. The Spanish physician Don Juan Manuel de Arejula, who encountered yellow fever at Seville in 1800 and at Alicante in 1804, claimed that cold bathing was among the most efficacious treatments, explaining its potency in physiological terms.[88] The French practitioner Victor Bally also claimed that cold bathing was useful during the first phase of fever when patients suffered from an 'exquisite sensibility' of their nervous system.[89] His compatriot, the military surgeon A. Mabit, likewise claimed that a French doctor named Fontanges was enjoying success with cold bathing in cases of fever in Port-au-Prince, where he may have met or heard of Jackson.[90] But bleeding, which had never really gone out of fashion in the French colonies,[91] was losing credibility at precisely the same time that its star was rising in the British Caribbean. The French writer Moreau de Jonnès recalled that an English physician who arrived on Martinique in 1802, at the time when an epidemic of yellow fever was at its height,

> pretended that he possessed a sure and speedy means of saving those who might be attacked with it. These means were no other than bleeding, and he employed it with such activity, that he lost twenty patients in eight days: so that I was on the point of forbidding his interference, when he himself was seized with the disease, he so confidently asserted he had the means of curing, and died either of its effects, or of those of his own remedy.[92]

In another curious twist, just as calomel was losing popularity in the British Caribbean, it was beginning to be taken up by the French. De Jonnès claimed that the practice had been introduced into the French West Indies by one Dr Amie in 1815. Having examined some of the doctor's patients, he acknowledged that some had shown an improvement but maintained that any salutary effects were not due to purging but more probably to the fact that it had excited salivation and urinary excretion.[93]

[87] e.g. Playfair, *De febre flava*, 17–18; King, *De febre flava*, 25; Watson, *De febre Bataviae*, 24.
[88] De Arejula, *De la febre amarilla*, 211.
[89] Bally, *Du Typhus d'Amérique*, 558–9.
[90] Mabit, *Essai*, 17.
[91] Ibid., 16–17.
[92] De Jonnès, *Monographie Historique et Médicale de la Fièvre Jaune des Antilles*, 130.
[93] Ibid., 134.

BLOODLETTING IN THE EAST

In British India, the biliary theory of disease and treatment with purgatives such as calomel were more deeply ingrained than they ever were in the West Indies, being sustained by a mixture of compulsion and faith. It is not surprising, therefore, to find that the shift towards a new therapeutic paradigm in India was more gradual than in the West Indies and that those who advocated a return to bleeding rarely did so to the total exclusion of mercurial drugs. Prior to 1800, bleeding had sometimes been used in military hospitals in India at the very beginning of fever to reduce inflammation but only in persons deemed especially plethoric. On the rare occasions that it was used, bleeding was performed in moderation and always preparatory to treatment with purgatives.[94] The first signs of a significant change in this respect came in Penang, in 1807–8, following a British military expedition from India to the Straits Settlements. There, the young military surgeon George Ballingall was investigating an outbreak of flux among the 1st Royal Regiment of Foot. All of those who died from the disease were dissected, showing evidence of inflammation of the large intestines, which he attributed to over-stimulation of the affected part, leading in time to 'loss of tone' and paralysis. In other words, this was an interpretation of the pathology of flux that was clearly derived from nervous physiology.[95] In an attempt to arrest the disease, Ballingall subjected a number of medicines to trial, including the common expedient of calomel. He found that the medicine had done little good, except possibly in the final stages of the disease, when it might contribute to the restoration of the healthy action of the affected parts. But this could happen only after any inflammatory symptoms had subsided, he claimed, and mercurial preparations had generally been used with little discrimination. Indeed, in Ballingall's view, they had probably done more harm than if the disease had been 'left to nature'.

Because of its power as a purgative, mercury could induce the very symptoms that Ballingall was attempting to combat,[96] although he later acknowledged that it could be used to good effect in cases of dysentery provided it was employed judiciously.[97] Opium was also given a fair trial, but again Ballingall enjoyed little success with it.[98] The only universally effective remedy, he maintained, was bloodletting, which he saw as particularly useful in 'florid'

[94] e.g. Surgeon General's Records, Madras, vol. 13A, from 1 January 1802 to 31 December 1802, p. 127, G 12450, Tamil Nadu State Archives.

[95] George Ballingall, 'Observations on the Flux which has prevailed in His Majesty's 1st Royal Regiment of Foot, 1808', Papers of Sir George Ballingall, WMS 6905/1, WL.

[96] Ballingall to David Barry, 1808 (no other date), WMS 6905/2, WL.

[97] Ballingall, *Practical Observations*, 80–1.

[98] Ballingall, 'Observations'.

young men recently arrived in hot climates. Importantly, it was an opinion grounded more upon observations made post-mortem than upon clinical experience; in particular, upon 'the ravages of inflammation, so universally apparent in the dead, than on any repeated or extensive experience of its effects on the living'.[99] When he first arrived in India he had found that the opinion of older practitioners was 'almost universally against' bloodletting and this made it difficult for him to conduct an extensive or systematic trial. But experience showed that bloodletting need not be dangerous, and Ballingall could see a clear rationale for the practice in nervous physiology. However, Ballingall did not refer to Jackson's work as the source of his ideas and his main debts appear to have been to the French physician Richerand, who recommended bloodletting to relieve inflammation, which he defined as the augmentation of vital power to an affected part. Richerand held that the circulation of blood through this part decreased in direct proportion to the degree of inflammation and that inflammation was produced by nervous debility, induced by extremes of temperature or intoxicating liquours. Bleeding was deemed salutary because it reduced inflammation.[100]

Ballingall remained in India until 1814, when he returned to Britain in ill health. Having recovered, he proceeded to Paris where he was part of the army of occupation after the defeat of Napoleon. After a period on half pay, he retired from the Army in 1818 and engaged in private practice in Edinburgh. In 1822, however, he was appointed Regius Professor of Military Surgery at the University of Edinburgh, being the second person to occupy this chair, which had been founded in 1806.[101] This appointment was something of a homecoming for Ballingall who had studied at Edinburgh, being particularly indebted to his teacher James Barclay, from whom he had acquired a taste for anatomy. Indeed, Ballingall's *Practical Observations on Fever, Dysentery, and Liver Complaints* (1818) was dedicated to his former lecturer. The publication of the book and the arrival of Ballingall as professor coincided with a flurry of Edinburgh MD theses on dysentery and fevers in tropical regions, most of which appear to have been written by former military and naval surgeons, lamenting the great loss of life which this disease had caused during recent campaigns. One of the characteristic features of these theses, like Ballingall's work, was that they relied heavily on morbid anatomy.[102] They also drew on the growing corpus of literature on the diseases of warm climates, making comparisons between their observations and those of practitioners in Spain and Greece for example.[103] Most stressed the

[99] Ballingall, *Practical Observations*, 67.

[100] Barry to anon., forwarding letter from Ballingall, undated, WMS 6905/5, WL.

[101] Kaufman, *The Regius Chair of Military Surgery*, chap. 3.

[102] e.g. M'Cann, *De dysenteria tropica*, 12–15; Rutherford, *De dysenteria Bataviae orientalis*, 12, 15–16; Allen, *Observations quaedem de febre remittente*, 18; Steel, *De febre insularum Indae Occidentalis*.

[103] e.g. Jameson, *De febris remittentis curatione.*

climatic origins of disease,[104] although predisposing factors such as fear and depression were also highlighted.[105] Like Ballingall, too, many stressed the benefits of venesection in the alleviation of fluxes and tropical fevers.[106] Hence, one doctoral candidate, Alexander Watson, advocated 'copious bleeding'.[107]

Military and naval surgeons who had returned to Edinburgh from the East Indies thus saw eye-to-eye with colleagues who had served in the Caribbean. In both cases, we can see a remarkable uniformity of outlook characterized by an emphasis upon climate, morbid anatomy, nervous physiology, and increasingly on the importance of letting blood in the treatment of tropical complaints. They differed markedly from those who had completed MD theses just a decade before. In his thesis of 1809, for example, James Watt had looked backwards to the work of Pringle and Cleghorn to find clues to the nature of dysentery in hot climates. Although he believed that it could become contagious, he also accepted the formerly dominant view theory that it could arise from accumulations of bile. Like most previous writers he also recommended a cure based primarily on purgation of the intestines rather than on bleeding.[108] In less than a generation, there had been a sea-change: purgation was not wholly out, but bleeding was definitely in.

This new conviction in the utility of bleeding in cases of tropical fever and dysentery was probably underscored by the publication of James Johnson's seminal work, the *Influence of Tropical Climates on European Constitutions* (1813), which became a veritable *vade maecum* for several generations of tropical practitioners. After he returned to Britain and founded the *Medico-Chirurgical Review*, Johnson had easy access to medical literature from around the world, much of which was incorporated into later editions of the *Influence* and other publications. Increasingly, the scope of Johnson's writing encompassed other hot countries and later editions carried as much on the West Indies and Africa as they did on India. Having grounded his system of medicine on nervous physiology as well as on pathological anatomy, Johnson felt able to make generalizations about the ways in which bodies responded to all hot climates, not simply India. Nevertheless, it was in India that Johnson was held in especially high esteem and it was there that his therapeutic observations probably had the greatest impact. When writing of fevers in general, Johnson helpfully reviewed all methods of treatment that were commonly used, giving something of their history and assessing their strengths and weaknesses. His own approach was pragmatic, relying solely on personal experience. In the treatment of the endemic

[104] e.g. M'Kinnal, *De dysenteria Indiae orientalis*; Fogo, *De febre flava*, 9, 14; Carter, *De febre endemica Indarium occidentalium*, 14–15; M'Cann, *De dysenteria*, 16–17; Rutherford, *De dysenteria*, 10; Allen, *De febre remittente*, 20.

[105] Carter, *De febre endemica*, 16.

[106] e.g. Cockburn, *De dysenteria Indiae orientalis*, 15–16; Steel, *De febre insularum*, 25.

[107] Watson, *De febre Bataviae*, 24.

[108] Watt, *De dysenteria complectens*, 16–20, 24, 27.

fever of Bengal, for example, Johnson explained: 'The impression made on my mind, by the dissection on one hand, and the perusal of Dr [John] Clark's case (Henry Pope) on the other, determined me to try venesection, notwithstanding the dreadful accounts which Dr C. himself gives of its fatal effects.' He did so with apparent success, although he recognized that this may have been due to the fact that his patients were newly arrived from Europe and otherwise in good health.[109] In fact, he believed that most cases encountered in India were likely to require a more discriminating form of treatment, beginning with bloodletting, but with something more 'to clear congestions of the head and the liver'. In such cases, he advocated treatment in four stages. Firstly, bleeding 'boldly and decisively till the head and praecordia are relieved'; secondly, to give half a scruple of calomel with the same quantity of opium to sedate the stomach; thirdly, to return to the lancet if dangerous symptoms such as intense headache or delirium continued; fourthly, to administer four to five grains of calomel combined with a half a grain of opium to the point of ptyalism (a fit) at which time febrile symptoms would be removed. Calomel combined with jalap could also be useful as a purgative, he claimed.[110]

Johnson's practice in fevers, as outlined in the earliest editions of his work, combined elements of treatments normally associated with both nervous and biliary theories. Cold bathing was also beneficial he claimed, but in India the practice owed little to the likes of Jackson and Currie, having been used since 'time immemorial, among the natives themselves'. He cited Captain Williamson, the author of *Oriental Field Sports*, who declared that 'the refrigerating principle, lately adopted by some of our leading physicians, owes its origin solely to the ancient practice of the Brahmans . . . of whom the generality affect to be deeply skilled in pharmacy'.[111] Johnson recommended bathing on very similar grounds, both in the treatment of fevers and more generally for the preservation of health in hot climates. Nor was he averse to employing other remedies commonly used by Indians, including local febrifuges. He noted that in Bengal the standard treatment used by the natives was first to purge the body of all bilious or sordid matter using a black purging salt called *bit-noben* or *kala neemuck*, and then to administer the kernel of the catcaranja nut (*Coesalpina bondicella*) which was intensely bitter, supposedly possessing 'the tonic or febrifuge powers of Peruvian bark in a very high degree'. These practices, he noted, had been adapted by a number of European practitioners in Bengal, where it had entirely superseded the use of Peruvian bark to complete the cure of intermittent fevers.[112]

In the treatment of that typically Anglo-Indian disease, hepatitis, Johnson advocated a similarly diverse array of remedies which were rationalized on principles derived from nervous physiology. According to Johnson, hepatitis was caused by the excessive perspiration of bodies ill-adapted to tropical climates.

109 Johnson, *Influence*, 1815 edn., 43–4.
110 Ibid., 45–6.
111 Cited ibid., 49.
112 Ibid., 58.

This led via 'sympathetic action' of the nerves to a 'loss of tone' in the system generally, causing bile to be secreted excessively in a manner that resembled perspiration. Much of this was based on Darwin's *Zoonomia*, which Johnson cited liberally at this point in his work. Darwin saw all excessive stimuli as detrimental to health and therapy therefore consisted in decreasing excitability, while simultaneously relieving symptoms. In patients who had been in India for less than a year, Johnson resorted to bloodletting in the first instance, both to relieve inflammation and to 'lower the tone of the constitution'. Once this had been completed, he returned to the more familiar Anglo-Indian practice of administering calomel, or a combination of opium and antimonials.[113]

Johnson was also willing to follow the usual Anglo-Indian practice in the treatment of dysentery, despite the fact that it was frowned upon back at home.[114] He thought that mercury worked in many instances, sometimes without the aid of other drugs; it was also a very practical remedy, unlike, some of those proposed by other writers on dysentery. Benjamin Moseley, for example, had argued that the best means of treating the disease was to use a mixture of sudorifics and emetics to excite the healthy action of the liver and bowels and to remove noxious substances. Johnson conceded that it might work in private practice or in a well-run hospital, but he thought the treatment utopian in fleets and armies. The spectacle of 'forty, fifty, or one hundred dysenteric patients, in a ship, wrapped up in blankets, beneath the burning skies of India, and spoon-fed with laudanum, antimonial wine, and warm balm tea' appeared ridiculous to him.[115] The best approach, according to Johnson, was to employ a variety of methods which brought rapid results, but they ought not to be mixed indiscriminately either. Treatment needed to follow a definite principle which was to restore a healthy perspiration and biliary secretion, together with equilibrium of circulation.[116]

Later editions of Johnson's *Influence* continued in the same pragmatic vein. On bloodletting, for example, Johnson wrote that 'the lancet has dispelled the mists of prejudice, the phantoms of debility and putrescency, with the delusions of the brunonian school; and bleeding is justly regarded as the paramount remedy, not only in symptomatic, but in most of the more violent and fatal idiopathic fevers, especially of hot climates'.[117] But there was still an important role for purgatives in the treatment of such diseases, he argued, not only to carry off morbid secretions of bile and other substances but also because they acted as stimulants, 'rousing the torpid circulation and excitability of the abdominal viscera'.[118] This applied to mercury no less than other remedies commonly used as purgatives and Johnson denounced those, especially followers of Jackson in the West Indies, who condemned the use of mercury in the treatment of fevers. He admitted that there were certain forms of inflammatory fever in the

[113] Ibid., 284–5. [114] Ibid., 361–2. [115] Ibid., 360–1.
[116] Ibid., 362–71. [117] Johnson, *Influence*, 1827 edn., 37. [118] Ibid., 41.

West Indies where hepatic congestions were rare, and where depletion of blood alone was probably the best means of treatment. But to draw a sweeping conclusion from this that mercury was useless, he warned, was erroneous. He insisted that his book was replete with examples of the febrifuge powers of mercury, which he explained on the Darwinian grounds that it acted as 'an equalizer of circulation and excitability'. Other types of remedy – emetics, diaphoretics, tonics, stimulants, and bathing – all had their place in Johnson's therapeutic arsenal, provided they were used according to a rational plan of treatment which took as its primary aim the restoration of nervous equilibrium.

Johnson's work had a great deal of influence even if there were some in the British profession, such as Thomas Wakley of *The Lancet*, who saw him as a ridiculous figure, who affected knowledge of classical scholarship. 'The truth is', the editorial went, 'that a blockhead, who attempts to palm himself upon the public for a man of learning, plays with penknives, and cannot chose but to lay himself open to derision.'[119] But this scorn probably had more to do with the fact that Johnson edited a rival journal than with matters of principle. Wakley's main objective was to discredit the *Medico-Chrurgical Journal* and its new incarnation, the *Review*: 'Meagre and insubstantial as was the quarterly farrago, the fortnight's fasiculus or bundle of rubbish, which has succeeded it, presents a wretched contrast even to its famished predecessor.'[120] But the transformation of the journal from a quarterly to a fortnightly review was a measure of its success. The size of each edition was growing and its leading articles and extended reviews were republished on the Continent and in America, where the opinions of its editor were becoming more widely known.[121]

As far as medical practice in the tropics is concerned, Johnson was definitely ahead of the game and his work – together with that of Ballingall – pointed to a new direction in the treatment of the country's diseases.[122] Within a decade of the publication of the first edition of Johnson's *Influence*, bleeding seems to have been fully rehabilitated in India as a treatment for dysentery and certain forms of fever. One of those who recommended it strongly in cases of dysentery was R. W. Bampfield, whose *Practical Treatise on Tropical Dysentery* (1819) advised bleeding in all cases of dysentery and even criticized Ballingall for being too cautious about bleeding 'old Indians'; that is, Britons who had long been in residence there.[123]

[119] Editorial on Johnson's quarterly journal, *The Lancet*, 8 March 1828, 854.
[120] Ibid., 850.
[121] 'A Sketch of the Life . . . of the Late Dr Johnson', 34–6.
[122] The young Assistant-Surgeon George Green Spilsbury, for example, wrote to his brother that 'Johnson's essay on the influence of tropical climates would give you a very good and clear insight into the principal diseases of this country'; 28 May 1819, MSS Eur. D.909, Spilsbury Letters from India 1811–1825, APAC, BL.
[123] Bampfield, *A Practical Treatise on Tropical Dysentery*, iv, viii, x.

But few authors with extensive Indian experience went quite so far as Bampfield. More typical was James Annesley who followed Johnson rather more closely. A surgeon on the Madras establishment, Annesley combined elements of the old biliary theory with newer concepts of disease grounded in nervous physiology. Like Johnson, he believed that there was a sympathetic connection between the skin and organs such as the liver, and that a dramatic change in climate caused the latter to secrete too much bile. Like Johnson, too, he recommended a combination of general bloodletting followed by calomel in common ailments such as hepatitis. In dysentery, he followed Johnson in advocating an initial purge with calomel, to remove morbid matter from the intestines, and then Ballingall (whom he cited) by using bloodletting to remove inflammation.[124] Annesley also followed a two-stage process in the treatment of fevers, with bleeding to reduce paroxysms, followed by emetics, calomel purges and bark, to prevent their return.[125] Indeed, by the 1820s, bleeding was again being used in the self-treatment of fevers by laymen, after decades in which they had been warned off the practice. In a letter to his sister, the Army officer Charles Wyndham wrote, 'I must tell you that I am become a great practitioner in physicking, bleeding and hot water; I breathe a vein as expertly as old Witcher or Blagden [presumably family physicians].'[126]

In Britain, too, bloodletting was far more popular than it had been for some time, partly because of the advocacy of Jackson and his followers, partly because of the influence of the French physician Broussais. But the revival of bleeding was accompanied by bitter controversy. In 1827, for example, the London Medical Society convened a meeting solely to discuss the practice of bloodletting in fevers, with a range of practitioners arguing passionately for and against. Its advocates justified the practice not only on the grounds that it had worked in their experience but with reference to post-mortem dissections which revealed inflammation in certain organs of persons deceased from fever. It was opposed on various grounds, not only because it was dangerous, but because bleeding was said to be incapable of cutting short fevers, which would always run a predetermined length.[127] The object of treatment, according to critics of bloodletting, was to support the patient until the disease had run its course, trusting to the *vis medicatrix naturae* much as contemporary economic theorists trusted to the logic of the market.[128] In both cases, intervention, however well-intentioned, was likely to make a bad situation worse.[129]

[124] Annesley, *Researches*, vol. 1, 297, 328; vol. 2, 272, 276.

[125] Ibid., vol. 2, 490, 496–7, 510.

[126] Charles Wyndham to his sister, Bombay, 13 November 1822, Wyndham MSS, Lilly Library, University of Indiana.

[127] Report of a meeting held at the London Medical Society, 19 December 1827, *The Lancet*, 22 December 1827. See also Ackerknecht, *Therapeutics*, 109.

[128] Halévy, *The Growth of Philosophical Radicalism*, 371–2.

[129] Atkinson, 'Popular Notions on Health and Disease Examined'.

Whatever their precise views on the treatment of fevers, most practitioners now understood fever primarily as a derangement of the nervous system. Over the next few years, British medical journals carried a number of articles speculating on just how depression of vital powers might affect certain systems or organs in the body. Although some practitioners regarded such speculation as useless, they did so largely on practical grounds rather than proposing an alternative pathology.[130] The only real challenge to the dominant view came from the margins of the medical profession, from notorious 'quacks' such as James Morison, who pedalled their patent remedies by appealing to older, humoral notions of the purity of the blood.[131] These evidently appealed to many laymen – including some who visited tropical climates[132] – but they were now regarded as outdated by the vast majority of practitioners in Britain and the Indies.[133]

By the 1830s, resort to bleeding and other forms of treatment predicated on nervous physiology dominated medical practice in India, although still not exclusively. In 1831, for instance, an extensive report published by the Medical Board of the Madras Presidency revealed that bloodletting was now used in the treatment of a range of diseases, together with stimulants and cold and warm bathing. In treating cases of cholera, Assistant-Surgeon J. Lawrence reported that the plan found most beneficial 'was of the most stimulating kind' and consisted in a combination of ether and laudanum, with calomel apparently given as a stimulant rather than a purgative.[134] Lawrence did not employ bleeding in cholera, but other Madras surgeons did, usually in combination with an opium-based stimulant regimen.[135]

Differences over cholera treatment seem to have hinged on the issue of whether the disease was caused by over-abundant bile or nervous prostration, not, as one historian has claimed, on whether it was an inflammatory disease.[136] Bloodletting was certainly used as a means of reducing inflammation, but

[130] e.g. Report of a meeting of the Westminster Medical Society, 4 March 1828, *The Lancet*, 8 March 1828.

[131] Morison made a deliberate pitch to those bound for the Indies and claimed in particular that his 'vegetable universal remedies' were of particular use in cholera. They worked, he claimed, by purifying the blood. He was ardently opposed to the use of the lancet and mercury. See James Morison, *The Practical Proofs of the Soundness of the Hygeian System of Physiology*; idem, *Morisonia*; idem, *Origin of Life and Cause of Diseases.*

[132] Col. Dickinson, Bombay, to his son, Sebastian Dickinson, Painswick, Gloucestershire, 3 January 1834: 'Having in a certain stage of my recent attack experienced the efficacy of that medicine, if it can be so called, would you kindly give me . . . two packets price 11 shillings 6 pence containing one box of No.1 and two boxes of No. 2 of Morison's pills or Vegetable Universal Medicine.' Dickson also requested a copy of *Morisonia*, amongst other medical books and remedies; 2 February 1834, D.6 F.173/2, GCRO.

[133] One of the few exceptions was the surgeon-orientalist T. A. Wise. See his 'Observations on the Vitality of the Blood'.

[134] Lawrence, 'Cases of Cholera with Observations', 75.

[135] Lister, 'Report of Cholera Epidemica', 5–9; Scarman, 'Observations on Cholera'.

[136] Durey, *The Return of the Plague*, 121–34.

inflammation was generally seen as a consequence of debility. In most nervous conceptions of fever, the distinction was one of sequence rather than of essence. Bleeding was employed by practitioners of many different persuasions, often as the preliminary to a long and varied course of treatment, that might or might not include other drugs formerly used to treat the disease in India, such as calomel and opium. The same was true of dysentery. Assistant-Surgeon W. Mortimer rated bleeding – general and topical – as the first treatment for the disease, followed by ipecacuanha and other remedies that calmed the abdomen. Bleeding worked, he explained, because it reduced inflammation.[137] Others, however, preferred to treat dysentery without resort to either the lancet or calomel, placing their faith in other drugs such as ipecacuanha or, in one case, in nitric acid.[138]

One of the most important breakthroughs in therapeutics during the early nineteenth century – sulphate of quinine – was also rationalized on the basis of its effects as a 'tonic' which restored tone and vitality to the nervous system.[139] Quinine had been isolated from the bark of the cinchona tree in 1817 by two French chemists: P. J. Pettelier and J. Caventou. It did not, however, immediately supplant Peruvian bark in medical practice, either in Europe or overseas. Rather, the next two decades saw extensive trials to determine its efficacy and safety, such as those conducted by the medical officers of the Madras Presidency in the late 1820s. One of these, William Geddes, who later went on to write *Clinical Illustrations of the Diseases of India* (1846),[140] claimed that he had studied the operation of quinine more extensively than any other medical officer in India, and averred that 'next to opium, I believe it to be the most valuable remedy which has been as yet presented to the profession'. Its arrival, he felt, heralded a 'new era, in the medical practice of this and other intertropical climates, from the peculiar powers it possesses of checking the tendency to paroxysmal exacerbations of disease, so generally evident in the disorders of such countries'.[141] It was useful not only in intermittent fever, he claimed, but also in remitting fevers and in the treatment of febrile symptoms attending diseases such as dysentery. He explained that quinine was effective because it had powerful tonic properties, capable of restoring vital power to bodies debilitated by long residence in hot climates or exposure to miasma.[142] Although quinine proved to be more effective in this regard than the Peruvian bark and a number of febrifuges indigenous to the East Indies, it is notable that their therapeutic properties had also, for some years, been justified on the basis of their ability to restore nervous tone, whereas formerly they had been

137 Mortimer, 'Observations on the Treatment of Dysentery', 89.
138 Geddes, 'Observations on Dysentery'; Coleman, 'Cases of Dysentery'.
139 Warner, *Therapeutic Perspective*, 69–70.
140 Geddes, *Clinical Illustrations of the Diseases of India.*
141 Geddes, 'Report on the Sulphate of Quinine', 201
142 Ibid., 205. See also Malcolmson, 'Report on the Use of Quinine in Fever'; Bell, 'Special Report upon the Sulphate of Quina'.

regarded as 'antiseptics' in Pringle's sense of the term.[143] This already betokened a shift from putrefactive theories of disease to those grounded in nervous physiology.

One distinctive dimension of therapeutics in early nineteenth-century India is the extent to which notions of race impacted upon medical treatment. It was still far from common for British practitioners to treat Indians as there were still only a handful of hospitals and dispensaries, most of which were located in the presidency towns and other large cities. For the most part, as in Britain, both in- and out-patients were drawn from among the poorest members of society, the numbers amounting to a few thousand annually in each of the large cities.[144] In the Army, too, it was still more common for Indian soldiers to be treated by Indian practitioners. For this reason, until the 1830s, most British works on medicine in India had little to say about the treatment of disease in Indians. But in that decade, practitioners such as William Twining, whose work lay primarily in the civilian domain, began to do so.

It will be recalled that Twining was a surgeon at the Calcutta General Hospital and an important figure in the city's medical circles. He was one of a number of practitioners, including his colleague Henry Goodeve, who were in the vanguard of medical reform. They were anxious to distance themselves from the biliary theory with its humoral associations, and eager to embrace the most recent developments in European medical science. Indeed, it is in Twining's work that we see perhaps the cleanest break with the therapeutic paradigm of the past. Previous writers on the diseases of India, according to Twining and his close associates, had mistaken effects for causes. Excessive bile was often to be found in cases that were dissected or vomited by patients suffering from diseases such as remittent fever, but it was a symptom rather than a cause of disease. Mercurial treatment of diseases such as fever and dysentery was therefore likely to do little good by itself, he argued. Twining was not wholly opposed to mercury but felt that it had been used indiscriminately and in excessive doses.[145] Such treatment was not only potentially harmful to patients but was based on erroneous principles, for the intention was to produce some change in the liver that would cause it to secrete less bile. To Twining, this was 'incomprehensible' because his post-mortem examinations showed that in dysentery cases, for example, the large intestines were diseased while the small intestines showed no little sign of damage, despite the fact that the bile must have passed through them, too.[146] In treating dysentery and most other diseases, his preference was

[143] See Maehle, *Drugs on Trial*, 264–75; Milman, *Enquiry*, 224, 226; Col. John MacDonald to Sir Joseph Banks, Fort Marlborough, 16 March 1795, MSS Eur. F.286/1, Papers of Col. John MacDonald, FRS, APAC, BL.

[144] Martin, *The History, Antiquities, Topography, and Statistics of Eastern India*, vol. 1, 48.

[145] Twining, *Clinical Illustrations*, 36.

[146] Ibid., 39–40.

for free and repeated use of the lancet, to reduce inflammation arising from local congestions produced by nervous debility.[147]

In deciding which modes of treatment were appropriate, Twining was guided by the evidence he claimed to find in post-mortem dissections such as those carried out at the hospital.[148] A couple of examples suffice to illustrate the way in which Twining utilized post-mortem evidence in his therapeutics. Dissection of patients who had suffered from dysentery revealed clearly to Twining that there was invariably some local inflammation or vestige of prolonged inflammation, such as an inelastic mesentery.[149] In view of these findings, he recommended liberal bloodletting, using both venesection and leeches, in order to reduce inflammation and the febrile symptoms that accompanied it.[150] For the same reasons, Twining came to recommend bloodletting in remittent fevers.[151] 'The closest attention to clinical observation, as well as the result of post-mortem examinations', he wrote, 'convince me that remittent fevers in Bengal are invariably connected with local congestions, which often run rapidly to inflammation.' These local manifestations of fever, he continued, were to be found principally in the stomach, intestines, the cellular structure surrounding the duodenum, and the root of the mesocolon; indications could also be found in the lungs, brain, liver, and spleen.[152]

But these were general recommendations, and Twining believed that they had to be modified according to the condition of each patient and according to their race. To an even greater extent than Annesley, Twining maintained that disease appeared differently in the bodies of Indians and Europeans. In the introduction to *Clinical Illustrations*, he informed his readers that each chapter would end with remarks on the 'modifications of disease, to which the Natives of the country are liable'. He explained that 'Such of their maladies as may be reasonably ascribed to high temperature, and the result of inflammation, are generally much slighter than corresponding diseases in Europeans; which is probably in a great degree owing to the peculiarities of their constitutions, adapted to the Climate.' However, he also believed that this diminished tendency to inflammation was, in some degree, due to their 'habits with respect to food and drink, which must be acknowledged in many respects to be more reasonable than ours'.[153] The same combination of constitutional adaptation and temperate lifestyle explained why Indians appeared to be exempt from certain forms of fever, such as the common continued fevers of Bengal, in which there was persistent inflammation.[154] 'In

[147] Ibid., 14, 558, 623, 625.
[148] Ibid., viii.
[149] Ibid., 13–14.
[150] Ibid., 14.
[151] Ibid., 625.
[152] Ibid., 623.
[153] Ibid., xxi.
[154] Ibid., 618. This opinion seems to have been generally held, although other writers were careful to differentiate between the anti-inflammatory vegetarian diet of high-caste Hindus and that of Muslims, which more closely resembled that of Europeans. See MacGregor, *Practical Observations*, 34.

the Dysentery of Asiatics', too, Twining claimed to observe a disease which was less marked by inflammatory symptoms.[155]

On account of these apparent differences, Twining felt that it was necessary to modify treatment to some degree. In the treatment of remittent fevers, for which he recommended a combination of copious bleeding, quinine, and cathartics in Europeans, he was inclined to be more moderate in the case of Indians. 'The Natives of Bengal, are very liable to suffer from remittent fever during the rainy season', he noted, and ordinarily 'the majority of cases occurring among Natives who are not in absolute poverty, are usually slight, requiring only a few mild purgatives, and the application of leeches to the temples, in the early stage of the disease, and small doses of Sulphate of Quinine in the intervals of the exacerbations.'[156] In other words, bleeding should be local and light in the case of Indians; and both general and local in the case of Europeans, who could be bled by venesection in addition to leeches. When Indian patients had been debilitated by poverty or fatigue, he refrained from bleeding altogether.[157]

It was much the same with cases of cholera: 'When Cholera attacks robust Asiatics, who are living in affluence,' he averred, 'they very seldom have that form of the disease which is at the commencement combined with pyrexia and inflammation: and that description of the disease which usually affects the poorer natives of Bengal, is still more rarely attended with febrile or inflammatory symptoms.' Post-mortem dissections also appeared to show that 'visceral disorders are seldom found to occur as its sequalae in natives.'[158] The predominance of this 'low' form of cholera among Indians meant that bleeding was seldom required, unlike in Europeans, where inflammatory symptoms were more likely. Rather, according to Twining, 'A tea-spoonful of laudanum with a spoonful of brandy . . . if given at the first moment of attack, very generally arrests the disease instantly.'[159] However, one ought not to forget that the treatment of Indians was also conditioned by *their* preferences. Bloodletting was used rarely in Indian traditions for the treatment of either cholera or fevers, except in only the most drastic of situations.[160] Indeed, the practice appears to have become the subject of bitter disputes between British and *Ayurvedic* practitioners. William Ward claimed that 'the Hindoo physicians profess to despise the Europeans: they charge them with destroying their patients by evacuations, and . . . prefer their own practice of starving away the fever'.[161]

The cultural and racial dimensions of treatment were not equally prominent in other contemporary works, but the basic assumptions which informed Twining's

[155] Twining, *Clinical Illustrations*, 122. [156] Ibid., 656. [157] Ibid., 657.
[158] Twining, *Practical Account*, 230.
[159] Ibid., 231.
[160] e.g. Martin, *History*, vol. 1, 473; vol. 2, 412; Royle, *An Essay on the Antiquity of Hindoo Medicine*, 52–3. Twining would have been aware of Indian medical practices from assisting George Playfair in his work on Indian *materia medica*. See Playfair, *The Taleef Shereef*, iv.
[161] Ward, *A View of the History, Literature, and Mythology, of the Hindoos*, vol. 1, 477.

therapeutics may also be found elsewhere: the belief that Indian constitutions were less robust than those of Europeans and that they were less able to bear violent purging or depletive remedies.[162] In other respects, however, it is difficult to generalize about therapeutics in either India or the West Indies in the years after 1830. Never again was the 'medicine of warm climates' dominated by a single remedy, as it was in the heyday of mercury. Bloodletting and bathing were certainly prominent in the therapeutics of the 1830s, 1840s, and 1850s but never wholly to the exclusion of mercurial therapies or substances such as opium.[163] The advent of an effective specific medicine in the form of quinine radically transformed the practice of treating fevers, but, again, not to the exclusion of other febrifuges. In these decades, most practitioners worked out a complex programme of therapeutic intervention that incorporated in some degree most of these elements. A cursory examination of the two or three decades after 1830s suggests a period free from bitter controversy, notwithstanding the British blood-letting disputes of the 1850s.[164] India and the West Indies were by no means unaffected by these, but bleeding continued to find prominent adherents much longer in the tropical colonies than in Britain itself. Having revised the sixth and final (posthumous) edition of James Johnson's classic *The Influence of Tropical Climates on European Constitutions* (1856), the eminent physician James Ranald Martin wrote of bloodletting:

> I am aware that a kind of fashion is at present moving against the practice . . . but those who are acquainted with the history of medicine, and who have seen and understood the nature of acute tropical diseases, will take fashion here at its proper value, and at no more.[165]

The typical sickroom of the 1830s and 1840s would thus have been littered with a wide array of instruments and medicines, not unlike like that described in the Anglo-Indian novel *Peregrine Pulteney*:

> On the table were two or three bottles of physic, a pill-box, and a number of blue powder-papers, a wine glass with the remains of a draft at the bottom and clinging to the sides, a few scraps of lint, a tea-spoon, which looked as though it had held a powder, and lastly a plate full of salt and blood, in which evidently a dozen leeches or so had lately been disgorging the sanguinary meals they had made.[166]

162 e.g. Norton, 'Intermittent Fever', 197.

163 See Dickson, *Prevalent Diseases of India*, 58–68, 89–101, 113–16, 130; Raleigh, *Observations on Idiopathic Dysentery*, 64–9, 71–3; Murray, 'Observations on the good and bad Effects of Calomel in some of the Diseases of India'; Morehead, 'Notes on the Treatment and Pathology of Intermittent and Remittent Fever'; MacGregor, *Practical Observations*, 10–13, 34, 46–9; Gordon, *The Principal Diseases of India*, 35–9, 51–2, 64–5, 77–8; Parkes, *Researches into the Pathology and Treatment of the Asiatic or Algide Cholera*, 205–40.

164 King, 'The Blood-Letting Controversy'.

165 Martin, *The Influence of Tropical Climates on European Constitutions*, 157.

166 Kaye, *Peregrine Pulteney*, vol. 2, 85.

CONCLUSION

The history of therapeutics in Britain's tropical colonies demonstrates that medical practices there became and, to some extent, remained distinctive. From the mid-eighteenth century, therapies in the Indies and other hot countries began radically to diverge from those then typical in Britain. Bleeding and other antiphlogistic practices were abandoned or used in a far more discriminating way than hitherto. According to contemporary disease theory, such treatments could be positively dangerous in tropical climates, where Europeans were likely to be weakened by prolonged exposure to an environment to which they were not accustomed. Therapeutics, in other words, mirrored the growing sense of the tropics as a distinct environment and of Europeans as exotic species within it. This sense of difference was exaggerated further at the end of the eighteenth century by the dominance of mercurial therapy, and the biliary theory of disease on which it rested. Yet this radically new application of mercury in the treatment of non-venereal complaints was ultimately to affect medicine in Britain itself. Many practitioners who had been stationed in tropical settlements later applied the experience they had gained in the treatment of diseases such as fever and fluxes to the varieties they encountered in Britain. The new infirmaries and fever hospitals, as well as the establishments of the Army and Navy, were among the key locations where colonial methods, such as mercurialization, were applied to British patients, albeit in modified form.

The case of Helenus Scott and nitric acid therapy further demonstrates the impact that colonial therapies could have on British medicine, but also the limits of that influence. Indeed, the fact that nitric acid continued to be used in the colonies long after it had been rejected in Britain (save perhaps in the Army), serves to illustrate the perceived distinctiveness of Britain's tropical realms. Lastly, the revival of bloodletting, and the emergence of other therapies based on nervous physiology, shows that therapeutic fashions in Britain and its colonies could sometimes emerge together, with independent developments in the colonies reinforcing trends deriving from Europe, particularly France. The period 1820 to 1850 is one in which there was a good deal of similarity between prevailing doctrines in the colonies and in Europe. This was, after all, a time when many colonial practitioners were eager to embrace the latest European developments and to distance themselves from what they regarded as vestiges of humoral medicine. In these three decades, differences certainly existed between tropical and temperate practice, but they were in the main differences of emphasis. It was only after 1850 that major differences in doctrine and method re-emerged, largely in relation to bloodletting and the therapeutic use of opium.[167]

[167] On the latter, see Moore, 'Is the habitual use of Opium in Moderation Injurious?'; da Cunha, 'Notes on the Treatment of Cholera and on the Opium Question'; Winther, *Anglo-European Science*

The professional identity of surgeons in the British colonies was not unlike that of the practitioners described by John Harley Warner in his study of early American therapeutics.[168] Like their counterparts in early nineteenth-century America, British colonial practitioners considered themselves men of action. Therapeutic intervention – often drastic – was their *raison d'être* and there was a good deal of similarity between the likes of Benjamin Rush and prominent British practitioners such as Charles Maclean and James Johnson. Indeed, they often contributed to the same journals, belonged to the same societies, and possessed similar outlooks on matters of politics. Many of the remedies which they used and advocated were the same, and their therapeutic practices were determined largely by the perceived centrality of climate and locality in disease. Until at least the 1820s, American medicine was marked by distinctive regional differences predicated largely on the peculiarities of disease, race, and climate, just like medical practice in the colonies. Heroic therapeutic practices – including mercury and bloodletting – were much in vogue in parts of America until the 1820s, when they began to be tempered by the empirically based scepticism of practitioners trained in or conversant with Paris medicine. The same is true in India and the West Indies: the distinctiveness of tropical practice and the tendency to heroic therapeutics gradually diminished from the 1820s, as practitioners in India and the West Indies began to embrace Paris medicine and distanced themselves from previous generations.

As Warner has suggested, this shift of opinion amounted to a revolt against the 'spirit of system': the victory of sceptical empiricism over the rationalistic system-building of the Enlightenment.[169] It is an interpretation that might seem to apply equally to the history of therapeutics in India and West Indies. And yet, the contrast evident in America before and after 1820 is less apparent in the case of Britain's tropical settlements. The putrefactive theory and its biliary variant which dominated medicine through to the early nineteenth century can certainly be regarded as systems, in which practitioners often had an uncritical faith. The same can be said of therapeutic practices such as mercurialization. But we ought not to forget that these therapies were seen by their proponents as empirically grounded, by contrast with the doctrinaire systems of Europe. Tropical practitioners in the mid- to late eighteenth century never ceased to point out that their practices were based on clinical observation and post-mortem evidence, and in some cases on systematic trials. In this sense, they were not so very different from the practitioners of the 1820s, 1830s, and 1840s, who often looked back at them with condescension. When it came to methodology, the difference between these generations was probably more rhetorical than real.

and the Rhetoric of Empire. However, Winther does not sufficiently acknowledge the extent to which opium continued to be regarded as a legitimate therapeutic agent in India.

[168] Warner, *Therapeutic Perspective*, esp. chap. 1.

[169] Warner, *Against the Spirit of System.*

PART III

ILLS OF EMPIRE

Introduction to Part III

Despite high death rates, many of those bound for the tropics during the eighteenth century held out the prospect of full acclimatization once their bodies had adapted to the seasonal rhythms of tropical life. Peacetime death rates among Europeans in the Caribbean were not much higher than in Britain,[1] and some writers even claimed that permanent residents lived longer than those who had never left their native land.[2] In India, too, for every newcomer who complained about the climate, another professed to find it congenial. The East India Company surgeon Francis Maxwell wrote to his father, after a year's service in India, that 'I have now experienced the Climate of a considerable part of India, and however different it may be in places, I find it everywhere agrees with me; in short, my constitution appears particularly well adapted to a warm climate.'[3] Some went so far as to claim that Europeans could take on the characteristics of native peoples and thereby enjoy a state of health equal to their kinsmen at home.[4] By the 1800s, however, a more pessimistic attitude prevailed.[5] The staggering losses caused by yellow fever in St Domingue eclipsed those of previous expeditions and left an immense tide of human misery in their wake. The deaths of thousands of soldiers and sailors left many families destitute, and those who returned alive were often rendered incapable of work by chronic illness.[6] These deaths were widely reported in the British press, and postings to the region were generally the cause of gloom and despondency.[7] Only a few, like Smollett's *Roderick Random*, heartily embraced tropical service – with its high wastage rates – as an opportunity for rapid advancement through the

[1] Chisholm, *Manual of the Climate and Diseases of Tropical Countries*, 8–9.

[2] Jameson, *Essays on the Changes of the Human Body*, 306–7.

[3] Francis Maxwell to father, Seringapatam, 2 June 1799, MSS Eur. C.101, APAC, BL. The belief in seasoning was also widely held in India, as it was in the West Indies. As Ensign George Clement, 18th Carnatic Btn. of Sepoys, put it in a letter to his parents: 'I believe this Country will now agree with my Constitution very well, having recovered from all the Disorders Europeans are liable to in it.' See letter of 29 May 1784, 31224(13)9(a), BRO.

[4] e.g. Curtin, *The Image of Africa*; Marshall and Williams, *The Great Map of Mankind*; Vaughan, *The Roots of American Racism*; Harrison, '"The Tender Frame of Man"'; idem, *Climates and Constitutions*; Wheeler, *The Complexion of Race*.

[5] This was also true of the French empire. See Jennings, *Curing the Colonizers*.

[6] Bewell, *Romanticism and Colonial Disease*, chap. 2.

[7] e.g. *The Times*, 14 August 1793, 3; 15 September 1796, 2.

ranks.[8] More typical was Capt. Richard Smith's comment that 'there is something in this climate very prejudicial to the Constitution of Europeans'.[9]

In the Caribbean, most Europeans counted themselves fortunate if they survived their first year: the period in which they would either become inured to the climate or succumb to one of the region's deadly fevers. But the worst location of all was West Africa. Hearing that her husband was about to embark for the Gambia, the wife of Capt. Harry Huntley, RN, cried:

> whilst you are in that horrid climate I shall ever be subject to much anxiety of mind. . . . I now sincerely hope that you can take care of your health! Repeated accounts reach me of the increased and universal unhealthiness of your post [Bathhurst colony] . . . the climate is noxious to many constitutions and you are not likely to spare yourself! You have not only yourself to think of now – but your wife and children![10]

Epidemics of 'tropical diseases' such as yellow fever in North America and the Mediterranean also raised the grim spectre of contagious pestilence spreading out from the tropics to infect more 'civilized' lands. Plague had reappeared in the Mediterranean, too, and cholera was creeping slowly over land from India to threaten Europe itself. Asiatic diseases thus marched hand in hand with the 'Asiatic influences' that some felt were corrupting political life in Britain.[11]

Growing unease about tropical service stemmed partly from these fears but also from deep and almost imperceptible shifts in the way in which Europeans understood themselves. Not the least of these was the growing tendency to think in racial terms. The emergence of new ideas of race at this juncture has been attributed variously to colonial conquests, the abolition of slavery, and Romantic nationalism,[12] yet none of these explanations is sufficient in itself. Historians have generally failed to recognize that the growing currency of racial ideas was part of a greater cultural transformation: the shift from an '*ancien regime*' of identity, as Dror Wahrman has termed it, to one that is recognizably modern. This entailed the abandonment of fluid notions of self for fixed categories of identity, grounded in what we would today understand as immutable biological differences.[13]

Wahrman has traced the origins of this change to the political revolutions that took place in America and France: an explanation which ignores equally momentous events in India and the Caribbean. But, whichever perspective one favours, there is much to be said for the idea of a revolution in identity that

[8] e.g. Richard Smith to William Barlow, 30 December 1827, Papers of Capt. Richard Barlow, Army Medical Department, D.6528/8/19/5, GCRO.

[9] Ibid.

[10] Anne Huntley to Capt. H. Huntley, 12 December 1840, 1 January 1841, C.8, D.48, GCRO.

[11] See Maclean, *Affairs of Asia*.

[12] See, for example: Banton, *Racial Theories*; Drescher, 'The Ending of the Slave Trade'; Stepan, *The Idea of Race*; Stepan, 'Biology and Degeneration'.

[13] Wahrman, *The Making of the Modern Self*.

simultaneously encompassed class, race, and gender. Identities were certainly becoming more rigid and combined to form a simplistic but powerfully effective referential grid.[14] Differences between races and classes, for instance, were invariably gendered, superiority often being ascribed to an abundance of 'masculine' characteristics.[15] By the early 1800s, susceptibility or resistance to disease had become an important marker of these differences, and anxieties about health and colonial service were commonly expressed as fears about racial decline and loss of manly vigour. The former was taken as a sure sign of the latter. Even those who had never left their native islands were deemed at risk from the baleful effects of an empire that corrupted their bodies and souls through an excess of luxury and nervous stimulation. Fears about declining martial prowess were compounded by the apparent political and medical threats posed by an urban working class whose pathogenic habits were equated with those of Britain's colonial subjects.[16] Writers such as James Johnson and Thomas Trotter feared these effects of industrialization and urbanization as much as they did the legions of 'tropical invalids' that congregated at Britain's spas. Furthermore, all these problems seemed to have a common origin in colonial expansion. It was Empire that fuelled the engines of commerce and industry, which drew ever greater numbers of Britons overseas, and which had created a consumer society that degraded the lives of all but the poorest. Colonial expansion, in other words, was eating away at Britain from the inside, destroying the very qualities that had made her great.

[14] For the relationship between ideas of race and class, see also Lorimer, *Colour, Class and the Victorians*. The increasingly naturalistic conception of sex and gender roles is stressed in Jordanova, *Sexual Visions*; Laquer, *Making Sex*.

[15] On the gendering of colonial landscapes in relation to disease, see Bewell, *Romanticism*.

[16] See Morris, *Cholera, 1832*; Durey, *The Return of the Plague*; Bewell, *Romanticism*, 49–51.

1

Invalids and entrepreneurs

The thousands of tropical invalids who began to gather at spa towns in Britain in the early 1800s presented tremendous opportunities for enterprising and occasionally unscrupulous practitioners. One of those who made a good living at the end of the eighteenth century by catering for well-to-do invalids was that renowned authority on liver diseases, William Saunders, Senior Physician at Guys Hospital in London. Saunders claimed that he had been:

> Frequently consulted by persons whose appetite and digestion have been much disturbed by a long residence in tropical climates; and who, although they have generally received much benefit by a sea voyage, and a gradual return to Europe, yet require the assistance of medicine, with a view to destroy the tendency to excessive secretion [of bile], and finally to restore strength and vigorous action.[1]

He believed that such complaints were best treated through a combination of mercurial medicines and mineral waters:

> I recommend it to my patient, every morning before breakfast, to dilute the contents of the stomach, by drinking half a pint of water of 90–114 degrees Farenheit. This may be done either in London or in Bath. . . . I do not, however, mean to discourage invalids from going to places of public resort, which may contribute, by their amusements, to restore a constitution enfeebled by a warm climate.[2]

On the whole, Saunders did not think spa waters superior to ordinary pump water in which had been diluted some neutral salts such as double tartar. However, he acknowledged that the Cheltenham waters were particularly well suited to persons returning from tropical climates as they contained an unusually large quantity of aperient salts, which were capable of removing large quantities of bile.[3]

Physicians normally recommended that invalids take a course of treatment that complemented the mildly purgative action of the waters. The remedy of choice for most invalids was some kind of preparation containing calomel,

[1] Saunders, *A Treatise on the Structure, Economy, and Diseases of the Liver*, 1795 edn., 136–7.
[2] Ibid., 137–8. [3] Ibid., 141–3.

following closely the methods devised for chronic ailments in India and the West Indies. Assistant-Surgeon W. Mortimer of Madras, for example, favoured blue pills to treat chronic dysentery, each containing three or four grains of calomel and two or three of ipecacuanha. These were to be administered two or three times per day, with the addition of tonic bitters and castor oil.[4] Calomel-based remedies were also widely advertised in newspapers and periodicals, with the express purpose of attracting the attention of tropical invalids. The *Cheltenham Chronicle*, for example, regularly carried advertisements such as the following, for the antibilious remedy of Samuel Dickson, who had worked as a surgeon in India with the British Army:

> As a mild and effectual remedy for all those disorders which originate in a vitiated action of the liver and biliary organs, namely, indigestion, loss of appetite, head-aches, heart-burn, flatulencies, spasms, costiveness, affections of the liver, etc, etc, DIXON's ANTI-BILIOUS PILLS have met with more general approval, than any other medicine whatever.
>
> In tropical climates, where the consequences of redundant and vitiated bile are alarming, they are an invaluable and efficient protection.

The pills were sold in boxes at 2*d.*, 9*d.*, 11*s.*, and 22*s.*, and were available at Butler's Chemists and all major bookbinders and druggists throughout England.[5] The advertisement of such remedies served to attract patients to physicians specializing in the treatments of tropical disorders, many of which tended to congregate around popular spas such as Cheltenham.

But if they sought the advice of physicians on their return, invalids ran the risk of dissipating whatever fortune they may have acquired in the colonies. The wife of Capt. Harry Huntley, RN, who had been governor of the British settlement at Fernando Po near the mouth of the River Niger, informed her brother-in-law that 'we are at present in a low ebb, but if Harry's life and health is spared they will I trust improve'. She continued: 'Harry has spent much of the money he derived from his regency at Fernando Po, in repairing his health, amongst the Doctors, he has never been quite well since his residence in that country, and is quite dependent upon Blue Pill for comfortable feelings.'[6] In a subsequent letter to her brother-in-law, a local clergyman, she was forced to request money to cover their debts: 'his Dress as Governor was very expensive, and he has also had to pay Mr Hinxman £200 with interest, which Mr H lent him to pay off sundry debts, before we came to you, a great part of which went to two Doctors.'[7]

At the lower end of the market, a host of practitioners peddled their wares, hoping to undercut the physicians. The most infamous of these was James

[4] Mortimer, 'Observations on the Treatment of Dysentery'.
[5] *Cheltenham Chronicle*, 26 October 1820, 1.
[6] Anne Huntley to the Rev. R. W. Huntley, Dunkirk, Glos., 30 March 1842[?], C.9, D.48, GCRO.
[7] Anne Huntley to the Rev. R. W. Huntley, 21 March 1843[?], C.9, D.48, GCRO.

Morison, self-declared 'hygiest' and president of 'the British College of Health'. As we saw earlier, Morison attracted criticism from orthodox practitioners for his opposition to the prevailing nervous physiology and his claims to be able to cure cholera.[8] His numerous books and pamphlets publicized a neo-humoral theory of disease, calculated to appeal to the 'common sense' views of the public, who were potentially wary of modish practices imported from Paris. And he appears to have read his audience well, for some of his publications went through several editions, helping to popularize his patent remedies, most of which were touted as gentle purgatives and blood purifiers. Morison went to great lengths to demonstrate that his 'vegetable universal remedy' would be of use to valetudinarians in the tropics and those that had returned home, hoping to displace their faith in mercurial preparations.[9] Writing of his vegetable remedies, Morison claimed that 'in cold weather, they will warm you, by allowing a more free circulation of your blood, which is the veritable warmer of life; and in hot sultry weather, they will cool you, and strengthen your powers of digestion, by ridding your body of those heated, acrimonious, bilious humours'.[10] The use of mercurial preparations, by contrast, had 'made more victims throughout the world than Buonaparte in all his campaigns'.[11] It is difficult to tell how popular Morison's remedies were, but they are mentioned from time to time in the letters of those serving in the colonies. For instance, Col. Dickinson, an officer in the Bombay army, wrote to his son in Britain that:

> Having in a certain stage of my recent attack experienced the efficacy of that medicine, if it can be called, would you kindly give me . . . two packets price 11s 6d containing one box of No. 1 and two boxes of No. 2 of Morison's pills or Vegetable Universal Medicine. . . .[12]

Ignorant of Morison's strictures on mercurial medicines, Dickinson was using the vegetable pills in conjunction with calomel and had recently undergone a 'long course of salivation', which had left him 'feeling better than I had done for years'. Indeed, Dickinson took quite an interest in self-medication, requesting a number of medical works to be sent to him in India, including Warren's *Discourse on National Dietetics*, Whitelaw's *Treatise on the Causes and Effects of Inflammation with Remarks on the action of the Vapour Bath*, as well as *Morisonia*.[13]

Medication was not the only remedy for the relief of tropical complaints. Bathing had been popular in the colonies as a restorative and precautionary measure since the seventeenth century and some West Indian islands were

[8] Morison, *Origin of Life*.
[9] Morison, *Morisonia*, 85–6.
[10] Ibid., 82.
[11] Ibid., 20–1.
[12] Col. Dickinson to Sebastian Dickinson, Painswick, Glos., 3 January 1834, D.6/173/2, GCRO.
[13] Col. Dickinson to Sebastian Dickinson, 2 February 1834, D.6/173/2, GCRO.

renowned for their hot springs. Thomas Trapham was among the enthusiasts for warm bathing, believing that it kept the pores open and that it restored vigour.[14] But by the end of the eighteenth century, it was cool bathing that was in the ascendant.[15] Whereas older treatments required the cleansing of corrupted humours, advocates of nervous physiology claimed that a cure could only be accomplished by an opposing stimulus to that of tropical heat. It was for this reason that Robert Jackson recommended cold bathing as the 'most important remedy in the cure of fevers of the West Indies; and perhaps of... all hot climates'.[16]

The proponents of pneumatic medicine also made an important contribution to discussions about hydrotherapy. Helenus Scott's vapour bath was employed by a number of practitioners including Colin Chisholm and Dr Ryan, Physician of the military hospital at Chatham, who used it to treat a range of diseases among tropical invalids, including chronic hepatitis. Chisholm explained its therapeutic power thus:

> According to Sir Humphry Davy, the muriate and sub-muriate of mercury, consist of metallic mercury, [and] combine with chlorine in various proportions. This combination acts much more powerfully on the system than simple chlorine communicated by absorption, through the medium of the bath. It is hence presumable that the former not only communicates the power inherent in simple chlorine, but also possesses a stimulant quality, which gives greater energy and greater efficacy to it.

Chisholm thus likened the bath to the action of calomel pills, in that the chlorine 'disengaged' by the nitro-muriatic bath appeared to be the same substance (oxygen) forthcoming from certain mercurial preparations, when received into the body through the stomach or skin.[17]

We can get a better impression of how these and other remedies were employed by examining the growing demand for such treatments in localities where invalids tended to congregate. From the 1790s until the middle of the nineteenth century, the principal resort for well-to-do invalids returning from the East and West Indies was Cheltenham. Cheltenham first acquired a reputation as a health resort in the early eighteenth century, when one Mr Mason discovered a peculiar spring on his land, to which pigeons flocked to peck calcareous particles, apparently as an aid to digestion. The spring water was found to possess purgative qualities and, in 1718, the spring was railed in with a view to commercial use. Mason's successor, Nash Skillicorn expanded the facilities, erecting a pump room in 1738 and placing an ornamental dome over the well; trees were also planted in parades to form avenues where invalids could take

[14] Trapham, *Discourse*, 140–1.
[15] Hillary, *Observations on the Changes of the Air*, vii.
[16] Jackson, *Treatise on the Fevers of Jamaica*, 245.
[17] Chisholm, *Manual*, 78–9.

the air. Soon afterwards, the spa attracted the attention of medical men, who subjected the water to chemical analysis. In 1740, Dr Short confirmed that the waters were rich in a 'purging chalybeate' (iron salts), the medicinal efficacy of which he praised highly, if taken in regular doses of between one and three pints. More such analyses followed, including those conducted by eminent London physicians like Dr Fothergill; as a result, the therapeutic property of the waters was widely discussed in popular and philosophical circles. By the 1770s, the fame of the waters was such that George III visited Cheltenham to drink them and ordered another well to be sunk for domestic use on the estate of his host, Lord Fauconberg. Here, more springs were discovered, including saline water of greater strength than the original spa. This well, popularly known as the 'King's Well', produced an abundance of water but began to dry up in the early 1800s and ceased altogether in 1819.[18]

The drying up of the wells disappointed many visitors to the town and marked the end of the first phase of the resort's development. The second phase began in 1802 when a Scottish physician, Thomas Jameson, who appears to have worked in Antigua and in India, established a practice in Cheltenham and searched for new wells on the southern side of the town, not far from the original spa. After drilling forty wells, Jameson found one that produced an abundance of saline water and obtained permission from Lord Sherborne, who owned the land, to erect a new spa upon what was then wasteland. In 1803, Jameson published a book that publicized his new venture, outlining his experiments on the soil, the discovery of the new springs, and the certainty that his new spa could supply Cheltenham with as much saline water as could be consumed by valetudinarians. The following year, a building was erected over the spa and it quickly acquired a high reputation.[19]

Jameson's success led other entrepreneurs to try their luck. Henry Thompson, who purchased a large piece of land from the De la Bere family in 1806, dug more wells in the corner of a field which became the fashionable district of Montpellier. Thompson also began to extract salts from the waters, which were packaged from 1811 as 'Cheltenham Alkaline Salts'.[20] The proprietor of the original well, Skillicorn, then opened what became known as the Orchard Well, while another was constructed about half a mile from Cheltenham at Alstone Villa. All these wells were purportedly different from spas in other parts of the country, in that their waters contained a higher proportion of what were known

[18] Jameson, *A Treatise on Cheltenham Waters and Biliary Diseases*, 9–11.

[19] Hembry, *The English Spa, 1560–1815*, 257.

[20] Brande and Parke, *A Descriptive Account of Mr Thompson's Laboratory at Cheltenham.* Thompson's enterprise was huge: he sank over seventy wells in order to provide sufficient water for the great boilers and evaporating machines housed at the Montpellier spa. The steam given off by the boilers was used to heat the baths owned by the proprietor. Thompson offered for sale six saline preparations, with 'No. 2', or crystallized, effloresced, and powdered alkaline sulphates, being recommended for use in the diseases of hot climates.

as Glauber salts,[21] whereas other spas usually derived their therapeutic qualities from Epsom or 'sea-salt'. Yet each of Cheltenham's wells was supposed to possess slightly different characteristics depending on the precise combination of minerals deposited near them; some contained more iron oxide and less saline, others contained concentrations of muriate (chloride), sodium, and magnesium.[22] A number of smaller spas efficacious in bilious complaints were also established in the vicinity of Cheltenham, at Tewkesbury, about ten miles distant and somewhat further afield at Malvern and Melksham.[23]

These waters were thought efficacious in hepatic and bilious complaints because they supposedly thinned the bile, thus preventing it from stagnating. By the late eighteenth century, such properties were generally explained using the fashionable idiom of pneumatic chemistry. According to James Johnstone, a physician at the General Infirmary in Worcester, these mineral waters owed their healing powers less to the metals and salts they contained, than to the 'volatile principles' united to them; these principles had purgative properties which were efficacious in the diseases of hot climates and most disorders of the endocrine and lymphatic systems.[24] How far these opinions were shared by other practitioners and those who frequented the spas is unclear, but the new discoveries in and around Cheltenham revived the resort's flagging reputation. By 1824, Dr William Gibney,[25] a former Army surgeon of relatively humble Irish origins, who now held the post of Physician at the town's Dispensary and the female orphan asylum, wrote that its population had doubled in the past fifteen years to around 12,000, excluding its floating population of invalids.[26] Many valetudinarians were now choosing to retire permanently to Cheltenham, including a large number who had served overseas in the Army, Navy, or East India Company. The spa waters were, of course, the principal attraction on account of the relief they were supposed to provide for the diseases of hot climates, but some were also drawn by Cheltenham's unrivalled facilities for cold and warm water bathing. According to Gibney, whose practice thrived in

[21] Hydrated sodium sulphate, named after the German-Dutch alchemist and chemist Johan Glauber (1604–68). These salts were used as cathartics and diuretics.

[22] Brande and Parke, 'Analysis of the Cheltenham Waters', cited in M'Cabe, *Observations*, 176–209; Jameson, *Treatise*, 2nd edn., 11–13.

[23] Johnstone, *Some Account of the Medicinal Waters, near Tewkesbury*; *Bath and Cheltenham Gazette*, 28 June 1820, 1. Johnstone was a friend of John Fothergill's and, like him and his circle, he took a strong interest in the medical applications of chemistry. His supporters claimed that he had been the first person to use chemical disinfectants to prevent fever, rivalling the claims of James Charmichael Smyth. Like Fothergill, Johnstone held an Edinburgh MD. See Hingston Fox, *Dr John Fothergill*, 380.

[24] Johnstone, *Some Account*, 22–4.

[25] Gibney entered the Dragoons as an Assistant-Surgeon in 1813 after graduating with an MD from Edinburgh earlier the same year. He served in the Army until 1818, when he retired on half pay, commuted in 1830. He was a Member of the Royal Medical Society of Edinburgh. See Ackroyd et al., *Advancing with the Army*, 125–8.

[26] Gibney, *A Medical Guide to the Cheltenham Waters*, 2.

Cheltenham for forty years,[27] the baths were 'fitted up in a style peculiarly elegant and commodious, not exceeded in any part of the kingdom. The patient may be supplied with every species of medicated, vapour, shower, dry douche, and other baths, at a moderate price.'[28]

The temperate climate of Cheltenham was also reckoned 'particularly well adapted for the invalid', being sheltered by hills to the east and sitting in the balmy but well-ventilated vale of the River Severn. The town's inhabitants were said to enjoy relative freedom from many common ailments such as consumption and their longevity was 'scarcely exceeded in any country'.[29] Such descriptions are strikingly similar to contemporary accounts of hill stations in India, which drew a causal connection between their favourable environment and the physical characteristics of native peoples. Thomas Jameson, who had a particular interest in the phenomenon of longevity, claimed that the climate of Cheltenham contributed not only to 'the preservation of the human system' but also 'a strength of stamina, which must be transmitted from father to son, and in series of successions, render longevity the inheritance of particular families, a circumstance extremely frequent in the valley of Gloucester'.[30]

By the 1820s, Cheltenham enjoyed such a 'degree of pre-eminence among towns, that its name ha[d] become as familiar in the British East and West Indies, as [it was] in London'.[31] Those who retired from the Company's service found the climate of Cheltenham reminiscent of the hill districts of India and a number of former Company officers bought land in Pittville, adjacent to one of the new spas. Later, in the 1850s, another Anglo-Indian community developed in the district of Battledown. Many of its inhabitants would have frequented Mr Brown's Coffee and Cigar Divan, 'where the fragrance of the Indian weed' could be enjoyed,[32] and they would have felt at ease amidst buildings constructed according to Indian style, including the façade of the old market arcade and the Cambray Spa, which opened in 1834. The names of some buildings, including a number of villas ('Malcolm Ghur' and 'Mosquito Ghur') and the Old Calcutta Inn, further displayed Cheltenham's Indian connections. Indeed, most of the major civic developments in the mid-nineteenth century owed something to Anglo-Indians. Cheltenham College, for instance, was the brainchild of retired Company servants, who envisaged the school as a preparation for the Army and the Indian Civil Service, while the first House Surgeon at the town's new

27 Ackroyd et al., *Advancing with the Army*, 246.
28 Gibney, *Medical Guide*, 4–5; Jameson, *Treatise*, 42, 53, 55.
29 Gibney, *Medical Guide*, 3.
30 Jameson, *Treatise*, 55. Jameson's interest in longevity stemmed from research into the physiology of ageing, conducted early in his career. He had lectured on the latter subject at the Medical Society of London in 1793 and, on the basis of further research, wrote a book dealing with the diseases relating to each age of Man, including the principal factors in longevity. See Jameson, *Essays on the Changes of the Human Body*.
31 Jameson, *Treatise*, 8.
32 Rowe, *Illustrated Cheltenham Guide*, 24.

hospital, which opened in 1848, was David Hartley, who had formerly worked in India.[33]

Hartley was merely one in a long line of Company and Army medics who decided to settle in Cheltenham. As the town attracted growing numbers of invalids and retirees from the colonies, great opportunities opened up for practitioners skilled in the treatment of tropical diseases and some of them, like Jameson, either became proprietors or worked closely in association with the spas. As a result, Cheltenham became the most important centre in Britain for the treatment of tropical invalids. According to Jameson, half of the invalids who visited Cheltenham were afflicted with bilious disorders contracted after long residence in hot climates or 'injurious treatment of their digestive organs'.[34] Many invalids also came to Cheltenham to obtain relief from an inflamed liver, a complaint common in both the East and West Indies, but somewhat less prevalent in the latter, supposedly on account of cooling sea breezes that afforded some relief from the heat.[35] The tropical heat was supposed to have a powerful influence upon the liver and this was sometimes aggravated by the large 'quantity of drink which is necessarily used in warm climates'.[36] While the onset of such diseases was often insidious, according to Jameson, they tended to become fatal if the afflicted remained in the tropics. But in Europe, by 'careful living', he explained, 'and occasional use of evacuating remedies, those invalids may live as long as if they had no such disease'.[37]

Explaining the apparent efficacy of the waters in a number of tropical complaints, Jameson drew a direct analogy between his practice in Cheltenham and his former practice in the West Indies, with Cheltenham waters being substituted for the purgative concoctions administered there:

> Medical practice in tropical countries, where fevers are always attended with excess of bile, consists almost entirely in the free use of bitter laxative drinks, to remove bile, and allay the febrile action of the system. The author had seventy patients every day under his care, in Antigua Hospital . . . who were either afflicted with Bilious fever, or dysentery, and as their stomachs could retain nothing solid for a minute, he followed the practice of that hospital, which was to give them . . . as much cold water, wherein a log of quasia wood had been steeped, as they could use. The effects of that portion of the bitter laxative, which remained upon their stomach, were to wash away the bile, and to invigorate the habit, sinking under the fatigue of perpetual vomiting.

Although he cautioned that the Cheltenham waters should not be used in acute fevers, his experience led him to conclude that they were useful in treating feverish states of the body that typically accompanied excess bile.[38]

33 Bailey, 'Cheltenham and the Indian Connection'.
34 Jameson, *Treatise*, 156.
35 Ibid., 160.
36 M'Cabe, *Observations*, x.
37 Jameson, *Treatise*, 163–4.
38 Ibid., 181–2.

Jameson insisted that the best time for treating invalids with the aperient waters of Cheltenham was during the summer season, from April to September, on account of the 'advantages derived from the co-operation of air and exercise with water'.[39] But before the waters could be usefully administered, the body had to be prepared so that the waters did not cause too much irritation to the stomach or brain. In line with received wisdom in the colonies, this normally entailed purging the system with calomel:

Invalids in the habit of using calomel, may begin with taking a small portion, in the form of a pill at bed-time, to be worked off next morning with a dose of water at the well. A dose of calomel, for three successive nights, to act as a purgative, with the assistance of Cheltenham water the next morning, will be sufficient for most bilious cases, without incurring the risk of its absorption, which ought never to be done without the advice of a medical practitioner on the spot, but as the use of calomel is not eligible for all patients, a preparatory pill of some other kind, may be taken over night, to quicken the action of the water next morning.[40]

Calomel was considered a valuable part of medical practice in Cheltenham because it supposedly emptied the bile ducts and alimentary canal more completely than any other cathartic. However, Jameson cautioned against its intemperate use, warning that too much mercury produced inflammation and excessive secretion of all bodily fluids, leaving the patient vulnerable to the onset of cold weather. Whereas calomel could be taken in large doses for months on end in tropical climates, those who persevered in such habits on their return to Britain faced ruin:

The author has known gentlemen in the East Indies, take calomel every night and morning for liver complaints until they had taken considerably above a hundred grains, without experiencing any inconvenience from it, who could not bear above twenty grains in this climate, without affecting the mouth; which is a symptom that generally renders confinement to the house a necessary expedient, to avoid the danger of getting cold.[41]

Yet many valetudinarians in Cheltenham continued to use calomel-based preparations indiscriminately and without medical advice.[42] The same was true of the waters themselves, which were often taken in such a way as to confer little benefit, or in a manner which was positively dangerous. Jameson claimed to have 'saved many persons from a fatal dropsy by preventing their drinking at the wells, when oedematous swellings appeared in their feet, accompanied with debility of the absorbent system'.[43] As might be expected, he stressed that it was best to take the waters as part of a personal regimen prepared by an experienced practitioner, the dosage depending on age, sex, constitution, and the patient's complaint.[44]

39 Ibid., 130. 40 Ibid., 131–2. 41 Ibid., 14. 42 Ibid., 13.
43 Ibid., 14. 44 Ibid., 133.

Similar regimes of treatment were recommended by other Cheltenham-based physicians with tropical experience. William Gibney also advised preparing the body with mercury, again using smaller doses than were used in India. This was necessary, he claimed, in order to clear the accumulation of hardened faeces that normally troubled those returning from hot climates. However, Gibney's use of purgative treatments was accompanied by measures to alleviate the plethoric condition of the larger viscera, which was common among tropical invalids. These measures included cupping over the affected part and the application of leeches to the anus, a practice which Gibney had witnessed in France. Apparently, the efficacy of the latter method depended upon 'applying the leeches as close as possible to the verge of the anus'.[45] Like Jameson, Gibney insisted that once the body was prepared, the waters should be given carefully in accordance with the patient's ailment and constitution, combined, if possible, with light exercise and an easily digestible diet from which fruit and vegetables were largely absent, on account of their acidity.[46] Gibney also stressed the advantages of bathing, especially for those whose constitutions had suffered from over-use of mercury in the colonies. He claimed that 'the nitro-muriatic bath, as recommended by Dr Scott, to be applied to the surface, will be of considerable utility, particularly in nervous constitutions, where morbid irritability exists, arising sometimes from those irregular effects often induced by mercury'.[47] It is impossible to say whether Gibney had met Scott, but he would have known him by repute and may have had contact with him in India. Gibney had also served at Waterloo and owed his rapid advance through the ranks to McGrigor, who held Scott and his bath in high esteem.

We gain further insight into medical practice among tropical invalids in Cheltenham from the publications of James M'Cabe and, particularly, the cases described in his *Directions for Drinking the Cheltenham Waters* (1823). It will be recalled that M'Cabe had been a military surgeon: a protégé of Jackson and McGrigor who had served in the Caribbean and other theatres during the Napoleonic Wars.[48] He retired from the Army on half pay in 1818, the same year as Gibney, another former Edinburgh graduate. In his description of Case VII, M'Cabe presents what had become the classic picture of a tropical invalid:

In the autumn of 1821, I was consulted by G.F.T.—— Esq. of the Hon. East India Company's Service, who had lately returned to England, after a residence of

[45] Gibney, *Medical Guide*, 61–3.
[46] Ibid., 121–33.
[47] Ibid., 61–2.
[48] M'Cabe entered the Army as a Hospital Assistant in 1810 and became an Assistant-Surgeon in the York Rangers in 1813; he was promoted to Surgeon in 1817 and retired from the Army on half pay in December 1818, which was commuted in November 1830. See Drew, *Roll*, vol. 1, 236.

five-and-twenty years in the climate of the East. During that period, he had suffered a great deal from the epidemics and endemics of India. He had had several attacks of what is called in India the 'Jungle Fever', – a kind of remittent, somewhat analogous to the yellow fever of the West Indies, and of the Coasts of the Mediterranean. He had also suffered from cholera, dysentery, and hepatitis; and his constitution was much impaired from the effects of these tropical diseases: countenance sallow, eyes suffused, appetite impaired, tongue furred (particularly in the mornings), a general restlessness and anxiety prevailed, and his bowels were generally constipated.[49]

M'Cabe claimed that he had treated this and other such cases successfully through a judicious combination of calomel pills and spa water, drunk three to four times daily. By having recourse to the waters every season since, his patient had enjoyed good health and his complexion and appetite had been restored.[50]

M'Cabe also treated a number of female patients, which is noteworthy in view of the increasingly pessimistic view taken of women's ability to adapt to tropical climates. Throughout the eighteenth century, there was no firm opinion on whether men or women were more or less likely to succumb to disease in hot climates, but it was often claimed that menstruation made women less plethoric and hence better able to withstand tropical heat. During the nineteenth century, however, women were increasingly regarded as weaker than men and more liable to become invalids. There is no more than a hint of this in M'Cabe's writings, but it is clear that the women he treated possessed no special advantage over their male counterparts. One such, a woman of thirty-two years, consulted M'Cabe after a long residence in the tropics, which had considerably impaired her constitution:

I directed, in the first instance, leeches to be applied to the abdomen, particularly to those parts which were the most tender to pressure. After which a warm bath, and some James's powder, and extract of hytosciamus, at bed-time, to be followed by a mild aperient in the morning, consisting of an infusion of senna, with manna, salts, and tincture of rhubarb. I enjoined perfect quiet, and prohibited animal food in every form, and desired that her diet should consist entirely of arrow-root, sago, and gruel. Under this treatment she recovered rapidly; and, in the course of a week, the pain and tenderness of the abdomen were completely removed; and she was able to take exercise in a carriage.[51]

The woman continued to drink one of the Cheltenham waters, as directed by M'Cabe, 'with the most considerable benefit'.

Like the rest of the Cheltenham physicians, M'Cabe insisted on the need for invalids to take the waters *in situ* and in accordance with medical advice. Although ostensibly a manual aimed at the layman, his *Directions for Drinking the Cheltenham Waters* is perhaps best seen as an advertisement for his specialist

[49] M'Cabe, *Directions for Drinking the Cheltenham Waters*, 50–1.
[50] Ibid., 52.
[51] Ibid., 66–7.

skills in treating a range of stubborn complaints. Each case is rendered in detail and the treatments differ greatly from one patient to another, thus emphasizing the desirability of a tailor-made regimen. M'Cabe seems to have made a good living from his books and his practice in the town, as is shown by his frequent changes of residence, from a modest cottage on the edge of town in 1820 to a fashionable terrace three years later. However, the claims made by M'Cabe and his colleagues in Cheltenham were subject to increasing scrutiny, and in the 1820s a number of practitioners publicly challenged the efficacy of the Cheltenham waters, including their use as a remedy for tropical invalids. The most damaging criticism came from Dr Adam Neale, a graduate of Edinburgh University, and formerly a Physician in the British Army and at the British Embassy in Constantinople; he had also been physician to the Duke of Kent and was a well-known authority on the history of the Peninsular War.[52] Although his military career had not progressed as far as he would have liked due to disagreements with McGrigor, Neale was a man of some standing and his words carried weight.

In 1820, Neale made the first of a series of attacks upon the efficacy of the Cheltenham waters and the misconduct of the town's medical practitioners. In a pamphlet addressed to a 'Professor of Medicine in the University of Edinburgh', Neale warned tropical invalids that they were probably wasting their time and money taking the waters:

> To those who resort to a watering place merely for the sake of amusement or fashion, . . . it must be a matter of little consequence to be informed that the fluid whereof they partake is stimulating or sedative, beneficial or injurious, factitious or natural. But to the real invalid, to the man who returns with a shattered constitution, from a long residence in a foreign and unhealthy climate, to spend the evening of life among friends and relatives, for whose sake, perhaps, he is anxious to prolong the close of a feverish existence; to such a man, I hold it to be some moment, that he should be warned against a blind confidence in an equivocal remedy, because he believes it to be a natural one.[53]

Neale claimed that the reputation enjoyed by the town's spas rested entirely on the proven therapeutic efficacy of the old well and that the new wells were merely 'weak brine springs', around which an elaborate edifice of pump rooms, walks,

[52] Adam Neale entered the Army as a Hospital Mate in 1796 but left to obtain an MD from Edinburgh University in 1802, whereupon he re-entered the Army as a Physician in July 1808, serving in the Peninsular War of 1809–13. His experiences in this campaign led to the publication of his *Letters from Portugal and Spain* in 1809. Neale retired from the Army on half pay in 1815, but re-entered in 1822, to retire once more on half pay in 1824. In 1821, he translated Assalini's *Treatise on Plague*, and published some accounts of his travels and a treatise on *Ergot of Rye* (1828). He became Medical Officer to the British Embassy in Constantinople and was Physician Extraordinary to the Duke of York; he died at Dunkirk on 22 December 1832. See *DNB*; Munk's *Roll*, vol. iii, 37; Ackroyd et al., *Advancing with the Army*, 227.

[53] Neale, 'A Letter to a Professor of Medicine in the University of Edinburgh respecting the Nature and Properties of the Mineral Waters of Cheltenham', in *A Collection of all the Papers, relative to the Alleged Adulteration of the Cheltenham Waters*, iii.

and plantations had been constructed to lure the credulous public.[54] He claimed that the observations of two respected chemists, Messrs Brande and Parke, showed that the new Montpellier spa differed greatly from the original well, as analysed by Fothergill and others in the eighteenth century. The quantity of aperient salts, or alkaline sulphates, in the Montpellier waters was not one half of that in the old spa, while the proportion of muriate of soda, or common sea salts was forty times greater. In order to remedy these defects, he claimed, the proprietors of the new spas had added minerals to their baths and drinking waters.[55]

Having established that the quality of the new spas was inferior to that of the old, Neale turned on the town's medical practitioners. He denounced them for their dishonesty and went so far as to claim that the new spa waters were positively dangerous to invalids returning from hot climates:

The cases which are generally sent to Cheltenham, are, as you well know, either people who have resided a long time in warm climates, and whose livers, and chylopoetic viscera have been injured by the influence of fevers and tropical heats; or such as have never travelled out of Great Britain, but whose abdominal organs have suffered excessive stimulation, from various causes. In neither of these two classes of patients, according to my experience, does a water containing muriate of soda, in excess, produce beneficial effects. In both, there is a tendency in the blood vessels to be rapidly and greatly excited into inordinate action, and many a torpid liver, which might have remained for years in a quiescent state, ... has been speedily thrown into violent inflammatory action, succeeded by suppuration, and the patient been hurried into the grave sooner by some years than would have happened, had he not been put upon a course of these stimulating waters.[56]

These allegations were potentially very damaging, not only to the reputation of Cheltenham's physicians who denounced them as tendentious,[57] but also to the economy of the town as a whole, which relied heavily on the business of invalids. In response, the proprietors of the new spas issued a hand-bill, which read:

To the Public

Dr Neale having returned, in a late publication, to insinuate without the slightest foundation ... that the proprietors of the Cheltenham Spas "possess a secret manner of adding to the strength of the waters, and thereby reap a rich harvest from the credulity of their visitors": and also to imply, that the waters are factitious. The proprietors feel called upon to offer a public refutation of this malignant and atrocious fabrication. They beg

[54] Neale, 'A Letter to a Professor of Medicine in the University of Edinburgh respecting the Nature and Properties of the Mineral Waters of Cheltenham', in *A Collection of all the Papers, relative to the Alleged Adulteration of the Cheltenham Waters*, iii, 9–10.

[55] Ibid., 12–13.

[56] Ibid., 16.

[57] Halpin, *Fact versus Assertion*; Newell, *A Letter to the Editor of the City Gazette upon the Misrepresentations contained in a Pamphlet recently Published by Dr Neale.*

leave to invite the most public scrutiny of their several wells and establishments, by which the falsehood of the insinuation will become apparent.

The bill went on to suggest that the matter be decided by a public meeting organized by its signatories: James Matthews, Henry Thompson, and J. Cossens.[58]

The meeting was held at the Assembly Rooms on 15 June 1820 and it was resolved that Neale should be authorized to nominate eight persons to a committee including fifteen others which would investigate the spa waters; the results of these investigations would then be published in the *Cheltenham Chronicle*. The meeting concluded after the proprietors swore affidavits to the effect that none of them had adulterated their spas with Epsom, Glauber, or other salts.[59] It then disbanded with Neale and his friend, one Capt. Smyth, being delivered in effigy into the hands of a mob, who burnt them in the Crescent amid the huzzas of between two and three thousand spectators.[60]

James M'Cabe also wrote a rebuttal of Neale's allegations. A former surgeon in the York Rangers and a graduate of Edinburgh, M'Cabe probably knew Neale before the controversy. There may already have been bad blood between them, as some former military surgeons had been angered by Neale's criticisms of regimental hospitals during the Peninsular War.[61] M'Cabe now condemned Neale's 'false' allegations and lamented the fact that he might deter the 20,000 to 30,000 annual visitors to Cheltenham from finding relief from their complaints. He argued that Neale's preference for sulphate of soda in the treatment of tropical diseases, rather than muriate of soda, was merely a personal opinion and that the most reliable test of the efficacy of the waters was the fact that thousands of visitors flocked to the town annually.[62] M'Cabe also cast doubt on Neale's motives in undermining the reputation of the newer spas:

The public is already in possession of the circumstances connected with this transaction, but to such as are not, it will be sufficient to inform them generally, that for the writing of the pamphlet, and his other exertions in favour of the 'Original Spa', the proprietor has acknowledged that he had given him one hundred pounds; and that he was afterwards to have a contingent interest in the concern, that is, that he should have a share of the surplus profits accruing to the Original Spa, from the magical influence of his pamphlet![63]

M'Cabe went on to add that Neale's allegations had made no impact on visitors that season, thanks to the oaths sworn by the proprietors of the Montpellier and Sherborne spas.[64] The flurry of other publications in the early 1820s, including

58 Cited in *A Collection of all the Papers*, 35.
59 Ibid., 37–8.
60 Ibid., 71.
61 Kelly, '"Not Surgeons Alone"', chaps 4–5.
62 M'Cabe, *A Reply to Dr Neale's Pamphlet*, 7–8.
63 Ibid., 11–12.
64 Ibid., 19.

Gibney's *Medical Guide to the Cheltenham Waters* (1824) should also be seen, in part, as an attempt to set the public's mind at rest in the wake of the controversy stirred up by Neale.[65]

The failure of Neale's attempt to undermine the reputation of the new spas is underscored by his decision, in 1822, to re-enter the Army, presumably having been unable to make a living from private practice. But the town's reputation received a further battering in 1821 from the radical journalist William Cobbett, who came to Cheltenham in the course of his *Rural Rides*. Cobbett described the town as a 'resort of the lame and lazy, the gourmandising and guzzling, the bilious and the nervous', its inhabitants and seasonal visitors being no more than 'vermin' and 'tax-eaters'.[66] These words did not endear him to the residents of Cheltenham, nor did similar comments made in the *Register* on 14 October 1826. When he returned to Cheltenham in 1830, to deliver a political speech, Cobbett was greeted by a riotous mob who forced him to flee the town. Finding the town too hot for him, the 'disappointed orator', as the *Cheltenham Chronicle* described Cobbett, 'prudently put himself into a post-chaise, and proceeded in the direction of Stow-on-the-Wold'. Unable to seize Cobbett, the mob contented itself with burning him in effigy.[67] However, Cobbett was not alone in remarking on the idleness and frivolity of Cheltonians. Catherine Sinclair declared, 'I never saw such resolute idlers with such a lounging indolent do nothing air.' Bernard Blackmantle, in the *The English Spy* (1826) also recalled life in Cheltenham as an endless round of 'Cards, cards, cards, nothing but cards from "rosy morn to dewy eve"'.[68]

Scepticism about the efficacy of the waters continued to be voiced in the years to come. The Company surgeon James Annesley wrote, for instance, that 'From misapprehension in such cases on the part of inexperienced physicians, many an unfortunate is sent to Cheltenham, or Bath, or Harrowgate, who would have derived much more benefit from a very different treatment under the salutory and natural influence of his own native climate.' 'We should not advise in every case to abstain from those valuable waters', he continued, 'but, it is certain, a very nice discrimination is required to ascertain when they are necessary.' There was also a growing feeling that spa-doctors were charging too much for their services. Lamenting the lack of affordable expert guidance for invalids, Annesley expressed the hope that the Company would one day provide a medical officer with experience of working in India to act as a physician for sick officers on their return to a land which had become strange to them.[69] In view of this, medical practitioners in Cheltenham felt the need continuously to demonstrate their

[65] Gibney, *Medical Guide*, v.
[66] Cobbett, *Rural Rides*, vol. 1, 40–1.
[67] *Cheltenham Chronicle*, 12 June 1830, 1.
[68] Hart, *A History of Cheltenham*, 194–5.
[69] Annesley, 'Medical Observations', 367.

credentials as experts in the diseases of hot climates. Dr Samuel Dickson, a former Army surgeon and protégé of McGrigor,[70] thus advertised his practice in Cheltenham through his books on the art of physic and the diseases of India.[71] Like other eminent physicians in the town, he was also careful to avoid accusations of quackery and emphasized that the Cheltenham waters ought to be taken only under the guidance of an expert physician. 'In the watering-hole where I now practise', he warned, 'their indiscriminate use is a source of emolument to the sexton!'[72]

[70] Dickson joined the Army as a Hospital Assistant in 1825, becoming an Assistant-Surgeon with the Royal Regiment the following year and full Surgeon in 1830. He resigned from the Army in July 1833. He obtained an MD from Glasgow University in 1833 and died on 12 October 1869, aged 67. See Drew's *Roll*, 276.

[71] Dickson, *The Fallacy of the Art of Physic*; idem, *On the Prevalent Diseases of India.*

[72] Dickson, *Fallacy*, 49–50.

2
The voyager returns

As we saw in the last chapter, the dyspeptics and hypochondriacs who congregated at Britain's spas had a seemingly insatiable demand for patent medicines and tonics. For many practitioners this was a matter for celebration, but for some it was a sad reflection on modern society and, in particular, on the new age of commerce and empire. One of those who were exercised by the problem of invalidism was the former naval physician James Johnson, who feared that a host of new diseases – which he dubbed 'curses of civilization' – would rend the fabric of British society if left to multiply unchecked. Johnson wrote not only of the diseases of hot climates but about the chronic ailments of Britons who had never left their country, who seemed to sicken as a result of luxury and over-stimulation. Britain's disease environment appeared to be changing: urbanization, commerce, and industry were producing new conditions and new ailments for which British practitioners were unprepared. But Johnson believed that the experience he had gained as a naval surgeon in many different parts of the world gave him unique insights into the afflictions of modern Britain. His experience as a naval practitioner sensitized him to issues related to occupational health while his travels overseas had demonstrated the power of diet and environmental factors in producing disease. On retiring from the Navy, it was these insights he set before his fellow practitioners and a lay public which seemed eager to receive his advice.

A few years after leaving the Navy, Johnson published his *Practical Treatise on Derangements of the Liver, Digestive Organs, and Nervous System* (1818), which was to be the first of several short treatises examining the causes of the gastro-intestinal complaints which now seemed to be widespread in Britain. The first section of this work was devoted entirely to 'The Influence of the Atmosphere, more especially the Atmosphere of the British Isles, on the Health and Functions of the Human Frame'. In the preface, Johnson drew attention to the fact that he had twenty years' experience in almost every climate of the globe,[1] and that his book was based on the theory of 'sympathy' that he had developed during his time in India and other tropical countries:

[1] *A Practical Treatise on Derangements of the Liver, Digestive Organs, and Nervous System*, 2nd edn., v.

> With the surface of the body some of the most considerable interior organs sympathize, particularly the lungs, the alimentary canal, and the liver. The sympathy between the functions of the last-mentioned organ . . . or in other words, between the functions of perspiration and biliary secretion, has not been noticed, as far as I know, by any author, till I traced it in my work on the 'Influence of Tropical Climates on European Constitutions'; though I trust it will not be overlooked by future observers.[2]

According to Johnson, the chief causes of digestive disorders in Britain were basically the same as those in the tropics: rapid changes of temperature. Although it was not subject to the great climatic extremes of India, Britain experienced rapid fluctuations in weather, often within the course of a single day. These, Johnson reasoned, were surely productive of disease. The relationship was most clearly evident in pulmonary conditions, which then killed around 55,000 Englishmen every year; equivalent to one-fifth of total deaths. Even consumption, or phthisis, could be attributed in large part to the weather, he claimed. Although he agreed with most practitioners that there was a hereditary predisposition to the disease, Johnson believed that this 'taint' was 'excited into action' by an external stimulus and, in four out of five cases, this appeared to be climatic.[3]

Next to the lungs, Johnson believed that the stomach was the organ most affected by climatic change, followed closely by the liver, which he saw as the seat of many physical and nervous disorders, including melancholy and hypochondria. Johnson's preoccupation with the liver owed much to his experiences in India, where that organ was accorded a central role in the causation of many fevers and bowel complaints.[4] Johnson's ideas about the relationship between the liver and various types of mental disorder echo those of Bichat and the anonymous author of a hand-written manuscript entitled 'An Essay on the Hypochondriac Disease', now in the library of the Royal College of Physicians of Edinburgh. Penned by a self-styled physician and valetudinarian, the manuscript is undated, although the ideas expressed in it suggest that it was written at the beginning of the nineteenth century. It is possible that Johnson was the author, although this is unlikely, given that he was not a fellow of the college and that there are slight differences in style. The identity of the author is, however, of secondary importance; its significance rests in the fact that it also exhibits concern about the incidence of nervous and digestive disorders in Britain at this time.

Like Johnson's work, the Edinburgh manuscript starts from the assumption that a sympathy exists between all parts of the body, the mind or 'soul' affecting

2 Johnson, *Practical Treatise*, 4–5.
3 Ibid., 17–18.
4 Ibid., 57.

the body, and vice versa.[5] It also notes that hypochondriasis is frequently accompanied by impairment of appetite and digestion, together with perspiration. The liver and spleen are singled out as the organs most frequently affected by hypochondriasis, being affected by pains, palpitations, and tension; other organs, such as the heart and lungs, are also said to suffer in similar ways.[6] As for the mental symptoms of the disease, hypochondriasis was supposed to manifest itself in 'a Love of solitude, an obstinate application to one particular study or employment, Sadness, Grief, Fear and other Passions akin to these as Chagrin, Difficulty, Suspicion, Jealousy, Despair, with an erroneous imagination springing from the suggestions of these'.[7] The author of the manuscript has little to say about the causes of the disease, but, like Johnson, recommends a light diet, regular exercise, and residence in a temperate climate as the best means of treating the disorder.[8]

Indeed, the relationship between liver diseases and climates was stressed in Johnson's comments on the diseases of Britain as well as of hot climates:

> If the high range of temperature in tropical climates . . . can produce such lesion of structure in the hepatic system, so in our own climate, the rapid transitions, the humidity, and the coldness of the atmosphere, operate most powerfully, though unsuspectedly on the functions of the liver. . . . The partial application of cold or wet to the body, and particularly to the lower extremities, when for any length of time continued, has a powerful influence on the biliary secretion, and consequently disturbing the functions of the whole intestinal canal.[9]

Herein lay the explanation for the prevalence of bilious disorders among the lower classes: their want of bedding and clothing, and the cold, damp conditions in which they often had to work. The next most important cause of such disorders was intemperance, to which Johnson believed all orders of society had become addicted.[10]

Of the various climatic conditions productive of disease, humidity was by far the worst, according to Johnson: an opinion he had formed during his tropical voyages. His experiences had convinced him that:

> The human frame, and particularly the English constitution can sustain considerable atmospheric vicissitudes with a great degree of impunity, when the air is dry, clear and elastic. But if these changes are accompanied with humidity or rain, every valetudinary, and many in health are sure to feel the effects.[11]

[5] 'An Essay on the Hypochondriac Disease', in a letter, Anonyma 16, RCPE, 25.
[6] Ibid., 26–34.
[7] Ibid., 31.
[8] Ibid., 45–79.
[9] Johnson, *Practical Treatise*, 72.
[10] Ibid., 73.
[11] Ibid., 6.

It followed, too, that the conditions that most resembled the lethal humidity of the tropics would be among the most dangerous in temperate latitudes, some of which were of Man's own making:

> In the overcrowded ball room, heated to a tropical temperature, the sensitive Belle and effeminate Beau carry exercise to the extreme of exhaustion, and, in this state, rush fearlessly forth under the gloomy skies of a hyperborean night! The ghastly train of consumptions which annually follow this imprudent conduct, have no premonitory effect in preventing a repetition of it.[12]

The effects of the atmosphere upon human health remained a central feature of Johnson's work and figured to a large extent in his writings on the preservation of health and on tropical invalids. Johnson's time in the tropics and at Walcheren left his body racked with fever and chronic dysentery; conditions which showed no sign of abating after he returned to England. As he put it: 'A return to Europe brought me no relief; on the contrary, by getting cold in my feet, while sitting in a dissecting-room in London, a few weeks after my arrival, a violent Hepatitis was induced, accompanied by the usual dysenteric symptoms.'[13] Although Johnson believed that a change of climate was the only hope for Europeans debilitated by tropical diseases, he warned that a sudden change of climate, or 'chill', could aggravate these conditions. He explained in his *Essay on Morbid Sensibility of the Stomach and Bowels* (1826) that:

> The powers of the constitution, however plastic, cannot immediately accommodate themselves to great and sudden changes of climate, even when the transition is from a bad to a good one; and the tropical invalid requires fully as much caution and patience in approaching the shores of England, as he did in landing at a former period, on the banks of the Ganges.[14]

Johnson believed that bodies became partially assimilated to and 'in some measure changed' by long exposure to a tropical climate. A sudden transition from a tropical to a cold climate, he warned, could therefore cause a 'determination' of blood to the organs weakened by tropical diseases, increasing the inflammation of the liver and mucous membranes of the bowels.[15] Chill could also lead to serious respiratory problems. Johnson averred that 'the mucous membrane of the lungs sympathises readily with that of the stomach, and thus produces what is called a stomach cough'.[16]

To prevent such unfortunate consequences, Johnson recommended that Europeans adhere to a strict dietary regimen on their homeward voyage:

[12] Johnson, *Practical Treatise*, 181.
[13] *Influence*, 308.
[14] *An Essay on Morbid Sensibility of the Stomach and Bowels*, 2nd edn., 117.
[15] Ibid.
[16] Ibid., 118.

It cannot . . . be too strongly impressed on the mind of the tropical invalid, that without a firm resolution to coerce his appetites into complete subjection . . . he will gain little by a return to his native skies; but, on the contrary, he will either confirm those maladies under which he already labours, or, what is perhaps worse, convert them into forms less formidable . . . in appearance, but effectually subversive of every enjoyment, mental or corporeal, which can render life desirable.[17]

He advised that tropical invalids should breakfast on ship's biscuits or stale bread, toasted and lightly buttered, with black tea or coffee, or chocolate taken with a little milk and sugar. There was to be no luncheon and the invalid was to eat nothing before an early dinner consisting of a small quantity of plainly cooked meat, again with the obligatory stale bread or ship's biscuit. Vegetables were to be avoided at all costs. 'This will be seen as a most terrible rule!' he acknowledged, especially after the luxuries of an oriental table, 'But let the invalid pursue it only till he passes the Cape of Good Hope, and then he has permission to change it, and adopt what system he pleases.'[18]

Though lauded by 'hermits and philosophers', vegetables, according to Johnson, were far harder to digest and thus more productive of irritation than meat. Best of all were farinaceous foods such as sago and porridge: 'We see whole nations, as the Hindoos and Scotch, live and thrive on food almost exclusively farinaceous', he observed, his own preference being for a 'good grit-gruel'. Another measure that might profitably be taken by tropical invalids was to break their homeward journey at Madeira or the south of France, where a warm but gentle climate would enable their bodies to adapt slowly to more temperate latitudes.[19] A number of physicians had already suggested Madeira as an appropriate place for tropical invalids,[20] and like some of these Johnson also recommended bathing. Depending on the nature of the complaint, warm or cold bathing would help regulate perspiration and, because of the 'sympathy' between the skin and internal organs, many digestive complaints could thus be alleviated. Johnson believed that the medicinal effects of bathing had been relatively ignored in Britain, notwithstanding the popularity of spa resorts. As a reminder of their medicinal uses, he pointed to the regular bathing practices of the Hindus, Russians, and Hungarians, as well as the ancient Greeks and Romans.[21] In addition to bathing, exercise was deemed necessary to improve digestion and counteract any depressing passions, such as those that might be attributed to an irritable bowel.[22] The tropical invalid, according to Johnson, was particularly liable to 'hypochondriacal despondency': a terrible affliction that could lead the

[17] Ibid., 120.
[18] Ibid., 126.
[19] Ibid., 79.
[20] e.g. William Lockhead to William Cullen, 20 September 1786, Letters to William Cullen, vol. 1, RCPE.
[21] Johnson, *Essay*, 181.
[22] Ibid., 73, 97.

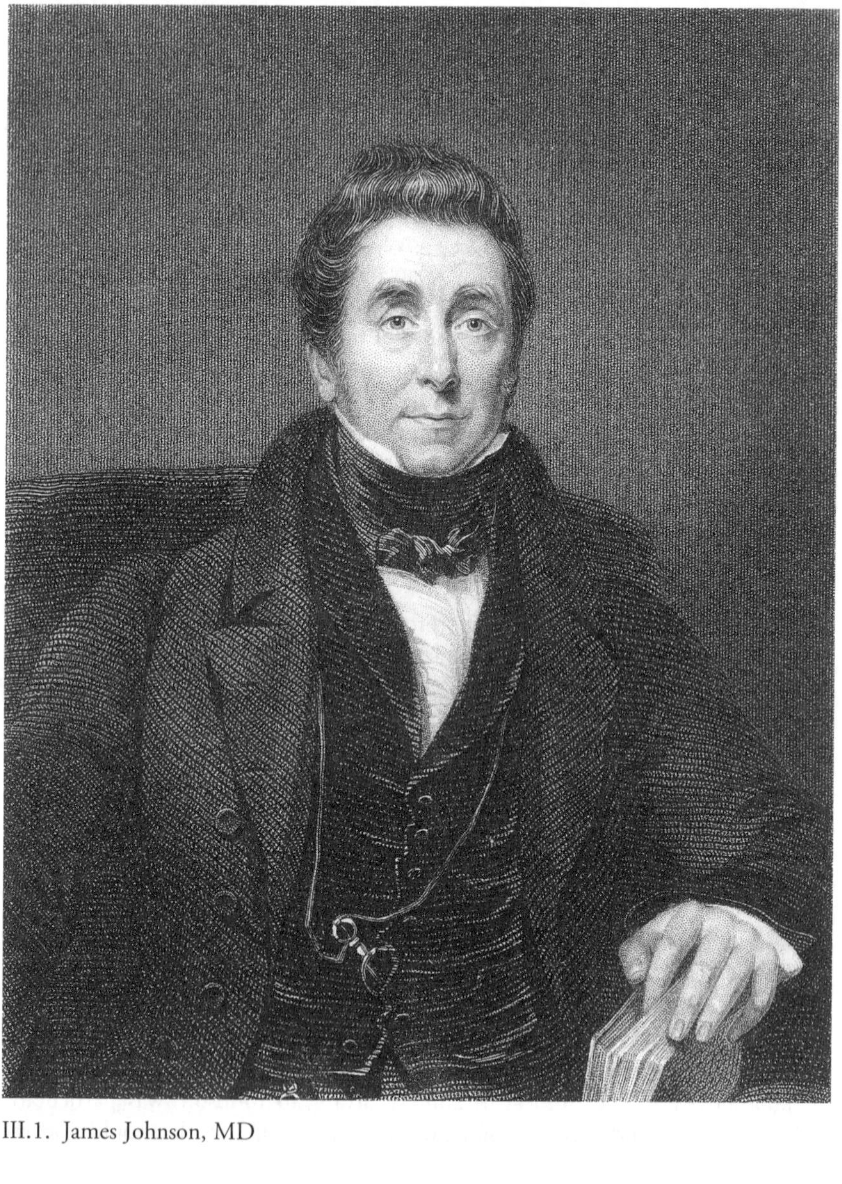

III.1. James Johnson, MD

sufferer to take his or her own life. Johnson referred not to an entirely imaginary complaint but a constant state of anxiety over one's health: a 'daemon' which drew its 'gigantic power and influence' from morbid sensibility of the digestive organs.[23]

It was a demon that had possessed Johnson himself. In the winter of 1822, the haemorrhoids from which he had suffered as a result of chronic dysentery had become so bad that he had to endure two operations to remove them. Although he recovered from these, his nerves became 'unstrung' and his digestive powers, which had been poor for some time, were now badly impaired. Gloomy images haunted him and in the midst of the London season, with his medical practice curtailed by illness, Johnson suffered a breakdown and retired to the seaside town of Margate, as he then thought, to die. But the sea breezes seem to have revived him and after a few weeks he returned to London as resolute as ever, his health much improved. This complaint – which had ruined his medical practice – was now to make him a fortune. His experiences led him to write his best-selling *Essay on Morbid Sensibility of the Stomach and Bowels*, which took London – or at least the dyspeptic part of it – by storm. Nearly every victim of indigestion possessed a copy or had borrowed it from someone else. It went through four editions in little more than nine months and eventually reached a tenth. It was reprinted in America and in translation in Germany and France; it received both public and professional acclaim. The book's success stemmed from its accessibility. Johnson wrote about what he had suffered and described it in plain and simple language; his emphasis upon a light diet in contrast to the 'farrago of tonics and stimulants' then popular for digestive complaints endeared him to many of those disillusioned with patent medicines.[24]

The great demand for Johnson's homely advice must have confirmed him in his opinion that Britain was becoming a nation of invalids.[25] Referring to the prevalence of hypochondriasis in Britain, Johnson wrote: 'The extent of this evil is so great in these isles that it has been suspected, and not without probability, that our tropical colonization has introduced and propagated, by hereditary descent, a strong disposition to stomach and liver affections beyond that which is observed in any other country.'[26] As we saw earlier, Johnson drew heavily on the evolutionary ideas of Erasmus Darwin, who advanced a theory in which environmental stimuli made a lasting impression on the nervous system, conferring characteristics that could be passed on to subsequent generations. Johnson attributed the growing number of nervous and digestive disorders in Britain to a

[23] Johnson, *Essay*, 120–1.
[24] Ibid., ii.
[25] For a stimulating discussion of such anxieties in early nineteenth-century Romantic literature, see Bewell, *Romanticism*, 8.
[26] Johnson, *Essay*, 121.

new range of stimuli peculiar to modern life, one of his chief complaints being the agitation that arose from speculation and commerce:

In this country, where man's relations with the world around him are multiplied beyond all example in any other country, in consequence of the intensity of interest attached to politics, religion, commerce, literature, and the arts . . . and where speculative risks are daily run by all classes, from the disposers of empires in Leadenhall Street [the East India Company], down to the potatoe[sic]-merchant of Covent Garden, it is really astounding to observe the deleterious influence of those mental perturbations on the functions of the digestive organs.[27]

These views were shared by other members of the profession. At his Cheltenham practice, James M'Cabe recalled treating a thirty-six-year-old man who complained of debility, languor, and poor concentration, which had arisen from his engagement in 'mercantile pursuits of a nature pernicious and fluctuating, and well calculated to keep the mind in a state of uncertainty and feverish anxiety – this, in speculations on the Stock Exchange'.[28] On the other hand, Johnson recognized the benefits brought by commerce: the roads, bridges, fine houses, and clothes, the improved diet of the working man. Bowel complaints and the nervous disorders that stemmed from them were the price that humanity paid for material and intellectual progress. 'This curse of civilization', he argued, 'is not confined to any age or any nation. Wherever the mind has been cultivated at the expense of the body, there hypochondriacism has prevailed. Aristotle informs us that all the great men of his time were hypochondriacs, or at least melancholics.'[29]

Johnson's ambivalence towards the age of enterprise reminds us of his rather uncomfortable position in matters of politics, professional and otherwise. He sat uneasily between the pugnacious radicalism of Wakley and *The Lancet* at one extreme, and the Tory Royal College of Physicians at the other. His editorship of the *Medico-Chirurgical Review* demonstrated a strong commitment to meritocracy but at the same time a veneration of ancient institutions and inherited wisdom, which Wakley lost no opportunity to ridicule.[30] Like many surgeons who had entered the Army or Navy, Johnson's career had catapulted him from his humble roots in rural Ulster to a metropolitan world which seemed to lack the moral certainties of his Protestant upbringing. Despite their success, men like Johnson were outsiders who looked nostalgically at the passing of agrarian society and its simple virtues. Their social marginality led them to cultivate the trappings of gentility,[31] but it also gave their work a critical inflection. They were beneficiaries of social change but at the same time alienated by it.

27 Johnson, *Essay*, 53–4.
28 M'Cabe, *Directions*, 39–40.
29 Johnson, *Essay*, 56.
30 See Desmond, *The Politics of Evolution*, 193–8, 238.
31 Inkster, 'Marginal Men'.

For the remainder of his life, Johnson wrote about how best to live in the brave new world arising from imperialism and commerce, with its host of 'modern diseases', as he termed them. Such diseases included 'irritability of temper', 'neuralgia', and other nervous complaints, 'nearly unknown to our forefathers', which were the product of 'over-excitement, . . . emulation, competition, ambition, anxiety, [and] tribulation'.[32] He wrote on the merits of various spa waters, the different modes of living necessary to maintain health at different stages of life, and developed some of his earlier theories about atmosphere and health. He became particularly enamoured of 'tours of health', that is, journeys to the more salubrious parts of Britain and Europe. These he recommended to all whose constitutions had been damaged by tropical service or a sedentary existence, especially in one of the larger towns. In the autumn of 1829, for example, Johnson made a lengthy tour of France, Switzerland, and Italy, which experiences were recounted in his *Change of Air* (1831). The book is in many respects typical of a new genre of literature in which travellers recounted their wanderings in Europe through the sensations of their bodies: a kind of valetudinary Grand Tour.[33]

But Johnson's account of his travels in Europe contains some interesting reflections on the dangers of urban civilization as well as remarks on healthful climates. While he applauded the fruits of urban civilization – manufactures, engineering, and the like – Johnson warned that pollution and feverish activity would take their toll on the human frame. The typical city dweller was characterized by his drawn expression, pallid complexion, impaired indigestion, and premature ageing: the results of what Johnson termed 'wear and tear'. This was a state of mind and body that lay somewhere between health and illness, though closer to the latter: a descendant of Cheyne's 'English Malady'.[34] Though this condition might be found in many modern towns, it was in London, the 'Modern Babylon', that it was most apparent. 'In London', Johnson quipped, 'business is almost the only pleasure – in Paris, pleasure is almost the only business.'[35] It was in London that 'the fury of politics . . . , the riot of dissipation, the madness of ambition, the thirst of gold, the struggles of competition, the cares of commerce' were most in evidence.[36] However, Johnson warned that the country as a whole was destroying its youth by forcing them through an intensively competitive system of education.[37] Again, he warned that the effects would be seen not only in the present but in subsequent generations: 'though

[32] Johnson, *Economy of Health*, 97.
[33] e.g. Matthews, *The Diary of an Invalid.*
[34] Johnson, *Change of Air*, 1–6.
[35] Ibid., 3.
[36] Ibid., 10.
[37] Ibid., 16.

acquired at first by external circumstance' they would 'in time, be promulgated from parent to progeny hereditarily'.[38]

In keeping with practices in hot countries, Johnson enjoined change of air as the sovereign remedy to the ills of modernity, together with 'rural relaxation' and physical exercise. Anything from a week in Margate to a tour of the Alps might suffice to restore the invalid's constitution to health.[39] In this and in so many other ways, Johnson's career shows the formative influence of colonial service on medical knowledge. His experiences in India and other tropical countries left him in no doubt that climate had a powerful effect on the human body and that many diseases were affected to a large extent by climatic factors. The theories he developed in India about the sympathetic relationship that existed between the surface of the body and its internal organs provided the physiological foundations for this strong conviction, which also underlay most of his work on the diseases to be found in temperate latitudes. But Johnson's experiences as an 'oriental voyager', as he had once styled himself, left a much deeper impression. It was not simply that he had been able to observe the effects of climate in and on the bodies of others: he had experienced them himself and had suffered from many of the maladies normally associated with tropical service. Like other tropical invalids, Johnson believed that his body had been transformed by prolonged exposure to such climates: not enough to make him fully acclimatized but enough to make it difficult for him to return to his native land. He was one among many thousands of Britons whose constitutions had been impaired by tropical service and who seemed likely to spawn another enfeebled generation. Furthermore, Johnson believed that the nervous anxiety that stemmed from commerce and speculation had created a host of new diseases. For good or ill, Britain's Empire was transforming its people: they were more prosperous than ever before but also more likely to suffer from nervous and digestive disorders. Johnson's remedy for these ills was self-control, as befitted the rather abstemious man that he was. But there is a deeper undercurrent in Johnson's work: a concern that the manliness of a proud and martial nation was being undermined. Whether it was produced by the jungles of Bengal, the ballroom, or the factory, invalidism was a feminizing condition that could be countered only by a robust assertion of masculine values.

[38] Darwin's work continued to be cited in justification of such views until the 1840s. See Armstrong, *The Influence of Climate.*

[39] Johnson, *Change of Air*, 10, 25.

3

Albion's coast is sick

The loss of manly vigour which Johnson touched upon in his writings figured prominently in much of the literature on 'diseases of civilization' at the beginning of the nineteenth century; nowhere more so than in the work of the naval physician Thomas Trotter (1760–1832). Writing against the backdrop of the Revolutionary and Napoleonic Wars, Trotter was one of a number of military and naval medics who mounted a trenchant critique of what they perceived as the mental and physical decline of the British nation. He claimed that the expansion of trade and manufacturing, which Thomas Addison had earlier celebrated in his famous essay on 'The Royal Exchange', had enriched the nation at the cost of indolence and vice. A growing taste for luxury, he warned, was consuming the nation's martial spirit, with dire consequences for its pre-eminence among nations. In formulating his critique of British society, Trotter drew, among other things, upon the ideas of eighteenth-century physicians such as his fellow Scot, George Cheyne (1673–1743), and the Genevan, S. A. A. D. Tissot (1728–97), who had both described new maladies which accompanied the process of civilization.[1] And, like his naval contemporary, James Johnson, he warned that the pathological aspects of modern life would become deeply ingrained, passing from one generation to another. But whereas Johnson had found an antidote to over-consumption in abstinence and modified behaviour, Trotter's remedy was less in tune with the individualism of the time. Attacking the root causes of Britain's afflictions, he denounced slavery and the tropical colonies, and sought to counter the effects of manufacturing and commerce by reinvigorating rural life. Trotter also believed that the Navy had a special part to play in stemming national deterioration. Like many critics of modernization, he saw the armed forces as a bastion of manly virtues. They provided a context in which the nation's youth could be nurtured to healthy manhood, uncorrupted by the vices of an effeminate and uncaring society. However, he warned that the moral and physical condition of the Navy was being undermined by the system of impressment from which the majority of naval manpower was traditionally

[1] Porter, 'Diseases of Civilization'.

raised in time of war. He held impressment responsible for problems of internal discipline and the Navy's poor performance during the American War of 1812. And, while he was not alone in making these criticisms, Trotter's *Practicable Plan for Manning the Royal Navy* (1819) was perhaps the keenest contemporary analysis of impressment and the most detailed manifesto for its replacement.

Thomas Trotter was born in Melrose, Roxburghshire, the third of five children (the second son) of John and Alison Trotter, a baker and his wife. He was educated at Melrose and Kelso Academy until 1777, when he left Melrose to study medicine at Edinburgh University. Like most of his contemporaries, Trotter lacked the means to study the entire degree course and was forced to abandon his studies after two years to take a post as a surgeon's mate in the Navy.[2] For an ambitious young man of modest means, the Georgian Navy seemed like a good prospect, offering a stable, if seldom remarkable, income, as well as adventure and useful professional experience. Some of the more ambitious surgeons attempted to cultivate patrons within the Admiralty who would further their careers, and a few counted aristocrats and members of the nobility among their patients. Those of a scientific bent also saw in naval service an opportunity to further their interests in new and sometimes exotic locations.[3]

When Trotter joined the Navy, the War of American Independence was at its height and his first posting was to the *Berwick*, in 1779: a vessel of the Channel Fleet in which he and the crew suffered badly from scurvy. After further active service in the Battle of Dogger Bank in 1781, and the relief of Gibraltar in 1782, Trotter was promoted to full surgeon. But with the conclusion of hostilities, he found himself unemployed and took a position as surgeon on board a Liverpool Guineaman, the *Brookes*, where he had medical charge of its cargo of slaves during the mid-Atlantic passage. A severe outbreak of scurvy on board the ship, together with his earlier experiences in the *Berwick*, formed the basis of his *Observations on the Scurvy* (1785). His spell as surgeon on board a slaving vessel also left him a fierce critic of the trade, which he denounced in several later works. After a spell in private practice in Northumberland, Trotter returned to Edinburgh, where he wrote an MD thesis on the subject of drunkenness, *De ebretate eiuque effectibus in corpus humanum* (1788), which was later published in English as *An Essay, Medical and Philosophical, and Chemical, on Drunkenness, and its Effects on the Human Body* (1804).

After leaving Edinburgh, Trotter resumed his career in the Navy, and was made physician of the *Barfleur* in 1788. Two years later, during the Spanish Armament of 1790, he was appointed surgeon to the flagship, the *Royal William*, and in 1793 was surgeon on board the *Vengeance* during its voyage to the West Indies. On the latter ship, Trotter gained further experience of the diseases of hot climates, and high rates of sickness and mortality among Britons in the

[2] Wallace, 'Thomas Trotter (1760–1838)'.
[3] Brockliss et al., *Nelson's Surgeon*, chap. 1.

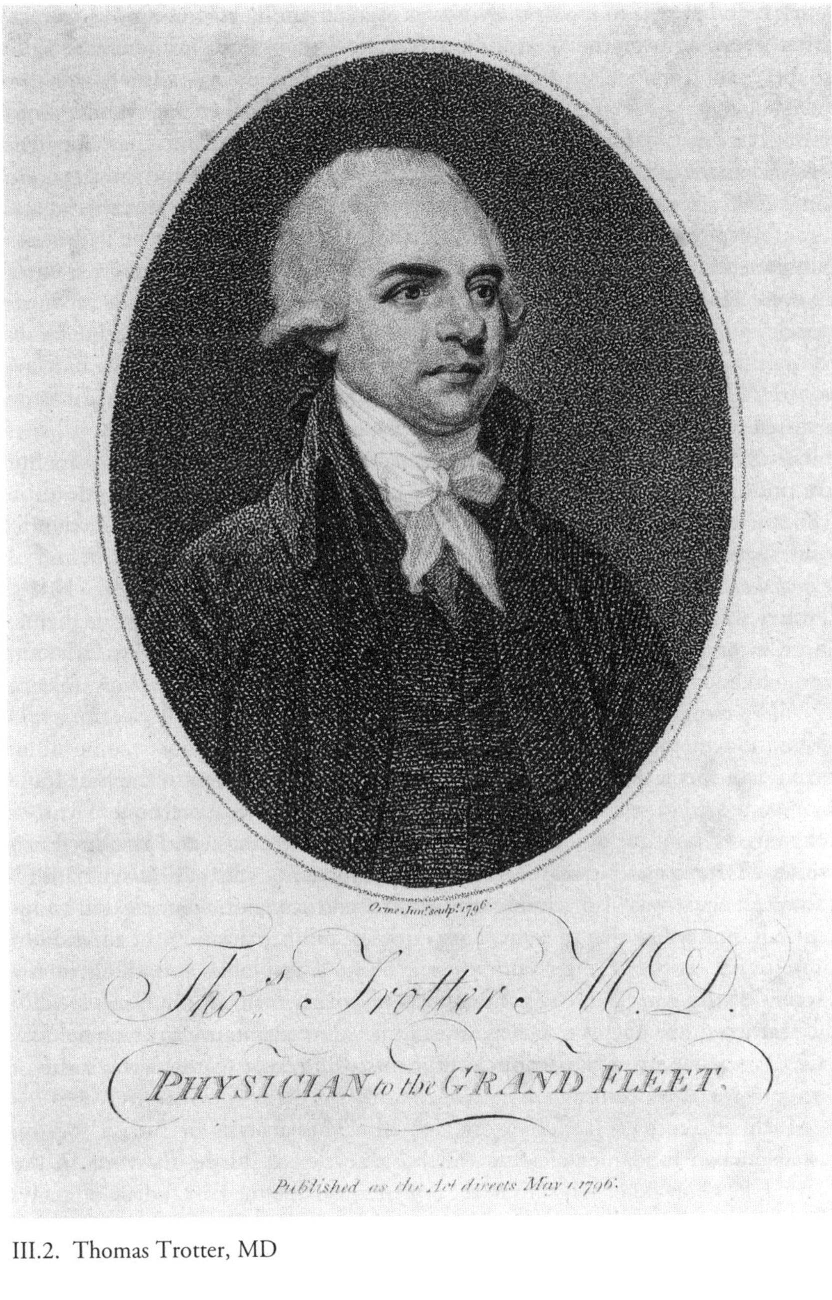
Thos. Trotter M.D.
PHYSICIAN to the GRAND FLEET.
Published as the Act directs May 1.1796.

III.2. Thomas Trotter, MD

Caribbean led him to doubt the wisdom of maintaining colonies in the tropics. After returning from the West Indies, Trotter was appointed in December 1793 to be Second Physician at Haslar, although the following April he left the hospital to take up the post of Physician to the Channel Fleet under Lord Howe. In this capacity, he served in actions against the French in the campaigns of 1794 and 1795, but his active service career was brought abruptly to an end in June 1795 after experiencing a rupture which left him incapable of service at sea. From then until 1802, when he left the Navy, Trotter wrote a large and subsequently popular book on medicine in the Navy, based on his experiences in the Channel Fleet. It was entitled *Medicina Nautica*, the first edition of which appeared in 1797, followed by others in 1799 and 1803. It was in this book that Trotter began to formulate his critique of contemporary Britain and its Empire.

After leaving the Navy with half pay, and what he regarded as a rather meagre pension, Trotter established himself in private practice in Newcastle upon Tyne. Finding his health unequal to medical practice, he retired after a few years but continued to write on naval and medical matters until shortly before his death in 1832. It was during this period that Trotter produced some of his most significant works, including his *View of the Nervous Temperament* (1807) and *A Practicable Plan for Manning the Royal Navy... without Impressment* (1819). Trotter was also actively involved in a range of interests outside of medicine. He was a member of the Literary and Philosophical Society of Newcastle and wrote frequently to local and national newspapers on a diverse range of subjects. It will be recalled that the Newcastle 'Lit and Phil' had a strongly reformist and Dissenting membership and that it claimed among its members some other prominent medical men, not least John Clark who had served in the East India Company's Marine. Although it has not been possible to determine Trotter's religious or political affiliations, his background, writings, and the circles in which he moved in Newcastle suggest nonconformity and radical sympathies. However, there was also a rather sentimental and Romantic complexion to his writings, not unlike that of some Tory critics of industrialization. In addition to professional works, Trotter composed a play, 'The Noble Foundling of the Hermit of the Tweed' (1812) and a book of poems entitled *Sea Weeds* (1829). The earliest of the poems – such as 'On a Learned Acquaintance Turning Soldier' (1798) – evince strongly patriotic sentiments, while later works reflect some of Trotter's social concerns.

Much of Trotter's medical work, including his analysis of British society, rested on two fundamental ideas which he developed during his years in the Navy. Like many other surgeons in the armed forces and the East India Company, Trotter enthusiastically embraced the pneumatic chemistry, first of Priestley and Black, and later of Lavoisier; indeed, his interest in the subject led him to develop a new theory of the causation and treatment of scurvy. During the 1770s, the naval physician Nathaniel Hulme, together with John Pringle, President of the Royal Society of London, had speculated that 'fixed air' (carbon dioxide) was necessary to prevent the 'putrefaction' of bodily humours which they thought responsible for scurvy. The beneficial effects of fresh vegetables and fruits – already well known to many surgeons and naval officers before Lind's famous demonstration[4] – were explained in this way; that is, on account of their possession of quantities of fixed air.[5] Trotter's theory of scurvy was different in two respects: first, in that he highlighted the role of 'vital air' (oxygen) as opposed to 'fixed air' and, second, in seeing scurvy as a *deficiency* disease. In the latter respect, he developed the insight of Gilbert Blane who had claimed in his *Observations on the Diseases of Seamen* (1785) that scurvy was due to 'a defect of nourishment' rather than a 'vitiated state of it'.[6] Trotter grew steadily more convinced of this so that, in the second edition of his *Observations on the Scurvy* in 1792, he declared that 'In the former [edition] I found the doctrine of putrefaction untenable, and in this I have deserted it altogether'.[7]

Trotter believed that scurvy was caused simply by the lack of one essential element – vital air – that was unusually abundant in citric acid. 'The lemon, lime, shaddock [grapefruit], and orange, in the manner we have set them down', he asserted, 'give out the citric acid in different degrees of purity. This genus of fruit has advantages above all others, for as it approaches to maturity, the acid is not attended for the worse, but rather purer than before.'[8] Extracts of the juices of these fruits had been used before on long voyages but Captain Cook and others had found them ineffective, much of their water content having evaporated; this was also the view taken by the Admiralty as a whole.[9] Trotter thought that the answer might lie in bottling the juice of citrus fruits immediately after squeezing them.[10]

Pneumatic chemistry was also central to the theory of contagion which Trotter was to develop some years later in his medical history of the Channel Fleet, *Medicina Nautica*. He was sceptical about claims that diseases such as typhus, which most contemporaries thought to be contagious, were caused by invisible 'animaluclae'. Although he accepted the probable existence of an unspecified form of contagious matter, Trotter believed that it could thrive and be transported only in an atmosphere which had already been corrupted by the breath of the sick. He asserted that 'they [gases] are the vehicle of it [the contagion]' and that they might even be the cause of contagion itself.[11] However, Trotter was wary of pronouncing with certainty on this matter, aware that his only evidence

[4] See Rodger, *The Wooden World*, chap. 3; Williams, *The Prize of All the Oceans*.
[5] See Carpenter, *History of Scurvy*, chaps 3–4; Lawrence, 'Disciplining Disease'.
[6] Blane, *Observations*, 3rd edn., 509.
[7] Trotter, *Observations on the Scurvy*, xxv.
[8] Ibid., 215.
[9] Williams, *The Prize of All the Oceans*, 225–6.
[10] Trotter, *Observations*, 223.
[11] Trotter, *Medicina Nautica*, 181.

for such a theory was that the breath of the sick smelled differently from that of the healthy, in some cases resembling a 'sulphurated-hydrogenous gas'.[12]

Despite the speculative nature of his theory, Trotter believed that it was more credible than one which rested solely on the hypothetical existence of invisible organisms, for the existence of discrete gases had after all been established. The gas theory also explained why contagious fevers such as typhus abounded in overcrowded and unventilated conditions, such as on board ships or in urban areas. The rising incidence of such 'crowd diseases' was, for Trotter and many other doctors, one of the most lamentable consequences of modern life: the inevitable concomitant of urbanization.

The other chief constituent of Trotter's medical theories was the notion of nervous excitability, which he seems to have developed largely from the work of Brown and Darwin. These men had pinpointed the nervous system as the seat of most bodily disorders; they had taught, as Trotter put it,

> that animal existence is endowed with a quality, called *Excitability* by Brown; *the Spirit of Animation*, or *Sensorial Power*, by the author of Zoonomia [Darwin]; on which the phenomena of life depend. Everything which supports life, exerts its influence on this principle: it is accumulated by the subtraction of stimuli, and is exhausted by excessive stimuli. . . . [A] due equilibrium between the exciting powers, such as heat, food, air, mental exertion, etc, and the sensorial power constitutes *health*; and every variation from either, is *disease.*[13]

Of the two, Trotter seems to have inclined more towards the doctrines of Darwin, declaring *Zoonomia* 'An inestimable work; and when physicians take the trouble to peruse it, it will probably supersede other systems'.[14] And, as we shall see, Darwin's notion of sensorial power underpinned – along with the pneumatic theory of contagion – most of Trotter's subsequent work on naval medicine, his criticisms of commercial and imperial expansion, and of the Navy's system of impressment.

Trotter's experiences on being appointed Physician to the Channel Fleet were such as to confirm his belief in the explanatory power of the two chief medical doctrines on which he based his practice. While typhus and other supposedly contagious diseases were rare in the Channel Fleet – which enjoyed remarkably good health by contemporary standards – they did occur on board certain transport ships and vessels which held men newly impressed into the Navy. The former were, according to Trotter, 'generally too small and generally crowded; soldiers with a number of women and children, the whole unaccustomed to sea';[15] while overcrowding on the latter, combined with the depressed

[12] Trotter, *Medicina Nautica*, 181.
[13] Ibid., 334.
[14] Ibid., 336.
[15] Ibid., 253.

spirits of the newly impressed, enabled typhus to spread with deadly effect.[16] It was the high incidence of contagious and other diseases among impressed seamen during the campaign that first led Trotter to condemn impressment as 'a most fatal and impolitic practice' and as the single greatest cause of ill health amongst seamen.[17]

An additional factor which favoured the spread of contagious diseases among impressed men was that, being unaccustomed to naval discipline and poorly motivated, they were given to slovenly and unhygienic habits. Among regular seamen, however, or 'thorough-bred seamen' as Trotter liked to call them, discipline was no longer a problem. 'In the present improved discipline of our Navy', he claimed, 'I have never found it a very difficult business to eradicate an infectious disease, provided my directions were duly complied with.'[18] It was to this new regime of discipline that Trotter attributed the lack of typhus in the Channel Fleet,[19] as well as the comparative absence of scurvy, formerly the scourge of many a naval campaign.[20] By 'improved discipline' Trotter meant the new forms of regulation and management which had been introduced on naval vessels since the 1770s, including the wearing of uniforms.[21] The most important of these was the divisional system, in which a ship's crew was divided into squads under the superintendence of midshipmen who inspected their clothing and personal cleanliness. By the 1790s, these and other procedures had been codified into regulations which aimed at ensuring health and order in all His Majesty's ships. The effects were dramatic, ushering in what Gilbert Blane later saw as a new era in the health of the Navy, in which death rates fell sharply, giving the Royal Navy an important edge over the French and reducing national expenditure.[22]

This new disciplinary regime had much in common with those instituted contemporaneously in factories and prisons. And, in this new order, medical men played a crucial role, managing the shipboard environment and inspecting the crew to ensure that they conformed to standards of dress and cleanliness.[23] By 1800, health, discipline, and efficiency were inextricably intertwined. However, naval surgeons did not see themselves simply as managers of health, unconcerned

[16] Ibid., 44.
[17] Ibid.
[18] Ibid., 225.
[19] Ibid., 253.
[20] Ibid., 405–13. The Channel Fleet was largely exempt from scurvy except for an outbreak which affected many ships during the winter of 1794, when extreme cold destroyed many of the vegetables grown around naval ports such as Portsmouth. After this attack, the Admiralty ensured that all vessels were liberally supplied with lemons and oranges, and such fresh vegetables as were available.
[21] Ibid., 48. Trotter, for instance, wrote that 'A uniform in all situations contributes so much to personal delicacy and cleanliness, that we are at a loss to conceive how our officers have neglected it so long.'
[22] Blane, 'On the Comparative Health of the British Navy'.
[23] Lawrence, 'Disciplining Disease'.

with the particularity of their men's circumstances. As Trotter emphasized on numerous occasions, the naval surgeon was uniquely placed to hear what he termed 'narratives of individual distress', and it was his familiarity with these that sustained him in his campaign against impressment.[24] The confined 'wooden world' of a naval vessel could thus foster relations between doctor and patient of a reasonably intimate kind.

Trotter's growing hostility to the system of impressment during the French Wars was driven not by concerns about liberty but by his conviction that impressed men were far more likely than regular seamen to fall ill. While this was due in part to their lack of discipline, and the insanitary conditions in which they were kept, it stemmed also from their depressed state of mind, which acted as a 'predisposing cause' of many disorders. Impressed men, he argued, were particularly subject to certain nervous complaints, such as bilious diseases and hypochondria; being poorly motivated, they were also far more likely to 'malinger' than men accustomed to naval service. Among the devices employed by impressed men to evade duty were the use of caustics to produce ulcers, inflation of the scrotum to give the appearance of a hernia, and drinking decoctions of tobacco to induce sickness, emaciation, and quickening of the pulse.[25] But Trotter's sympathy with the plight of impressed men led to him advocate 'patience and discernment on the part of the officer and the surgeon'. Such behaviour, he counselled, should rarely be an occasion for punishment, whereas a 'well-regulated ship soon reconciles all disaffection'.[26]

We shall return to the subject of impressment in a moment, but the growing incidence of 'spasmodic' or 'nervous' affections in the Navy during the French Wars was also a symptom of what Trotter believed to be the degeneration of British stock. Referring to his naval experience and to his civil practice in Newcastle after retiring from the Navy, Trotter claimed that such disorders were becoming more common every day, sapping the vigour of a formerly proud and manly nation. In 1733, Cheyne had estimated that one-third of all maladies in England were of the 'nervous' type,[27] but in 1807, Trotter went so far as to claim that 'nervous disorders now constitute two-thirds of all disorders'.[28] Once the preserve of the nobility, nervous maladies had descended the social ladder to afflict practically the whole of society.[29]

Trotter's designation 'nervous disorders', and that of Cheyne before him, included not only manifestly nervous complaints such as 'low spirits' and irritability, but also corporeal afflictions related to over- or under-stimulation

[24] Trotter, *A Practicable Plan for Manning the Royal Navy*, 16–17.
[25] Trotter, *Medicina Nautica*, 40–1.
[26] Ibid., 41.
[27] Cheyne, *The English Malady*, ii.
[28] Trotter, *Nervous Temperament*, xvii.
[29] On the 'democratization' of nervous disorders, see Foucault, *The History of Sexuality*, vol i, 122–7; Risse, 'Hysteria at the Edinburgh Infirmary'.

of the nervous system: for example, gout, bilious disorders, indigestion, and liver complaints. Cheyne had reckoned these to be diseases primarily of the 'better ranks', but Trotter claimed that they now afflicted the poorer classes from among whom the Navy recruited its seamen.[30] He believed that the British were particularly prone to such disorders on account of the dampness and variability of their climate, but also because of their 'political institutions and free government', which they enjoyed uniquely among the European nations, not to mention the country's 'vast wealth, so diffused among all ranks of people'.[31] In Trotter's opinion, the expansion of commerce and manufacturing industry since Cheyne's day had accustomed even the lower ranks to a life of luxury and comparative indolence which threatened to sap their bodily and mental vigour.

These views were shared by other medical practitioners who saw over-consumption as a disease of modern society.[32] They included fellow naval surgeons such as James Johnson and Leonard Gillespie, but also the radical physician Thomas Beddoes and the Army surgeon Robert Jackson, who lamented the 'state of luxury' in the country and the 'depraved' appetites of the English.[33] It is surely significant that military and naval surgeons were among the most trenchant critics of social change and in one sense this is easy to account for. A military or naval career, particularly one which took men away from the country for long periods of time, was particularly conducive to the type of social criticism in which men like Trotter engaged. Protracted absence from Britain and the privations of service life threw into sharp relief the comforts enjoyed by many civilians, especially the new-rich; a theme which comes through strongly in Gillespie's correspondence, for example. The camaraderie of life in the armed forces also contrasted sharply with the selfish individualism of the new consumer society.

Of the medical authors just mentioned, Trotter's critique of British society was perhaps the most trenchant and his remedies the most radical. His *View of the Nervous Temperament* is a secular version of Man's fall from grace: from a state of nature in which his wants and diseases were few, to a state of civilization and abundance in which he had become sickly and enfeebled. The book begins with an account of the lives of hunter-gatherers whose demise was generally the result of war, accident, or 'the decay of nature', rather than of excess or debauch. In both these states, moral and physical health was inextricably intertwined: 'It is notorious', he wrote, 'that all the savage tribes of the new continent [America], when compared with European manners are observed to be chaste, temperate, and abstemious.'[34] The feudal system, he claimed, was also 'highly favourable to vigor of the body, and by consequence to health', on account of both sexes

[30] Trotter, *Nervous Temperament*, xvii.
[31] Ibid., xvii–xviii.
[32] Porter, 'Consumption'.
[33] Jackson, *Treatise on the Fevers of Jamaica*, 409.
[34] Trotter, *Nervous Temperament*, 20.

working in the fields and enjoying pastimes which prepared their minds and bodies for the fatigues of war.[35] The benefits of a simple temperate existence, he reminded his readers, were also enjoined by the biblical patriarchs, as well as in the *Iliad* and *Odyssey* of Homer.[36]

But with the progress of civilization, humanity had become corrupt and increasingly sensitive to pain and misfortune. 'The timid dispositions', he wrote, 'are apt to increase in proportion to delicacy of feeling and debility of frame. We see the truth of this as we recede from the country to the town; from the occupation of the husbandman and farmer, to that of the artisan and manufacturer; and from the rustic exposed to all the vicissitudes of weather and season, to the recluse life of the citizen.'[37] The rustic also enjoyed a simple and healthy diet, which, unlike his modern urban counterpart, was not 'inflamed or vitiated by highly seasoned dainties'. Consequently, the rustic's constitution was never, unlike his urban cousin, 'raised to excess by inordinate stimulation'. He also enjoyed the benefits of a clean and invigorating atmosphere and of vigorous exercise, which ensured that 'all his motions are performed with strength and agility'.[38]

The belief that occupation and environment moulded one's mind and body was common in the early nineteenth century. However, Trotter went into far more detail in his 'medical analysis' of society than most commentators, describing seven distinct social and occupational pathologies. Firstly, he examined the afflictions of 'literary men' who, on account of their sedentary, indoor existence, were characterized by a 'sallowness of countenance', flabbiness, weak lungs, debility, dyspepsia, melancholia, and hypochondria.[39] 'Men of business' were prone to similar complaints, but especially those, such as corpulence and gout, which were produced by over-indulgence.[40] The next group considered were 'the idle and dissipated', who were 'subjects of diseases which originate chiefly from excess and debauch', leaving them prey, if not to an early demise, then to premature senility and decrepitude. Like the literary and business community, the debauched were concentrated primarily in towns and cities, 'where all the vices that more particularly enervate the constitution and injure health, can be . . . practised long without suspicion or restraint'.[41] Many of these problems were associated with drunkenness, which Trotter considered (unlike the vast majority of doctors) to be a disease rather than a vice. In his *Essay on Drunkenness*, Trotter viewed it as a 'psychological' and medical problem, outlining the

[35] Jackson, *Treatise on the Fevers of Jamaica*, 22–3.
[36] Ibid., 23–4. The equation of prelapsarian innocence with physical health was common throughout the eighteenth century. See, for example: Oliver, *Practical Essay*, ii–iii.
[37] Trotter, *Nervous Temperament*, 25.
[38] Ibid., 27.
[39] Ibid., 41.
[40] Ibid.
[41] Ibid., 43.

chemical changes produced in the body by excessive consumption of alcohol, as well as the causes of drunkenness, among which he included fashion (amongst the rich) and compensation for disappointment (amongst the poor). In cases of drunkenness, he wrote, the doctor should attempt to identify those aspects of a patient's lifestyle that drove them to drink.[42]

The growing class of 'artificers and manufacturers' was another a cause for concern according to Trotter, for these men were often debilitated by the effects of a sedentary life, as well as from many hazards peculiar to their trade.[43] Thus miners were exposed to 'choke damp' and other noxious gases,[44] and iron workers to the fumes of their furnaces. Those employed in labouring and drudgery, however, fared somewhat better, especially if they laboured out of doors. With the exception of diseases attributable to drunkenness, to which they were prone, the afflictions of this class were as likely to be diseases of want rather than of excess. According to Trotter, the former were easier to cure, for they could be remedied simply by supplying that which was deficient, whereas diseases of excess often damaged the body irreparably.[45] Such persons were also liable to the contagious fevers that thrived in overcrowded parts of manufacturing towns such as his own city Newcastle, and it is notable that Trotter was a subscriber to and a member of the committee of the Fever Hospital, which had been founded by the former Company surgeon John Clark. However, it is unclear whether Trotter and Clark were acquainted. Although they were both members of the city's Literary and Philosophical Society and its Medical and Physical Society, Clark died shortly after Trotter appears to have settled in Newcastle.[46]

To his list of occupational categories, Trotter added persons who had returned from the colonies and women, regardless of their particular circumstances. The former had been often been debilitated by long residence in the tropics, which confirmed Trotter in his belief that the possession of colonies might be a mixed blessing to say the least.[47] Women were considered separately, for they were liable to follow current fashions which encouraged them to cultivate refinement and delicacy.[48] The effects of fashion, urbanization, and the expansion of empire and commerce, were such, according to Trotter, as to endanger Britain's

[42] Trotter, *An Essay, Medical, Philosophical, and Chemical, on Drunkenness*. For an excellent introduction to this volume, see Porter's Introduction to Trotter's *Essay... on Drunkenness*.

[43] Trotter, *Nervous Temperament*, 46.

[44] Trotter wrote specifically on this subject in his *A Proposal for Destroying the Fire and Choak Damp* (1806).

[45] Trotter, *Nervous Temperament*, 47–8.

[46] 'Report of the State of the Institution for the Cure and Prevention of Contagious Fever in Newcastle and Gateshead, for the Fourth Year, ending April 30 1808', 3, 15, Hospital Archives 58; Minutes of the Meetings of the Newcastle upon Tyne Medical and Philosophical Society, 'List of Members', Hospital Archive 15, Special Collections, Robinson Library, U of N.

[47] Trotter, *Nervous Temperament*, 48.

[48] Ibid., 49.

pre-eminence among nations. Like Cheyne,[49] he drew an analogy between the demise of Britain and the fall of ancient civilizations:

> The arms of imperial Rome subdued the world; and made that city the emporium of wealth and grandeur, drawn from all other nations. Luxury, crimes and irreligion, were soon the consequences of power overgrown, and riches abounded. And this haughty, wicked people, when they had lost their moral virtue and dignity, and with these, their physical strength, became a prey to barbarous hordes; who, undebauched by refined pleasures, found the enervated Romans an easy conquest. Let Great Britain look to this example. The East and West Indies at this moment, are a theatre of oppression and slavery, to gorge her with commercial wealth; and a district of Africa, larger than Europe, is made a field of blood, to purchase the natives for cultivating her colonies, whose produce only tends to weaken her manly character, and overwhelm her with nervous infirmities.[50]

The sickly condition of Britain was epitomized not only by the institution of slavery but by that 'puddle of corruption, the Stock Exchange', which fuelled imperial expansion and filled the nation with 'degenerate fears, apprehension, and hypochondriacism'.[51] This general state of anxiety, which the British people in their greed had brought upon themselves, compounded the physical evils of the towns, with their overcrowding, contagious diseases, and fashionable pleasures. 'Under these circumstances', Trotter warned, 'the human frame must degenerate in both body and mind, as we see in Egypt, Turkey and Italy. Thus flourishes the commercial town or state, till its wealth and effeminacy weigh it down, when it falls like Tyre or Alexandria, like Corinth or Carthage, to be a retreat to robbers; and a den to wild beasts.'[52] The problem of social degeneration would admit of no easy solution, for as Trotter emphasized, degenerate traits became more firmly entrenched as nervous disorders were passed from one generation to another.[53]

Like James Johnson, who also believed that acquired characteristics could be inherited, Trotter's views owed much to a reading of Darwin's *Zoonomia.* At this point in time, such opinions were only rarely articulated in medical texts, but within the next few decades they were to become more common, as concern

[49] Cheyne, *English Malady*, 56: 'The antient Greeks, while they lived in their Simplicity and Virtue were Healthy, Strong, and Valiant: But afterwards, in Proportion as they advanced in Learning . . . and distinguished themselves from other Nations by their Politeness and Refinement, they sank into Effeminacy, Luxury, and Diseases, and began to study Physick, to remedy those Evils which Luxury and Laziness had brought upon them. In like manner, the Romans fell from their Bravery, Courage, and heroick Virtue, which had gain'd them the Empire of the World.'

[50] Trotter, *Nervous Temperament*, 143–4.

[51] Ibid., 147–8. Here, Trotter was referring to the tendency of the City to over-react to news of even the most minor set-backs in the war against France, despite the country being free from the prospect of invasion since the Battle of Trafalgar in 1805.

[52] Ibid., 146.

[53] Ibid., 166.

mounted over the effects of industrialization on the urban poor. In 1842, the report of the Poor Law Commissioners noted that the 'assembled masses in our manufacturing towns' suffered from stunted development, their musculature impaired by work that required dexterity rather than strength, and their constitutions wrecked by impure air, poor housing, and bad food. 'This acquired constitution of body is transmitted to the offspring', the report concluded, and 'This permanent deterioration in the qualities of the race, has been clearly proved by their disqualification for those offices, where a certain standard of size and strength is required.' In other words, the military capacity of the nation was at stake: an opinion shared by Sir James McGrigor, who stated that 'A Corps levied from the Agricultural districts in Wales, or the northern counties of England, will last longer than one recruited from the manufacturing towns.'[54] In the opinion of some commentators, it seemed that the urban poor had degenerated to the point where they were indistinguishable from the 'savage' peoples of tropical lands. These analogies extended beyond the realm of behaviour to that of physique. Indeed, a number of Victorian theorists followed Blumenbach in observing resemblances between the skin colour or cranial measurements of beggars and other 'degenerates' and those of 'Ethiopians' and 'Hottentots'.[55]

But Trotter differed from many later commentators on the health of the urban poor in locating the causes of their ills firmly within the system of industrial capitalism. The architect of sanitary reform, Edwin Chadwick, tended to ascribe the causes of fevers to conditions incidental to industrialization: to filth and ignorance rather than long hours, low wages, and the drudgery of factory labour.[56] Whereas Chadwick's programme was to focus narrowly on sanitary works, Trotter's aimed at the heart of the system itself. He did not advocate merely ameliorating the ills of commercial society, as Johnson advised, but sweeping them away altogether. His starting point was nothing less than the abolition of slavery and liberty for Britain's tropical colonies, which he viewed as sources of moral and physical decay. However, he was equally concerned with the root causes of poverty and illness at home and aligned himself with influential figures who were attempting to reinvigorate rural life. In his *View of the Nervous Temperament*, Trotter applauded Sir John Sinclair's attempt to 'regenerate the physical strength of the country by recalling mankind to agricultural life', and drew attention to a society he had formed for that purpose.[57] However, Trotter was not calling for a return to feudalism; rather, he saw political freedom as being the 'hereditary right' of every Briton,[58] and more importantly, he was an advocate of agricultural modernization. Like Sinclair, who was the first president

[54] Cited in Armstrong, *Influence of Climate*, 10–11.
[55] Weber, 'Science and Society in Nineteenth Century Anthropology'.
[56] See Brown, 'Making Sense of Modernity's Maladies'; Hamlin, *Public Health and Social Justice*; Pickstone, 'Ferriar's Fever to Kay's Cholera'; idem, 'Dearth, Dirt and Fever Epidemics'.
[57] Trotter, *Nervous Temperament*, 149.
[58] Trotter, *A Practicable Plan*, 30.

of the short-lived Board of Agriculture,[59] he sought to revive rural life by harnessing and developing the most recent innovations in farming. To this end, Sinclair had formed a society including several noblemen and members of Parliament, and the President of the Royal Society, Sir Joseph Banks, to establish eight experimental arable and livestock farms in different parts of Britain, with two further upland breeding farms for the improvement of mountain sheep, and the purchase of 5,000 acres of woodland for an experiment in scientific forestry.[60] As well as advancing the standard of agriculture, the society aimed to regenerate village life by building model cottages for labourers, and providing each community with a school and playing field for children. The money for this scheme – the not inconsiderable sum of £80,000 – was to be raised by selling shares in the enterprise.[61]

Another bastion against social decay, according to Trotter, was the Navy itself:

> Amidst the general effeminacy of manners, that is rapidly consuming the manly spirit and physical strength of this age, and what may ultimately annihilate all that is great in the character of Britons, it is somewhat consoling to observe, that the seamen of the navy, that bulwark of our liberties, will be the last of the community to feel the effect of those enervating customs. The naval officer and seamen embark in their profession while boys, before they can be acquainted with the softening arts of the day.[62]

Much the same opinion was expressed by Gilbert Blane, who claimed that 'There is . . . something in the harsh sensations from the objects which seamen are in use to see, hear, and handle, which so modifies their constitutions and hardens their nerves as to make them little liable to what may be called the diseases of excessive refinement.'[63]

As the backbone of the nation, it was imperative that the Navy's strength should not be diluted by the system of impressment which was the root cause of most of its problems with discipline and disease. According to Trotter, impressment was to blame for the 'Obstinate and incurable rheumatisms' – which were one of the prevailing diseases of seamen – and for the 'contagious typhus fever' prevalent in the home station. It was among impressed men that all its predisposing and exciting causes were to be found: 'Dejection of spirits . . . exposure to

[59] For Sir John Sinclair (1754–1835), see *DNB*; Colley, *Britons*, 373–4; Hammond and Hammond, *The Village Labourer*, 36, 59ff.,74, 83ff., 157. Any affinity which Trotter may have had with Sinclair as a fellow Scot and advocate of rural regeneration may have been underpinned by Sinclair's interest in naval matters, which formed the subject of his maiden speech to Parliament in 1780.

[60] Sir John Sinclair, *The Plough, Joint Stock Farming Society*. Sinclair's interest in agricultural improvement and the reinvigoration of the Highlands stemmed from a long-standing interest in the position of the poor in British society and in public finance. See Langford, *Public Life and the Propertied Englishman*, 266, 365.

[61] Sinclair, *The Plough*, 3.

[62] Trotter, *Nervous Temperament*, 153.

[63] Blane, *Observations*, 190.

cold... sleeping on deck without a bed, no change of clothing, closed and confined lodging... and air vitiated by respiration, to a certainty give birth to contagion... such is the constant history of all crowded tenders and receiving ships.'[64]

Trotter also believed that the callous treatment of impressed men, and even of regular seamen, was the reason why many sailors took to the bottle. Slavery and commercial greed, he argued, had dulled the nation's moral sensibility: 'Has the avaricious spirit of trade so hardened the human heart in Britain, that her seamen shall plead in vain for the privileges of national beneficence?'[65] It was an ungrateful nation that spurned its heroes in this manner: how quickly were the battles of Trafalgar and the Nile forgotten on seeing a sailor stagger from a tavern. 'Here, indeed, is a lesson of humiliation to human pride', he wrote, 'for after having performed the noblest services to his country, when his purse comes to be emptied, he is thrust from the presence of his landlord like a felon, and common pity for the wretched denied him.'[66]

It was to this neglect and, in particular, to the system of impressment, that Trotter attributed the mutiny that occurred in the Channel Fleet at Spit Head in 1797. 'The founders of the mutiny', he observed, 'were men of about the middle age, married and had children. Their families were daily claiming relief from them; provisions for the two preceding years... had been enormously high [in price], and they found themselves starving. These families contrasted their situation with that of other more fortunate seamen, who had escaped impressment and were receiving from the merchants four and five pounds per month.'[67] Such events would recur, he argued, if steps were not taken to end impressment and to find a fairer method of enlistment in wartime, with pay and conditions that compensated for any loss of liberty. Peacetime conditions, too, he argued, should be made more attractive, so as to maintain a sufficient establishment of 'thorough-bred' seamen.

The potential dangers of impressment were further underlined by the difficulties faced by Britain in the war against America in 1812; a point also made by an earlier critic of impressment, Thomas Urquhart. Urquhart had argued that the Navy had been lax in recruiting good seamen in the days since Trafalgar and that it had only been shocked out of a false sense of security when it again came into contact with a navy staffed by regular seamen during the American War. Unlike impressed men, regulars were well motivated and had time to acquire the requisite technical skills. He therefore advocated a system of voluntary enlistment, in which men would be attracted to the service by fixed terms of employment,

64 Trotter, *A Practicable Plan*, 43–4.
65 Ibid., 15.
66 Ibid., 32.
67 Ibid., 22–3.

better pay and conditions of service.[68] Urquhart's pamphlet caused quite a stir, but Trotter's was the more the eloquent and the more detailed, in terms of both its analysis of the problem (which was informed by his unique insight into the condition of the men as a naval physician) and in its proposals for change.

Trotter's scheme of recruitment was based on a short-lived Act of Parliament introduced by Pitt in 1795, which set limits to the number of merchant seamen and landmen that could be impressed into naval service: one out of every seven merchant seamen or, alternatively, two landmen. The recruitment of landmen was the responsibility of the justices of each parish who were left to their own judgement as to the exact mechanism to be used. It was anticipated, however, that the system would follow closely the ballot system used for recruiting men to the militia.[69] Trotter's plans aimed at ensuring a peacetime establishment of 20,000 seamen, including marines, and a further war establishment of 93,000. The peacetime establishment was to be enlisted for fixed periods of three or five years depending on age, with the option of signing on for a further term. The landmen of the wartime establishment were to be raised like the militia by a ballot system, as under Pitt's Act, while the number of seamen that could be taken from merchant service would number no more than one in three. Those on the war establishment were to be engaged with a bounty for a period of five years, with the option of a further term and half the original payment in bounty. He also set age limits for service: a maximum age of forty-two for seamen and an age range of seventeen to thirty-six for landmen and marines.[70] This efficient, well-motivated navy would be a match for any in the world: a protector of liberty and a beacon of moral and physical health.

The impressment issue probably had wider significance for Trotter than for most others who opposed the system. Like Urquhart, he condemned impressment for reasons of naval efficiency and because he felt it to be, like slavery, an affront to humanity. Indeed, both Trotter and Urquhart drew direct parallels between impressment and slavery, and drew attention to the apparent blindness of philanthropists when it came to the plight of their own countrymen; a theme that was to resurface in the 1840s in criticisms of antislavery operations along the West African coast. Where Trotter seems to have differed from other critics of impressment is in seeing the system as a symptom and a cause of a general moral malaise. In his view, commercialism and the growth of industrial towns were undermining all that had made Britain great: the yeoman and seafaring stock which had traditionally formed the backbone of the armed forces was being driven into penury and corrupted by sensual indulgence. Trotter was thus deeply pessimistic about the direction in which modern society was heading, but he was no Rousseauian. He sought, rather, to revive the sources of Britain's prowess by

[68] Urquhart, *Substance of a Letter to Lord Viscount Melville.*
[69] Trotter, *A Practicable Plan,* 47, 56.
[70] Ibid., 61–2.

modernizing agriculture and improving conditions of service in the Navy. Whilst he had much in common with other critics of urban, industrial society, Trotter went further than most in stressing the consequences of hereditary degeneration. If drastic action were not taken, he warned, the pathological aspects of modern society would become indelibly imprinted upon the minds and bodies of the British people. By raising the spectre of irreversible degeneration, Trotter was among the first to warn of the dark possibilities of human evolution and of the moral and physical ills that would befall Britain if it retained its tropical colonies. It would seem that Alan Bewell was correct in observing that fear of 'colonial disease' shaped British culture 'to a degree that has not been adequately recognized'.[71]

[71] Bewell, *Romanticism*, xiv.

4
The prospect of invasion

The writings of Johnson, Trotter, and other military and naval surgeons evince growing unease about the influence of commerce and empire on British society. Their critiques of luxury, of the slave trade, of unaccountable and predatory imperialism, were accompanied by dire warnings about the rise of new diseases. But fear of decay from within was matched by fear of invasion from without. From the 1790s, as yellow fever took a heavy toll among British troops in the Caribbean, concern began to be expressed about the disease returning with invalids and prisoners of war. The spread of yellow fever along the eastern seaboard of the United States and the terrible epidemic in Philadelphia – much reported in Britain – provided some justification for these concerns. Even more alarming was the arrival, apparently for the first time, of yellow fever in Europe. The epidemic at Cadiz, in 1800, was the first of many outbreaks of yellow fever along the Mediterranean coast over the next two decades. The plague, too, was once again a credible threat to Western Europe. British and French troops dispatched to Egypt were badly affected by the disease, particularly the French army which lost around 2,000 men. In the early 1800s, plague also began to spread from the Levant, affecting a number of Mediterranean islands including Cyprus and Malta, which were now of strategic importance to Britain. Finally, there was the threat posed by entirely new diseases: first, a mysterious eye infection (ophthalmia), which spread in Britain following the return of troops from Egypt;[1] second, the dreaded 'Asiatic Cholera' which had already claimed the lives of thousands of Britons in India. Cholera did not arrive in Western Europe until 1831–2, but during the 1820s, concern mounted as the disease spread inexorably across Asia towards Europe, killing thousands in Russia and the Ottoman Empire.

All of these diseases were linked in some way to colonial expansion; to slavery, commerce, and imperial rivalry. Just as her wealth threatened to undermine Britain from the inside, her position at the centre of an expansive commercial and imperial network left her vulnerable to invasion from disease. The threat was

[1] See Kelly, '"Not Surgeons Alone"', chap. 3.

real enough, but anxiety about a return of pestilence to Albion's shores also had roots in the ambivalence, if not hostility, with which some Britons had come to view their place in the world. Commercial intercourse and war had long been associated with the arrival of disease, and pestilence now loomed as a judgement on the sins of men, whether they were greed or unprincipled aggression.

Medical practitioners with first-hand experience of exotic diseases had much to say on these matters and, as the perceived dangers to Britain increased, their professional colleagues, the government, and the public at large, began to take note of what they had to say. They did not, however, speak with one voice. The question of whether or not yellow fever was a contagious disease, and thus of whether it was likely to appear in Britain, was one of the most divisive issues in British medicine from the 1790s to at least the 1850s. Debates over the communicability of plague and cholera were equally heated, not least because they, too, were politically charged. All issues within medicine are political in the sense that they are inseparable from questions of professional authority and that was certainly true of debates over contagion, which pitched the surgeons of the military and naval establishments against elite metropolitan physicians. The contagiousness of yellow fever, cholera, and plague were, however, political issues in a more obvious sense. For practical purposes, the issue of contagion was inseparable from that of quarantine: Britain's traditional defence against epidemic invasion. The tension between safeguarding public health and fostering commerce made quarantine inherently controversial and, in an era of revolution and reform, it was regarded by many as oppressive and inhumane.

Practitioners who had witnessed epidemics of these diseases did not always agree about their aetiology or how to prevent them. But the net effect of their intervention in these debates was to shift professional opinion against contagion, at least in terms of the free transmission of disease between human beings and merchandize. If they regarded such diseases as contagious, the majority saw contagion as contingent upon other factors, particularly climate. Most colonial practitioners were of the opinion that epidemics behaved in a law-like way and that they could be understood just like other natural phenomena. Their first-hand knowledge of diseases such as plague and yellow fever suggested a more 'rational' alternative to quarantine: the possibility of preventing epidemics either by manipulation of the environment and/or forms of personal protection.

Some historians have argued that these 'anticontagionist' views were closely aligned with political ideologies. That those of a liberal disposition, champions of free trade, opponents of political and professional tyranny, were among the most ardent critics of quarantine and the doctrine of contagion. Authoritarian governments and their medical officials, by contrast, favoured quarantine as a means of upholding the integrity of their borders and enhancing the power of the state.[2]

[2] Ackerknecht, 'Anticontagionism'.

Opposition to quarantine and the theory of contagion certainly harmonized with liberal politics and the objectives of some manufacturing and mercantile groups.[3] Indeed, there was a fairly strong association between attitudes towards contagion and political views.[4] But professional and political opinions did not always coincide; nor were political affiliations the only factors that may have had a bearing on the vexed issue of contagion. Anticontagionism was a badge of professional identity as much as a political statement; it set out the knowledge claims of practitioners who had spent their formative years in the armed forces and, more often than not, overseas. The challenge to the doctrine of contagion was therefore symbolic of the attempt by colonial practitioners to establish the primacy of experience – of direct observation – over what they regarded as the speculative hypotheses of metropolitan physicians. In this, the final chapter of the book, we explore these debates through a case study of yellow fever: a disease which provoked impassioned debate in British medicine, much as it did in France and the new American republic.

In the early eighteenth century, it was common to think of 'yellow fever' as a contagious disease. Like plague, it appeared in epidemics that were relatively infrequent, making it easier to conceive of the disease as alien and imported. When epidemics of a peculiarly malignant kind raged in the West Indies, quarantine was sometimes imposed against vessels sailing from there to North America and Britain, just as it was against ships from plague-infected ports in the Mediterranean.[5] But surgeons posted to tropical regions during the Seven Years War began to express doubts about the contagious nature of yellow fever and many came to see it as merely a severe form of remittent fever: a disease said to be common in all hot climates. This shift in opinion is clearly illustrated by the trajectory of James Lind's writings on the nature of yellow fever. In his essay on the diseases of seamen, published in 1757, Lind declared that the common fever that affected all hot countries was 'extremely different from what is called the Yellow Fever or black Vomit, which is rare, and takes places only among a Few, on their first Arrival in the West Indies'.[6] In this and in the second edition of his book, Lind did nothing more than to acknowledge received wisdom on the disease and shared the prevailing opinion that it was contagious, particularly in confined spaces. Although he did not equate yellow fever with plague, he conceived of it as contagious in the manner of other putrid fevers in jails, ships, and hospitals. In other words, it appeared to be spread by the breath of the sick.[7] Within a few years, however, Lind had changed his mind. In his pivotal *Essay on Diseases Incidental to Europeans in Hot Climates* (1768), published five

[3] See Baldwin, *Contagion and the State.*
[4] Cooter, 'Anticontagionism'.
[5] Slack, *The Impact of Plague*, 342.
[6] Lind, *Essay*, 1808 edn., 49–51.
[7] As in the work of Pringle, Huxham, and Cleghorn, among others. See Part I.

years after the end of the war, he was 'now of opinion, that the remarkable dissolution of the blood, the violent haemorrhages, the black vomit, and the other symptoms which characterize the yellow fever, are only accidental appearances in the common fever of the West Indies'. According to Lind, these symptoms proceeded from a 'peculiar unhealthfulness of the air', aggravated by constitutional factors and immoderate behaviour.[8] 'Yellow fever', in other words, was neither a distinct disease, nor a contagious one.

Lind's opinions changed after his appointment as Physician to the naval hospital at Haslar, where he treated large numbers of invalids returning from campaigns in the Caribbean. By the 1760s, the conviction among military and naval surgeons that most of the diseases they encountered were climatic in origin had made an impression on Lind, who valued experience and careful observation over theory. One of those who insisted that yellow fever was not a separate disease was Dr Huck, who considered the malady to be a variety of the common autumnal fever which affected most regions to some degree. However, in tropical countries he believed that it was rendered more inflammatory and more putrid by the intensity of heat, especially in confined localities where the air was of poor quality.[9] In his Edinburgh MD thesis of 1764, James Makittrick also stressed the atmospheric causes of yellow fever, attributing it to air which was humid, stagnant, and corrupt.[10] Makittrick's was one of the more influential Edinburgh MD theses of the period and was considered to be a reliable guide to the pathology and aetiology of yellow fever, if not always to its treatment.[11]

In the two decades after the Seven Years War, most of those who wrote about yellow fever on the basis of personal experience insisted that it was not contagious and that it was difficult to distinguish from common varieties of fever.[12] This belief in the underlying unity of fevers and their climatic origins continued to dominate medical literature on the West Indies during and after the American War of Independence. The military surgeon John Hunter, for instance, claimed that there was an 'intimate connection' between the fevers of all climates and that there was often 'interchange' between them. He therefore concluded that all fevers 'seem to depend on the same cause, perhaps differently modified'; that is, on exhalations from low and marshy ground.[13] Benjamin Moseley, whom later writers such as Trotter credited with having given the best clinical account of the malady, also maintained that yellow fever was not a contagious disease, finding

[8] Lind, *Essay*, 128, 133, 136.

[9] Huck communicated these views to Pringle, shortly after his return from the West Indies. Papers of Sir John Pringle, annotations on Hillary's *Observations*, ff. 430–1, 2 October 1762, RCPE.

[10] Makittrick, *Dissertatio medica inauguralis*, 24–6.

[11] Comments of Dr Macnamara on Makittrick's *Dissertatio*, March 1769, f. 272, Papers of Sir John Pringle, RCPE.

[12] e.g. Blicke, *Essay*, 1, 5.

[13] Hunter, *Observations*, 15.

accounts of its introduction into the West Indian islands implausible because of the apparent immunity of long-standing residents.[14] To the extent that yellow fever was considered contagious, most authors granted personal contact a minimal role, claiming that the disease could be spread only within confined spaces by the breath of the sick.[15] Pringle, Cleghorn, and Huxham all took this view,[16] as did William Cullen, who taught many of those practitioners entering the military and naval services.[17]

The mid- to late eighteenth century, then, brought a growing interest in the subject of yellow fever, largely as a result of its consequences for military and naval expeditions. Most of the literature on yellow fever at this time tended to minimize the role played by contagion, even if it did not reject it altogether. After 1793, yellow fever figured even more prominently in medical discussions following the heavy losses sustained by the British and French armies in the Caribbean, not to mention the epidemic in Philadelphia. James Bryce, formerly of the East India Company's Marine, was among many who recalled the depressing effects that the disease had upon the morale of soldiers and their families, who, 'instead of cherishing the hope of seeing them return with victory and honour, think of them merely as so many victims, devoted to disease and death'.[18] As might be expected, the epidemics of yellow fever also exercised the naval reformer Thomas Trotter who declared that:

> The ravages which this fatal Disease have made, during the present war, in our fleets and armies, are beyond all precedent.... It has offered the severest obstacles to military operations, which the history of modern warfare can produce: the chief victims of its fury being the young, the robust, and those free from other diseases; by which means a campaign in the West Indies is now considered as little better than a *forlorn hope.*[19]

Elliot Arthy's *The Seaman's Advocate* (1798) was devoted precisely to this problem and he warned of its implications 'To a nation like Great Britain', which was

> dependent on the number, the goodness, and the valour of her seamen, for her protection from foreign enemies, and whose commerce extends into almost every known part of the world, the increase and preservation of her seamen must be, at all times, very highly desirable and necessary, but now that the nation is engaged in war with all the greatest maritime Powers of Europe, and actually threatened with invasion, they become... objects of immediate and most serious concern to every honest Englishman.[20]

[14] Moseley, *Tropical Diseases*, 1789 edn., 390–1, 401.
[15] e.g. White, *De febre remittente*, 3–4.
[16] Huxham, *Essay on Fevers*; Cleghorn, *Observations*, 121–2.
[17] Lectures of William Cullen, f. 114, Cullen Papers, 29, RCPE.
[18] Bryce, *An Account of the Yellow Fever*, 1–2.
[19] Trotter, *Medicina Nautica*, 322.
[20] Arthy, *The Seaman's Advocate*, i.

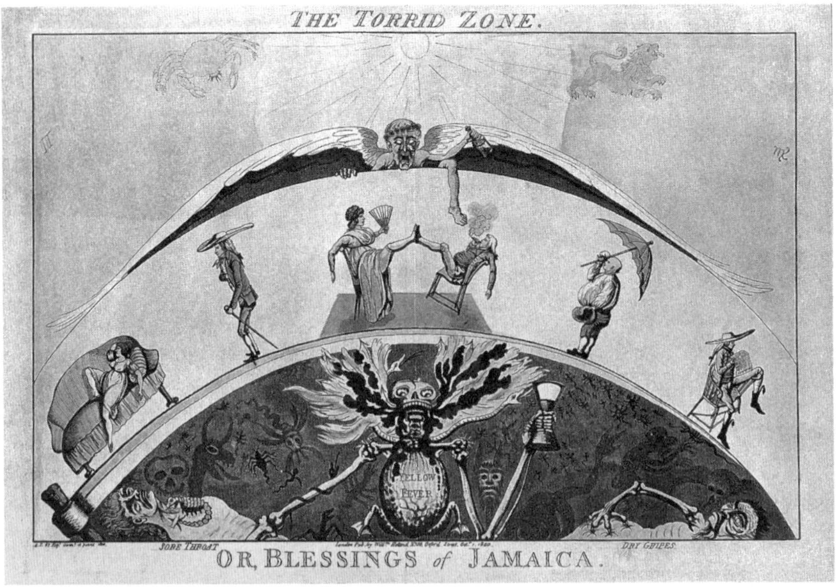

III.3. The Torrid Zone

According to Arthy, yellow fever claimed the lives of 5,000 seamen annually, if both the Navy and merchant marine were taken into account. This is a truly staggering figure, even by contemporary standards, and yet these losses were largely preventable, he insisted. In his opinion, yellow fever was not a disease in its own right, but a deadly variety of the remittent fever found throughout the tropics. It was not contagious, he argued, but arose from the action of climate upon tropical vegetation. The resulting miasma acted powerfully upon men whose constitutions had been impaired by fatigue, intemperance, poor discipline, and lack of skilled medical attendance.[21] Like Trotter, he argued that if the Navy were to abolish the system of impressment and improve its conditions of service, it could do much to prevent sailors dying from the disease.[22]

Arthy's views were typical of much of the literature on yellow fever over the next two decades, which continued to articulate climatic theories developed earlier in the century. But a powerful minority continued to insist that the disease was contagious and this included some of the most senior officers in the Army and Navy medical departments; men such as Sir Gilbert Blane and Sir James McGrigor. Through these men and some of the authors they championed, we can gain some useful insights into the mindset of those who upheld

[21] Ibid., 1–5, 20.
[22] Ibid., 154–5, 219.

the doctrine of contagion in respect of yellow fever and who saw quarantine as the preventive measure of choice. Perhaps the most important observation which can be made of their views is that they were compatible with those of the ruling elite. Support for quarantine was often espoused in the same breath as patriotic sentiments and was firmly entrenched among the ruling coalition of king's friends, Old Whigs, and Pittite Tories that dominated British politics at the turn of the nineteenth century.[23] For this reason, a robust stance in defence of quarantine was a prerequisite for appointment to the highest medical offices.

Like his patron, the Duke of Wellington, McGrigor was a Tory, as were many other military surgeons who benefited from their patronage. While this is by no means true of the Army's medical establishment as a whole, many of those served in the French Revolutionary and Napoleonic Wars can be aptly described as 'conservative progressives': firm believers in a social hierarchy tempered by meritocracy.[24] Patriotic sentiments may have fostered social unity, but they also generated expectations for change; even if only for a more porous and accommodating elite.[25] Although he was never a member of the Royal College of Physicians and had benefited from the removal of its placemen on the old Army Medical Board, McGrigor's opinions on the issue of contagion put him well within the bounds of respectable opinion. As far as most fellows of the College were concerned, this meant a commitment to quarantine and the doctrine of contagion. Indeed, McGrigor's opinions on contagion strengthened as his career progressed. In his *Medical Sketches on the Expedition to Egypt* (1804), he favoured the view that plague was contagious and recommended a range of preventive measures which included quarantine and the isolation of victims. But as a comparatively junior surgeon, he shied away from controversy, stating 'I have no intention of entering on the discussion of theories of contagion; an obscure subject on which I do not presume to think that I can throw any new light.'[26] He was later to become more definite in his opinions about contagion and became a stalwart defender of quarantine, perhaps because he had ascended to circles in which such views would have been dominant if not *de rigueur*.

Blane was of a similar persuasion. Though not a fellow of the Royal College, he was very much a society physician and possessed an enviable list of aristocratic patients. The dukes of Devonshire, Manchester, and Richmond, the Earl of Malmesbury, and Lord Chatham were among his many distinguished clients.[27] Blane was prominent in court circles, too, and in 1785 he was appointed Physician-Extraordinary to the Prince of Wales and later became Physician-

[23] For a recent survey of scholarship on the decline of radicalism in Britain following the advent of war with France, see Macleod, 'British Attitudes to the French Revolution'.

[24] Ackroyd et al., *Advancing with the Army*, 198–202, 318.

[25] Colley, *Britons*, 318–19.

[26] M'Gregor, *Medical Sketches*, 68.

[27] See Gilbert Blane to James Harris, the 1st Earl of Malmesbury, 22 June 1801, 9M73 183/75, Hampshire County Record Office.

in-Ordinary to the king's household. On the accession of George IV, he was appointed Physician to the king. In part, these appointments were due to good fortune: he had met the Duke of Clarence while serving in the Navy. But they also owed something to his upbringing. Compared with most naval surgeons, Blane was from a relatively well-to-do background, the fourth son of a wealthy Ayrshire merchant. His religious orientation also appears to have been Church of Scotland rather than one of the Dissenting sects from which Scottish surgeons typically hailed. However, his religious views were somewhat unorthodox and it seems that he declined a career in the Church on religious scruples. Switching to medicine, he excelled as a student at Edinburgh University, where he was elected president of the students' medical society. He left Edinburgh without a degree but moved to Glasgow University, where he took his MD in 1778. At Glasgow, he was a protégé of William Cullen, who recommended Blane to William Hunter in London. Through Hunter, Blane was able to secure a position as private physician to the statesman Lord Holderness and then to Admiral Lord Rodney, accompanying the latter to the West Indies when he took command of the naval squadron dispatched there in 1780. Blane's background and his mode of entry into naval service were therefore different from most surgeons' and his connections enabled him to rise rapidly in his chosen profession. It was largely through Rodney's influence that he was appointed to the position of Physician to St Thomas's Hospital and, in 1796, to the head of the Navy Medical Board.[28]

Moving in these exalted circles, Blane was well placed to influence the actions of government. It was Blane, for example, who devised the quarantine regulations under which the Army was allowed to return from Egypt following the plague epidemic there.[29] He was also a staunch advocate of quarantine in the case of cholera, the spread of which, he observed, closely followed routes of overland and maritime trade. On this matter he corresponded with the Duke of Richmond, who endorsed Blane's contagionism and who formulated directions for the Board of Health created to deal with the impending emergency in 1831.[30] Both Blane and McGrigor could also use their positions to advance or retard the careers of ambitious young surgeons and this helps to explain the bitterness with which disputes over contagion and quarantine were usually conducted. Some protagonists would have been in the invidious position of having to choose between their professional convictions and their career.

The intense debates over the contagiousness of yellow fever which raged through the 1790s and early 1800s can be traced to the publication in 1794 of two treatises which had come to very different conclusions. The most famous of

28 Wallace, 'Blane'.
29 Ibid.
30 Blane, 'Warning to the British Public against the Alarming Approach of the Indian Cholera', 9–21; Blane to the Duke of Richmond, 18 October 1831, 28 November 1831, 30 November 1831, 6 January 1832, Goodwood MSS 1450; Richmond to Blane, 17 October 1831, 18 October 1831, 18 January 1832, Goodwood MSS 1486, West Sussex Record Office.

these is Dr Benjamin Rush's book on the fever that afflicted Philadelphia, shortly after the arrival of French refugees fleeing the slave revolt on St Domingue.[31] Rush's treatise did not rule out the role of contagion altogether but declared that its role was minimal, the disease being spread only at close quarters and in unventilated conditions. The chief cause of the outbreak, he argued, was not importation but the mouldering of coffee left on the city's wharves. Abnormal weather had caused the coffee to putrefy, giving rise to a noxious miasma.[32] The other book was Dr Colin Chisholm's account of the yellow fever epidemic which he witnessed while a surgeon with the Royal Artillery in Grenada, in 1793. Unlike Rush, Chisholm considered yellow fever to be new to the island and attempted to prove that the disease had been imported from Bulam, on the west coast of Africa. One of the key facts adduced by Chisholm to support his argument was the immunity of those who had survived an initial attack, which he likened to immunity from smallpox: a disease almost universally regarded as contagious.[33] Unlike Rush, who saw no need for quarantine, Chisholm saw it as a wise precaution, taking much the same view as the prominent physician Patrick Russell in his recent *Treatise of the Plague* (1791). Like his younger brother Alexander, Patrick Russell used his direct experience of the disease in the Levant to caution against the removal of quarantine in Britain.[34]

Several historians have commented on the close relationship between Rush's view of the Philadelphia epidemic and his political beliefs. An Edinburgh graduate, Rush was a close associate of several Edinburgh alumni who were noted for their radical politics as well as their attacks on quarantine, contagion, and other prevailing orthodoxies in medicine.[35] He took a keen interest in the British literature on fevers and admired the work of Jackson, Pinckard, and M'Lean. All these writers viewed 'yellow fever' as a variety of the common remittent fever of the West Indies and therefore as non-contagious.[36] Rush was also a signatory to the Declaration of Independence,[37] and believed that quarantine was not only medically unjustified but an attack upon liberty and free trade. He shared this position with British and American contributors to such journals

31 See Powell, *Bring Out Your Dead*; Coleman, *Yellow Fever.*

32 Rush, *An Account of the Bilious Remitting Fever.*

33 Chisholm, *Essay.*

34 Russell, *A Treatise of the Plague.*

35 Shortly after graduating from Edinburgh, Rush was introduced by Dr Huck to the small circle surrounding Pringle in London. He afterwards maintained a correspondence with a number of British reformers, often on the subject of quarantine. These included some non-medical men such as the prison reformer John Howard. Most of Rush's correspondents shared his opposition to quarantine against yellow fever, with the notable exception of John Coakley Lettsom. See letters to Howard and Lettsom in Butterfield (ed.), *Letters,* 14 October 1789 and 13 May 1804, vol. 1, 527; vol. 2, 880.

36 Rush to John Syng Dorsey, 23 May 1804, and to James Craik, 26 July 1798, in Butterfield (ed.), *Letters,* vol. 1, 883; vol. 2, 880.

37 Haakonssen, *Medicine and Morals in the Enlightenment,* 214–16.

as New York's *Medical Repository* and the proceedings of the *Manchester Literary and Philosophical Society*, an organization of which he was a member.[38]

The position taken by Rush was that of the majority of his fellow Republicans, as the infant republic began to cleave into what became the first party system.[39] Their opponents, the Hamiltonian Federalists, blamed the epidemic on the arrival of French refugees, whereas the vast majority of Republican practitioners opposed the theory of importation.[40] With Rush, the latter insisted that the disease had resulted from miasmas in unsanitary areas around the docks. Party leaders exploited the medical controversy, the Federalists using contagion as a pretext to back demands for the exclusion of French immigrants, who were supposed to harbour revolutionary sympathies. Republicans and their many allies among the city's merchants also believed that the importation theory was a ruse to wreck their lucrative trade with the Caribbean. It was the Federalist position that ultimately won the day, perhaps because the Republican alternative – a home-grown plague – offended patriotic sensibilities.[41] Northern cities such as Philadelphia, Baltimore, and New York, which had removed quarantine restrictions thus reintroduced them, although the severity of their regimes varied considerably, remaining considerably more lenient in Baltimore than in New York, for example.[42]

Chisholm, by contrast, seems to have had no connection to radical societies and did not espouse overtly political views. After graduating MD from Aberdeen in 1793, he worked in Grenada for several years and owned a plantation in Demerara. In 1796, he was appointed acting surgeon to the Army in Grenada and appears to have become Inspector-General of Hospitals in the West Indies. After Demerara returned to Dutch sovereignty in 1801, Chisholm moved to Bristol, where he established a lucrative private practice. In the course of his career, he became a member of several prestigious learned societies in Europe and North America, including the Royal Society of London, the Physical and Natural Historical Society of Geneva, the Helvetic Society for the Promotion of Science in Switzerland, and the Medical and Natural Societies of New York and Philadelphia.[43] His last years were spent in Geneva, where he wrote his final book,

38 See, for example, Rush's correspondence with Thomas Jefferson, James Madison, and John Adams: 6 October 1800, 23 June 1801, 14 August 1805, in Butterfield (ed.), *Letters*, vol. 2, 826, 835, 901. Rush was an honorary member of the Manchester Literary and Philosophical Society and sent papers to its meetings. See *Memoirs of the Manchester Literary and Philosophical Society*, vol. 2 (1785), 506–7; vol. 3 (1790), x–xi.

39 e.g. Academy of Medicine of Philadelphia, *Proof of the Origin of the Yellow Fever.*

40 e.g. A Philadelphian, *Occasional Essays on the Yellow Fever.*

41 Pernick, 'Politics, Parties and Pestilence'.

42 Duffy, *A History of Public Health in New York City*, 97–150; Coleman, *Yellow Fever*; Travis Howard Jr, *Public Health Administration and the Natural History of Disease in Baltimore*, 56–62; Baltimore City Health Department, *The First Thirty-Five Annual Reports*–see especially reports of 1825, 1827, 1828, 1829, 1830.

43 Goodwin, *rev.* Reznick, 'Chisholm, Colin (c. 1747–1825)'.

A Manual of the Climate and Diseases of Tropical Countries (1822), in which he reiterated his belief in the contagious nature of yellow fever and the need for quarantine to protect cities in Europe and the eastern seaboard of America. He credited the quarantine laws introduced in New York in 1805 with having protected that city from epidemics, whereas ports without quarantine, such as Charlestown, South Carolina, continued to be affected.[44]

Chisholm's career is in many ways typical of those men who reached the higher echelons of medicine in Britain without the benefit of an Oxford or Cambridge degree, and who were therefore excluded from fellowship of the Royal College of Physicians. By the early 1800s, several practitioners from the Army and Navy had achieved notoriety through their military exploits and publications; some, like Lind and Johnson, had even become royal physicians. Chisholm did not join that charmed circle, but he made a good living for himself after leaving the Army and was widely esteemed in Britain and overseas. His advancement may have owed something to his relationship to McGrigor – also a graduate of Aberdeen – who is one of the people to whom his book was dedicated; the other being Frederick, Duke of York, was Commander-in-chief of the British Army. Many practitioners dedicated their monographs to McGrigor but, in this case, the dedication reveals a deeper relationship reflecting their similar outlook on the causes of yellow fever and plague. McGrigor was one of several physicians who offered support for Chisholm's contention that yellow fever was contagious and that the disease was a form of typhus. In 1796, he wrote to Chisholm affirming that 'I myself entertain no doubt that the fever which I saw in Grenada in the year 1796, and which proved so destructive to the army there, was communicated by contagion.'[45] Chisholm also received support from Dr Wright, another physician on the staff of the Army in the West Indies from 1793 to 1798,[46] but McGrigor's support was crucial because of the position that he was to attain after serving with Wellington in the Peninsula. McGrigor was a valuable source of patronage and Chisholm remained close to him and the Army long after he had retired.

Chisholm's career is typical in the sense that his support for contagion assisted his professional advancement. His views were therefore compatible with official attitudes towards quarantine and with the stance of the Royal College of Physicians. By the early 1800s, the opinions of the College were by no means uniform, but they still tended towards contagionism in yellow fever and plague. At any rate, to insist on the contagiousness of these diseases did no harm to a practitioner's career and was probably essential for anyone aspiring to rise to the top of the Army medical department or any official position in civilian life. Epidemic disease was synonymous with disorder and the importation of alien

[44] Chisholm, *Manual*, 24–5.
[45] Quoted ibid., 191.
[46] Ibid., 190.

maladies was feared for much the same reasons as 'alien' revolutionary ideas. When William Pitt, who had presided over the wars against France and the repression of dissent in Britain, died in 1806, the inscription upon his monument at London's Guildhall read: 'In an age when the contagion of ideals threatened to dissolve the forms of civil society, he rallied the loyal, the sober-minded and the good around the venerable structure of the English monarchy.' Whether ideological or epidemiological, contagion was regarded as a serious threat to social order and needed to be eradicated using drastic means if necessary. The anti-combination legislation of the Pitt era and the reactionary conservatism of the Liverpool administration of 1811–27 was the government's answer to the former. Its ready resort to and defence of quarantine was its answer to the latter. As well as seeming to be justified by Britain's long freedom from plague, quarantine provided a means of controlling the movement of peoples across and within national borders. Conservatives were therefore instinctively attracted to it and it was anathema to most radicals for the same reasons.

In the Navy, however, the situation was rather more complicated. Most of its senior physicians, like Blane, believed yellow fever to be contagious and approved of the use of quarantine to prevent its spread. But its operations were sometimes adversely affected by quarantine and the view that yellow fever was easily communicable was, to say the least, inconvenient. As we shall see in a moment, this left scope for the promotion of non-contagionists to some senior positions within the medical department, while placing some of those who believed yellow fever to be contagious at odds with the Lords of the Admiralty. A measure of concern over the contagious nature of yellow fever is the discussion which took place at the Admiralty in 1796. In August of that month, Dr Johnston, the Commissioner for Sick and Wounded Seamen at Portsmouth, informed the Admiralty of the alarm raised in the neighbourhood from the dread of yellow fever and other infectious diseases being introduced by prisoners expected to arrive from the West Indies, following the conclusion of operations on St Domingue.[47] The Admiralty responded by ordering that a report be sent to them as soon as ships carrying prisoners arrived off of Portsmouth, so that the necessary precautions could be taken. In the event, the Admiralty was reassured that there were no cases of 'violent contagious disease' among the prisoners and that all cases of fever were of a 'mild and common type'.[48] The fear of infection from without may have been particularly pronounced in 1796 because of heightened fears of a French invasion. In that year, detailed plans were made for the defence of southern England, marking the first of a number of invasion scares which fuelled an atmosphere of suspicion and dread, but also of stolid patriotism.[49] But public concern over the importation of yellow fever from

[47] In letters from the Sick and Hurt Board, 19 August 1796, ADM/F/27, NMM.
[48] 26 October 1796, ADM/F/27, NMM.
[49] Bryant, *The Years of Endurance*, 166, 221–9, 234–5, 341–2; Philip (ed.), *Resisting Napoleon*.

Africa and the Caribbean outlasted war with the French. In ports which had regular contact with the Caribbean, such as Portsmouth and Southampton, there was periodic unrest sparked by rumours of yellow fever on board visiting ships for the remainder of the century.[50] Apart from the immediate danger of infection, yellow fever scares may have expressed anxieties about the transgression of the implicit boundaries which were beginning to define British identity and which ordered the new imperial world.[51] In view of this, it is not surprising that the populations of port cities in regular contact with tropical lands should have continued to lean instinctively towards quarantine despite growing opposition from mercantile elites.[52] At a popular level, then, as well as in government circles, there was a sense that yellow fever was in some sense contagious. Indeed, in the 1790s, opposition to contagion and quarantine outside of the medical profession seems to have been confined largely to sections of the mercantile community and some humanitarian reformers, such as John Howard, who drew attention to the inefficiency of and abuses perpetrated in lazarettos, especially those in the Mediterranean.[53]

Howard did not advocate the abolition of quarantine but campaigned for the reform of institutions in accordance with humane and rational principles. Hostility towards France and the Mediterranean powers may also have contributed to discontent with present arrangements. From the enactment of Britain's first plague statute in 1711, opponents had equated quarantine with despotic Continental regimes and some had claimed that the doctrine of contagion had been fabricated by the papacy to exclude certain delegates from the Council of Trent. This convenient fiction, as they saw it, had been perpetuated by the Catholic powers to justify oppressive measures from which they profited at the expense of British merchants.[54] Some of these writers, notably Dale Ingram, drew an analogy between plague and yellow fever, and insisted that both were due primarily to atmospheric factors. Such diseases could be communicable under certain conditions, he admitted, but the colder climate of northern Europe formed a barrier which ensured that it would seldom be invaded, except under exceptional meteorological conditions. A surgeon and man-midwife, Ingram had practised medicine in Barbados for six years, where he observed that the diseases affecting Europeans were due largely to the effects of putrid effluvia on constitutions unsuited to the climate.[55]

[50] e.g. *The Lancet*, 22 January 1853, 99.

[51] In this sense, anxiety over yellow fever was not dissimilar to that expressed about leprosy some decades later, although it lacked the latter's close association with moral and physical degeneration. See Edmond, *Leprosy and Empire*.

[52] Baldwin, *Contagion*, 198.

[53] Howard, *An Account of the Principal Lazarettos in Europe*.

[54] e.g. Manningham, *A Discourse concerning the Plague*.

[55] Ingram, *An Historical Account of the several Plagues*, 68–70, 73–4, 99–100, 119, 139.

Rush's work on the epidemic at Philadelphia appeared at a time when sections of the British public were growing accustomed to reading attacks on contagion and quarantine, and his arguments received favourable mention in some organs of the non-medical press.[56] The initial reaction of the medical profession, however, was to avoid siding with either Rush or Chisholm; largely, it seems, in order to deflect accusations of partisanship or *a priori* judgement. This was particularly true of practitioners who had returned from St Domingue, such as the surgeon James Clark. Clark stressed that he had been 'cautious not to peruse any of the publications which have appeared on the same subject' and that his opinions were the result of twenty-five years' of constant practice in the West Indies.[57] Nevertheless, his conclusions were broadly similar to those of Rush, in that he denied that yellow fever had ever been imported. During epidemics of the disease, he observed, many had been exempt from it, including those that had attended the sick. If the disease had become contagious it had done so only in peculiar circumstances, in which there was a high concentration of vitiated air.

In accounting for the epidemic on St Domingue, Clark drew on the pneumatic chemistry of the French natural philosopher, Fourcroy, who stressed the role of what he termed 'mephitic gases' in disease.[58] The severity of the epidemic, he argued, was due to rarefaction of the air, which had caused the 'vital' part of the atmosphere to rise above the heavier or 'mephitic' stratum, which was unfit for respiration. Into this deranged atmosphere came thousands of men already suffering from exhaustion, who were kept crowded together in air contaminated with mephitic exhalations.[59] Clark speculated whether such concentrations of mephitic gas might, in future, be purified by the burning of brimstone or other combustible substances in the holds of ships, hospitals, and other confined spaces.[60]

A slightly different approach was taken by the military surgeon Hector M'Lean. M'Lean was thoroughly conversant with recent literature on yellow fever, but maintained that the disease on St Domingue was quite different from the epidemic in Philadelphia or the Bulam fever described by Chisholm.[61] The fever that had ravaged St Domingue, he insisted, was neither highly pestilential nor contagious; rather, his experience had convinced him that it was merely 'the common Remittent Endemic of that Country, applied to the English constitution, and accompanied occasionally with yellowness, as an accidental symptom'.[62] The assumption that the disease was contagious, he warned, had

[56] Review of Rush's *Account of the Bilious Remitting Fever*, *Gentleman's Magazine*, 64 (1794), 838–40.
[57] Clark, *Treatise on the Yellow Fever*, v–vi.
[58] Fourcroy, 'Preliminary Discourse', *Elements of Natural History*.
[59] Clark, *Yellow Fever*, 61–2.
[60] Ibid., 68.
[61] M'Lean, *Enquiry*, v–vi.
[62] Ibid., viii–ix.

harmed recruitment to the Army, 'by terrifying young men from enlisting in any West India regiment'.[63] The main cause of the epidemic, he insisted, had been miasmata entering the human body, perhaps through the skin, or perhaps through the lungs or saliva, where it had a depressing effect upon nervous vitality. As nervous power diminished the vascular system became weaker, causing an irregular determination of blood to the organs and the head.[64] M'Lean took the view that noxious vapours had a more detrimental effect upon Europeans than on African slaves. Young men, who had the most plethoric and irritable dispositions, were particularly liable to their influence and the typical soldier's diet tended to aggravate the problem. As a preventive measure he recommended anything calculated to reduce inflammation, including a diet low in meat. Incoming troops fed on such a diet – preferably over the age of thirty-five and 'seasoned' *en route* at Gibraltar – had little to fear, he argued, provided they were housed in clean, dry quarters and prevented from mixing with troops already stationed on the island.[65] Where the latter had occurred, it had tended to produce indiscipline and intemperance, both of which were productive of disease.[66]

The message of surgeons returning from St Domingue thus tended to be reassuring; the heavy toll taken by 'yellow fever' was not the result of some capricious contagion but the effects of climate upon bodies ill prepared to withstand it. As such, the great mortality experienced by British troops was largely preventable provided that due attention was paid to selection of men and the preservation of their health. But practitioners with West Indian experience did not always agree. The eminent physician William Wright, a Fellow of the Royal College of Physicians of Edinburgh and of the Royal Society of that city and of London, had been asked to report on the disease by the London physician Maxwell Garthshore. His report confirmed the position taken by the majority of physicians, but unlike them, Wright had many years experience in the West Indies, where he had been a Physician to the Army. Contradicting those who claimed that diseases in tropical countries were never contagious, Wright claimed to have seen many such instances and insisted that the 1793 epidemics were a case in point. 'Dr Rush has classed this disorder with remittents', he observed, 'but every one who has practised in the West Indies, knows for certain, that the remitting fevers of warm countries are not contagious.' In Wright's view, there was no doubt that yellow fever was not a species of remitting fever but a kind of typhus, 'exalted to a great degree of virulence from climate, situation, and other adventitious circumstances'.[67] 'All the letters I have had from my medical

63 M'Lean, *Enquiry*, ix.
64 Ibid., 24, 27.
65 Ibid., 13, 37, 39–40, 186–7.
66 Ibid., 192–200, 202–3.
67 Wright, 'Practical Observations', 6–7.

friends agree', he wrote, 'that this fever is highly contagious, and that new comers are most subject to it.'[68]

Wright's friends were untypical, however, and his opinions on yellow fever bore more resemblance to those of the Royal College of Physicians than the medical establishment of the Army. The yellow fever epidemics of the 1790s therefore left British practitioners as divided as their American counterparts. As in America, these divisions sometimes coincided with political affiliations. However, they tended even more strongly to reflect the ongoing friction between fellows of the Royal College of Physicians and surgeons from the Army, Navy, and East India Company who were asserting their independence from the metropolitan elite. During the French Revolutionary Wars, these tensions came to a head as surgeon-apothecaries intensified their campaign for legal protection. The outcome was the Apothecaries Act of 1815, which stipulated that the Society of Apothecaries should become the licensing body for all medical practitioners who lacked an MD or a diploma from the Royal College of Surgeons. The Society had the power to confer a licence on any practitioner who had followed an apprenticeship and had attended classes in certain subjects.[69] Army and naval surgeons were not immediately affected by the new legislation, but it was symptomatic of the gradual erosion of the unique status formerly enjoyed by the royal colleges.[70] Another reason for the heightened tension between physicians and this new breed of general practitioner was that the end of the wars threatened to swamp Britain's medical market with a host of practitioners who had gained valuable experience overseas. During the French Wars, the medical services of the armed forces and East India Company had expanded massively. Some 2,850 surgeons had been recruited to the Army alone.[71] The debate over the nature and causes of yellow fever in Britain was thus bound up with wider disputes over professional authority. Both sides accused the other of faulty reasoning and poor judgement, which were symptomatic of other social vices. 'Though the contagion of yellow fever may prove to be a fiction', noted Robert Jackson, who had returned with the Army to the West Indies in 1795, 'the contagion of fear has so impressed the minds of men, that things are seen through a false medium, and common sense cannot obtain a hearing.'[72] According to Jackson, such a state of mind had existed in England, where ill-founded fears of the contagiousness of yellow fever had 'paralized [sic] the vigour and appalled the courage of the English nation'. The same was true of St Domingue, where the arrival at New Providence of a number of men in an impaired state of health created great alarm, leading the sick to be needlessly

[68] Ibid., 8.
[69] Holloway, 'The Apothecaries Act 1815'; Loudon, *Medical Care*, chaps 6–7.
[70] Ackroyd et al., *Advancing with the Army*, 57.
[71] Ibid., 17.
[72] Jackson, *Outline of the History and Cure of Fever*, 223.

quarantined on an island to the great detriment of their health.[73] Their disease, he insisted, had been nothing more than the endemic intermittent fever of the island. Contrary to Wright, he claimed that 'It was perfectly well known, that contagion did not exist in the hospitals of St Domingo.'[74]

For Jackson, the unfounded fear of contagion betokened a general malaise which could be ascribed to modern lifestyles, particularly the steady erosion of the rural society which had been the bedrock of Britain and its Army. Like Trotter, he believed that the growth of manufacturing towns had sapped physical endurance and that the factory system had broken the organic bonds of society, leading men to become weak, fearful, and self-interested. The cramped conditions of the new towns had likewise given rise to a range of endemic and contagious fevers which thrived in crowded spaces and which contributed to the sickliness of those recruited to the Army.[75] For this reason, Jackson's book was addressed not just to the medical profession but to 'statesmen and generals', and in a manner that dispensed with professional courtesies in an effort to arrive at the truth. In placing his evidence before laymen, Jackson was reaching above the heads of established professional authorities such as the Royal College of Physicians and some of his peers in the Army with whom he had had violent disagreements. In doing so, he insisted upon the primacy of experience and direct observation, experience which had led him to change his own mind about the nature of yellow fever. Whereas he had originally supposed it to be a separate disease, he now admitted that his time in Jamaica had been insufficient to gain accurate knowledge of it. His subsequent encounters with yellow fever on St Domingue, by contrast, had convinced him that the disease was simply an aggravated form of the endemic remittent fever of the West Indies.[76]

In the first decade of the new century, the nature of yellow fever remained as contentious as ever. Thomas Dancer of Jamaica, for instance, vigorously defended Chisholm's conclusion that the disease was contagious in the sense that it arose, like typhus, from human effluvia; that is, emanations proceeding directly from the sick body or substances imbued with them. Like Chisholm, he believed yellow fever to be a distinct malady, on the grounds that diseases differed in genera according to their remote causes. Outbreaks of yellow fever in Jamaica, he insisted, had always occurred following the arrival of seamen or soldiers from outside the island and were thus imported: a conclusion widely held on the island, despite assertions to the contrary.[77] The contagious nature of yellow fever was also attested by Gilbert Blane. Blane had always insisted that yellow fever was a disease distinct from the bilious remittent fever of hot climates,[78] and restated

[73] Jackson, *Outline*, 224–5.
[74] Ibid., 224.
[75] Ibid., 109–11, 350–2.
[76] Ibid., 6.
[77] Dancer, 'Observations on the Contagiousness and Importation of Yellow Fever'.
[78] Blane, *Observations*, 396–8.

his opinion in an essay 'On the Yellow Fever', in which he speculated that the disease had originally been imported into the Caribbean on board slave ships from Africa.[79]

Yet others continued to reject Chisholm's importation hypothesis. The miasmatic origins of the disease were affirmed, for example, by Dr George Davidson of St Vincent (who had conducted eudiometrical experiments there), Dr Joseph Comstock of Rhode Island, Dr Ffrith of Calcutta, and, of course, by Benjamin Rush. All insisted that yellow fever was not derived from a specific contagion and that it was always generated by putrefaction. Some, like Rush and Ffrith, extended this observation to plague, which they also regarded as a disease of putrefaction, rather than a disease susceptible of importation. Indeed, one of the most interesting features of the literature on yellow fever at this point is the extent to which practitioners working in different parts of the world found common cause, often sharing their opinions in journals like the *Medical Repository*. Ffrith, for example, drew analogies between the 'yellow fever' and malignant fevers in Africa and Asia, and Rush cited the opinions of the East India Company surgeon John Clark. Another common theme in this literature was the benefits to be gained from rejecting the doctrine of contagion: of reducing the expense incurred by detention and fumigation of goods, of delays caused by quarantine, and of delivering people from the danger of being confined in lazarettos. As Rush insisted, it was more effective and enlightened to look to environmental improvements; to the drainage of marshy ground and the removal of other sources of impure air. It was to such improvements, rather than to quarantine, that he attributed the long absence of plague from the countries of northern and western Europe.[80]

All these writers went to great pains to portray Chisholm as a lone voice crying in the wilderness. This was by no means true, for he continued to attract influential supporters; and yet the majority of writers on yellow fever attacked his theory of importation, either directly or implicitly. Many of his critics were relatively young men who had spent the formative years of their career in the armed forces, and it is significant that yellow fever was one of the most popular subjects of MD dissertations at Edinburgh University in the first two decades of the nineteenth century. The majority of these were written by men who had recently been demobilized from the Army or Navy and were hostile to the concepts of contagion and importation, preferring to ascribe epidemics to the

[79] Blane, *Select Dissertations*, 285.

[80] Mitchill, 'Thoughts on Quarantines and Lazarettos'; Rush, 'Facts intended to prove the Yellow Fever not to be Contagious'; Eckard, 'Correction of Chisholm's Misstatement respecting the Prevalence of the Malignant Fever at St. Thomas's'; Davidson, 'Practical and Diagnostic Observations on Yellow Fever'; Comstock, 'Remarks on the Bilous, or Yellow Fever'; Ffrith, 'Practical Remarks on the Similarity of American and Asiatic Fevers'; Rule, 'Considerations on the Origin, Causes and Character of Yellow Fever'.

action of the heat upon European constitutions and/or the effects of miasma arising from putrescence.[81]

Participants in the debate over yellow fever were aware that their failure to agree on a matter of national importance was potentially damaging to their profession and sometimes to their own careers. The former Army physician Edward Bancroft showed sensitivity to this in his *Essay on the Disease called Yellow Fever* (1811) and endeavoured to place his own conclusions 'beyond the reach of future controversy'.[82] Bancroft entered the Army as a physician in 1795, after taking an MB degree from St John's College, Cambridge, the year before. He served in the Windward Islands and in Portugal, and was in Lord Abercomby's expedition to Egypt in 1801. After the Peace of Amiens, he left the Army on half pay and took an MD from Cambridge in 1804, becoming a Fellow of the Royal College of Physicians the following year. In 1806, at the comparatively young age of thirty-six, he was invited to give the prestigious Gulstonian Lectures, which he delivered at the Royal College of Physicians in 1806 and 1807.[83] On the strength of these lectures, which formed the basis of his *Essay*, he was convinced that he had 'done more than enough to convince every candid and judicious reader' that yellow fever possessed no contagious power and that labelling diseases on the basis of their symptoms was erroneous.[84] In his view, the disease popularly known as yellow fever was generated by the 'joint influence of marsh miasmata, and of an atmosphere unusually and sufficiently heated upon persons habituated to a cold or temperate climate'.[85] The 'yellow fever' was thus nothing more than an aggravated form of remitting fever and consequently 'devoid of contagion'.[86]

Bancroft's *Essay* was first published in 1811, the year in which he was re-appointed as a Physician to the Army and dispatched to Jamaica, where he was to remain until his death in 1842. In it, he attacked Chisholm's 'unfounded assertion' that the fever which struck Grenada in 1793 had been imported from the west coast of Africa. His own opinions were based both on direct observation and on the views of a variety of modern and ancient authors. Together, these attested to the fact that the so-called Bulam fever was not unique but merely a form of remittent fever which was common in all hot climates. Bancroft made particular use of Hippocrates, Galen, and other ancient authorities to bolster commonly held opinions about the role of marsh miasmata which had not been mentioned by Sydenham, who resorted to occult explanations for the morbid effects of different

[81] e.g. Veitch, *De methodo tratandi, et praevendi, febrem flavam Indarium occidentalium*, 20–9; Woodcock, *De febre flava Indarium Occidentalium.*
[82] Bancroft, *Essay on the Disease called Yellow Fever*, vi.
[83] Creighton, *rev.* Reznick, 'Bancroft'.
[84] Bancroft, *Essay*, vi–vii, 5.
[85] Ibid., 275–6.
[86] Ibid., 282.

seasons.[87] Like other opponents of quarantine, Bancroft complained of the 'expensive delays and embarrassments, by which useless quarantine laws shackle the commerce, and naval operations of a great maritime country'.[88] But quarantine, in his opinion, was also socially corrosive. It was notorious, he wrote, 'that during the late epidemics in the south of Spain, an unfortunate exercise of civil authority, occasioned the loss of many thousands of lives, by compelling the inhabitants of the towns, where it prevailed, to remain in their morbific atmosphere'.[89] He warned:

> Few in this country have heard or can conceive how often, and to what extent, the strongest and best ties which unite and benefit mankind, have been cruelly broken, within the last twenty years, in some parts of America and Spain, by persons acting under the terror of imaginary dangers; and driven by it, to abandon their homes, their occupations, and even their nearest relatives and dearest friends in the hour of sickness.[90]

He cited the opinions of Spanish doctors who had witnessed many deaths among persons abandoned to starve in their beds, or shot while trying to find asylum.[91] It is important to point out, however, that Bancroft differed from many others who denied the contagiousness of yellow fever (Rush, for example) in that he did not extend this claim to plague. He had experienced the disease in Egypt in 1801, where he claimed to have seen ample evidence of its being communicated to military surgeons attending the sick in pest houses, like the one in which he worked in Aboukir.[92]

Among the many books on the subject of yellow fever in the wake of the epidemics in the Americas and the Mediterranean, Bancroft's stood out among the British offerings in that it was one of the few anticontagionist tracts penned by a fellow of the Royal College of Physicians. As such, it attracted a great deal of attention and was singled out for particularly hostile criticism from those who defended the 'doctrine' of contagion. Bancroft's two principal antagonists were Sir James Fellowes, who had been Physician to the Army in St Domingue and later in Cadiz, and another senior military physician, William Pym, who had also experienced yellow fever and plague in the Caribbean and Mediterranean. Fellowes' *Reports of the Pestilential Disorder of Andalusia* (1815) contradicted the opinions of Bancroft, claiming that yellow fever was a specific disorder propagated by a 'specific contagion'. He had come to this conclusion partly because the disease seemed to be spread by the sick and partly because it shared certain characteristics with diseases such as smallpox and measles which were generally accepted as contagious; in particular, those who survived appeared to be

[87] Ibid., 277.
[88] Ibid., 492.
[89] Ibid., 493–4.
[90] Ibid., 494.
[91] Ibid., 495.
[92] Ibid., 578.

protected from further attacks.[93] In this sense, the disease was quite different from the miasmatic causes of intermitting and remitting fevers, which had the capacity to attack the same body more than once.[94]

In his book, Fellowes set out simply to provide an account of the fevers he had witnessed, bringing together personal observations with the testimonies of Spanish physicians and evidence from Spanish medical and historical literature. He avoided speculation and hoped that the facts would speak for themselves.[95] Bancroft was the only practitioner singled out for criticism,[96] and although he felt strongly that Bancroft was wrong, Fellowes openly admitted that he was himself unsure about the origins of the disease. While convinced that it was contagious, he admitted that there was no clear evidence that it had been imported from Vera Cruz or Havana, as some practitioners claimed. Indeed, he speculated that the disease might have originated locally, a 'combination of peculiar circumstances' causing the disease to become contagious.[97] It is not altogether clear from Fellowes' account what these circumstances were. Heat is mentioned as a factor on one occasion, although he had earlier dismissed the relevance of meteorological data, stating that he had included an appendix containing such information 'more out of compliance with custom than from any conviction . . . of the utility of meteorological observations . . . with regard to the cause of pestilential fevers'.[98]

In view of his uncertainty over the origins of the fevers he had encountered in the West Indies and Spain, Fellowes stopped short of recommending that quarantine be imposed against them, although he believed that it was an understandable precaution. In fact, he remained deliberately vague about this controversial method of prevention, postponing discussion of it to some future publication.[99] One method which Fellowes explicitly rejected was fumigation with various acid-based gases. These had apparently been subjected to rigorous trials by the Spanish physician Dr Arejula and had been found wanting.[100]

In some respects, Fellowes' cautious empiricism resembled the approach of the military surgeons placed under him as Physician to the Forces and Inspector of Military Hospitals during the Peninsular War. However, in apparently rejecting the relevance of meteorological data he went against the grain of opinion in the Army's medical establishment and, as we learned in Part II, he had made himself rather unpopular with military surgeons in Spain by prohibiting post-mortem dissection in cases of yellow fever. Although Fellowes had done so on the grounds

93 Fellowes, *Reports of the Pestilential Disorder of Andalusia*, xxii–xxiii.
94 Ibid., xxii.
95 Ibid., x, xiv, xxii.
96 Ibid., xix.
97 Ibid., 403.
98 Ibid., 403, xix.
99 Ibid., 401–2.
100 Ibid., 395.

that dissection was likely to spread the disease, surgeons claimed that he was merely deferring to the opinion of the Spanish authorities and elite physicians.

Whether or not this was actually true, it is easy to see why most military surgeons would have been wary of Fellowes. He had been born into a well-to-do and well-connected family. His father was Physician-Extraordinary to the Prince Regent and a brother of Rear-Admiral Sir Thomas Fellowes. After finishing his education at Rugby school, Fellowes decided to follow his father in becoming a physician, but before he embarked on formal education he entered the Army as a surgeon's mate in 1794. No more than a year had elapsed before he was appointed Physician to the Army and dispatched to St Domingue. Such rapid promotion can only have occasioned jealously on the part of the surgeons who now served under him, many of whom would have been a good deal more experienced. Having returned from the Caribbean, Fellowes went up to Gonville and Caius College, Cambridge, graduating an MB in 1797 and MD in 1803, later becoming a Fellow of the college. Although he subsequently attended lectures in medicine at Edinburgh, he had little in common with the majority of military surgeons and was not welcomed when he was sent to Gibraltar to investigate an outbreak of yellow fever among the garrison there. After returning to England, he became a Fellow of the Royal College of Physicians in 1805 and was knighted by George III in 1809. Shortly afterwards, he was appointed chief of the Army's medical establishment in Spain, where he witnessed further epidemics of yellow fever.[101] Having had the opportunity to observe the disease at close quarters, Fellowes received a request from the Army Medical Board in 1810 to inquire into the nature of the disease and to submit a report on whether or not it was similar to yellow fever in the West Indies. However, the Board seemed to have already decided that the disease was contagious and ordered that steps should be taken to separate the sick from the healthy. This may explain why Fellowes came to a similar conclusion in his own report, despite his lack of certainty over importation. If so, it was a course of action which did no harm to his career. In 1813, he became the Army's Inspector of Hospitals, a powerful position from which he would have been able to dictate medical practices and dispense patronage.

Bancroft's other chief antagonist was William Pym, who had served with the 35th and 70th regiments of foot and, from 1794 to 1796, with the Army in the West Indies. He had been in medical charge during an epidemic of yellow fever in Martinique and had also served in Sicily, Malta, and Gibraltar, where he acted as medical adviser to the governor, the Duke of Kent. Pym was appointed Deputy Inspector-General of Army Hospitals in 1810, and in 1811 was made President of the Board of Health in Malta, where he had responsibility for quarantine. In September 1816, he was promoted to Inspector-General of Army Hospitals, after

[101] Moore, *rev.* Herrick, 'Fellowes, Sir James (c. 1771–1857)'.

having returned to Malta during an epidemic of plague. Pym was close to McGrigor and shared his opinions on quarantine and contagion, in respect to both plague and yellow fever;[102] he had also met Fellowes on at least one occasion, during the epidemic on Gibraltar in 1804. Pym saw Bancroft's contribution to the debate over the latter as highly damaging, no doubt because, as a Fellow of the Royal College, his words carried weight. He explained that:

> The principal object I have in view, is to counteract the influence which the opinions of Dr. Bancroft have had upon the minds of the public as well as of the profession, by bringing forward evidence to prove, that it is a different disease from the Bilious Remitting Fever of warm climates; that it is not produced by, nor in any way connected with Marsh Miasmata; that it has not been a constant resident in the West Indies; that is Contagious, and capable of being imported to, and propagated in any country enjoying a certain degree of heat.[103]

Potentially, this included many European countries, not only those in the Mediterranean, but also countries to the north, including Britain, during the right season.

Pym's position was that the epidemics which he had witnessed in the West Indies and in the Mediterranean were caused by a disease wholly different from the yellow fever of the Caribbean islands, which he saw as a kind of non-contagious bilious remittent fever, the bile giving rise to the characteristic yellowness of its victims. Pym thought that the term 'yellow fever' was misapplied to the fever he had witnessed and, like Chisholm, insisted that it be termed 'Bulam fever' on account of the supposed origins of the disease on the West African coast. Part of Bancroft's problem, according to Pym, was that he had misidentified the disease in question: 'He has taken a great deal of unnecessary trouble to prove what, I believe, has not been doubted for a great many years, the non-contagion of marsh fevers.'[104] For Pym, like Fellowes, one of the key facts determining the contagiousness of the disease they had witnessed was that it conferred immunity upon those who had survived it. Pym claimed to be the first person to take note of this, although he was not. However, he did use this insight to practical effect and, on Gibraltar, proposed that all the men who had been in the West Indies or had recovered from the disease be employed in hospital duties caring for the sick.[105] These measures were based on the knowledge he had gained of the disease in the West Indies and the quarantine regulations which he had devised in Spain in 1800 and 1803, which he credited with having protected his garrison.[106]

[102] Pym, *Observations upon the Bulam Fever*, v, vii.
[103] Ibid., 1–2.
[104] Ibid., 2.
[105] Ibid., 26.
[106] William Pym to the Hon. William Windham, Secretary of State for the Colonies, 16 May 1806, Wentworth Woodhouse Muniments, Sheffield City Archives [hereafter, SCA].

Although Fellowes was rather ambivalent about quarantine in his published work, Pym advocated it strongly, stating emphatically that the only effective means of preventing the disease was 'the establishment of Quarantine and a good Police'.[107] On Gibraltar, he ordered all the sick to be placed in hospital and anyone in close proximity to be placed in quarantine. While he regretted that the quarantine had been imperfectly implemented in Gibraltar, he credited it with having saved the lives of at least 1,200 soldiers in the British garrison. By contrast, only 28 of the 14,000 civilians on the island escaped the fever and, of those, 12 had previously had the fever in the West Indies.[108] For Pym, this was conclusive proof that the disease was contagious and that quarantine worked.

It is not surprising that Pym, as a staunch supporter of quarantine, both within Britain and in its Mediterranean dependencies, later found employment as Superintendent of Quarantine with the Privy Council, which was the department of government responsible for such measures. In this capacity, he continued to defend the practice of quarantine against numerous critics, and to insist that the fever which most still referred to as yellow fever was a contagious disease. He was mindful of the naval and commercial advantages of free navigation, but believed that it was necessary to balance these against those of public health. He was not opposed to the liberalization of quarantine, but only if it could be demonstrated that there would be no additional risk to health, and provided that it did not invite retaliation from other countries. Such opinions placed him squarely within official opinion through to the late 1840s and explain his long tenure in office; he was knighted in 1831.[109]

In 1815, however, there was no consensus on the contagiousness of yellow fever, and the heightened controversy within the medical profession, together with the possibility of the disease arriving in Britain, led the government to involve itself in what had hitherto been a purely medical controversy. The Privy Council examined Pym's work and considered the contrary opinions of Bancroft, whereupon they solicited an opinion as to their relative merits from the Royal College of Physicians.

There had been a similar approach in 1804, following the outbreak of an apparently contagious fever on Gibraltar. On that occasion, the government requested that a Board of Health be established in London, to be comprised of fellows of the College who would communicate with medical officers in Gibraltar and the West Indies regarding yellow fever. Pym had corresponded with the Board from Gibraltar and then visited London, where he gave the Board the benefit of his views on the causes and spread of the Gibraltar fever, with the result

[107] Pym, *Observations*, vii.
[108] Ibid., 26.
[109] In this post, he became embroiled in a series of controversies over the nature of yellow fever and the utility of quarantine, his main antagonists being Sir William Burnett and Alexander Bryson, both naval medical officers. Power, *rev.* Herrick, 'Pym, Sir William (1772–1861)'.

that he appears to have been offered the position of Superintendent General of Quarantine in England. This position, which was very similar to the one he would later hold with the Privy Council, would have entailed visiting the quarantine stations of England and reporting to the Board any measures he considered necessary for their improvement.[110] However, the Board was dissolved in 1806 following the death of Pitt and the formation of a new administration.[111]

This time, however, the majority of the Royal College of Physicians concluded with Pym that the disease was contagious and that those who survived were exempt from future attacks. As he later explained, few fellows then had any knowledge of the disease and were able to judge only on the basis of second-hand reports.[112] However, the College's report stressed the provisional nature of the evidence it had considered and warned that medical opinion was always subject to revision.[113] This small concession left the Privy Council in a quandary, inducing it to take the unprecedented step of appealing beyond the usual sources of medical authority to the Army Medical Board and its naval equivalent: the Commissioners for the Service of Transports, Sick, and Wounded Seamen. This is highly significant because the move implicitly recognized the claims of military and naval practitioners to expertise in such matters as fever, in much the same way as the Apothecaries Act had recognized those of civilian general practitioners the year before.

Neither of these reports appear to be extant but their conclusions were summarized by Bancroft. The naval report was drawn up by Dr Harness, the Medical Commissioner and his assistants, Dr Gray, Physician at Haslar, and Dr Tait, Physician of Yarmouth Hospital, after a review of opinions held by their surgeons. Bancroft was given access to the naval report and McGrigor, recently appointed Director-General of the new Army Medical Department, permitted him to see the various documents submitted to him on the subject of yellow fever. It is not clear whether Bancroft was able to see the report itself or how he managed to gain access to the testimonies of military surgeons. It is possible that he received a copy of the report via military surgeons based in Jamaica, where he was then living, or through a contact in London. It is highly unlikely that McGrigor would have released the information to Bancroft himself, as there was no love lost between them. Just a few years earlier, they had been involved in a bitter dispute over the relative merits of general and regimental hospitals. McGrigor, Robert Jackson, and other military surgeons favoured the latter, on the grounds that general hospitals were hot-beds of disease and indiscipline,

110 Pym to Windham, 16 May 1806, SCA.

111 Pym, *Bulam Fever*, vi.

112 Bancroft, *Sequel to an Essay on the Yellow Fever.*

113 Statement of the Royal College of Physicians, 15 November 1813, published in the *London Medical Repository*, September 1816.

whereas Bancroft vigorously defended general hospitals.[114] General hospitals were traditionally the domains of military physicians, and Bancroft saw the attack on them as an attempt to assert the primacy of regimental surgeons. He wanted to uphold the traditional distinction between physicians and surgeons, and the former's precedence in the military-medical hierarchy.[115] The dispute may also have reflected anxieties about the relative positions of surgeons and physicians in the event of a cessation of hostilities, when hundreds of the former would spill out into civilian practice. Bancroft certainly lost no opportunity to question the competence of military surgeons, in both the British Army and in the East India Company.[116]

The evidence respecting yellow fever which had been collected by the Army included testimonies from several authorities on yellow fever, including Dr William Fergusson, the Inspector of Hospitals in the Windward Islands. It also included the replies given by medical officers in the British garrison on Gibraltar, which had recently suffered an outbreak of the fever. Bancroft flattered himself that their opinions vindicated his own stance against the attacks made by Pym and Fellowes.[117] However, McGrigor's strong opinion in favour of contagion contradicted the statements of Ferguson and other non-contagionists, and would have done little to resolve the dilemma faced by the Privy Council or debates among medical practitioners themselves.

The bitter controversy over the nature of yellow fever revived again in the early 1820s, following further outbreaks of the disease along the eastern seaboard of the United States and the Mediterranean coast of Spain, all of which were widely reported in the British press.[118] Having witnessed the epidemic in Cadiz, the military surgeon Thomas O'Halloran declared that the disease had not been imported; neither could it be attributed to 'germs' which had lain dormant from the epidemics of 1800 and 1819. Rather, he attributed the outbreak to warm south-easterly breezes which had caused drought and increased noxious exhalations from swamps, lakes, and marshes, and, above all, malignant emanations from decaying animal and vegetable matter. Although occasioned by peculiar atmospheric conditions, yellow fever was thus, to some degree, a filth disease.[119]

O'Halloran's conclusion clashed with that of some authors who had recently written on the Spanish yellow fever epidemics and notably, and somewhat surprisingly, with the opinions held by McGrigor. Like other military surgeons seeking to curry favour with the Director-General, his work was dedicated to

[114] M'Grigor, *A Letter to the Commissioners of Military Enquiry*, 2, 4, 6–7, 14–15.

[115] On this dispute, see Ackroyd et al., *Advancing with the Army*, 32–5; Kelly, '"Not Surgeons Alone"'.

[116] Bancroft, *Exposure of Misrepresentations by Dr. McGrigor and Dr. Jackson to the Commissioners of Military Enquiry*; idem, *A Letter to the Commissioners of Military Enquiry*.

[117] Bancroft, *Sequel*, xv–xvi.

[118] e.g. *The Times*, 21 September 1819, 2; 3 November 1819, 2; 13 October 1820, 3.

[119] O'Halloran, *Remarks on the Yellow Fever*, 179–82.

McGrigor, 'with the author's most respectful compliments'.[120] However, in O'Halloran's case, this gesture may also have been an attempt to detract from the volume's contents, with which McGrigor would certainly have disagreed. In his book, O'Halloran took issue with the eminent French physician Étienne Pariset, who had drawn attention to the coincidence of epidemics in the Caribbean, North America, and the Mediterranean. In Pariset's view, this strongly suggested that the disease was imported and that France, too, might be at risk from yellow fever. Quarantine of some sort was therefore necessary, he argued, although it ought to be made more systematic and less open to abuse than present arrangements.[121] However, the measures taken by the French government were, according to critics, anything but enlightened. Merchants (foreign and domestic) and reformers within the medical profession argued that they were unnecessary and damaging to trade, and pointed to the abuse of the 'sanitary cordon' marshalled along the border with Spain.[122]

Like fellow critics of quarantine in France, such as Valentine, Devèze, and Chervin, O'Halloran stressed the importance of basing all preventive measures upon facts. This entailed accurate observation of the nature of disease, preferably at first hand, as well as an analysis of historical trends. While he appears not to have ruled out the utility of quarantine *per se*, O'Halloran concluded that it was unnecessary in the case of diseases such as yellow fever, for which there was no evidence of contagion. In such circumstances, he argued, 'quarantine restrictions are futile in the main point, and they are injurious, or even destructive in others. If the cause of the disease be local, it must be considered as barbarous... to prevent the people from leaving the destructive locality.' Making a more general point about the role of medicine in statecraft, he continued:

> If the lights of science were permitted to direct the health arrangements of states and kingdoms, there are grounds to believe, that the alarm, misery, and destruction, which attaches to the appearance of contagious or epidemic diseases, would be much diminished, indeed, that the common business of life would be scarcely interrupted. Such change of measures may be wished, but can scarcely be expected. Power is self-sufficient, and does not permit humble science to enter its threshold; but until it grants this indulgence, the affairs of human life will be fluctuating, tumultuous, and without permanent prosperity.[123]

These sentiments, which appear prominently in the introduction to O'Halloran's monograph, encapsulate the position of most of those who opposed quarantine

[120] See the discussion of dedication and patronage in Ackroyd et al., *Advancing with the Army*, 308–9.

[121] Pariset, *Observations sur la fièvre jaune*, i–ii, 96–7, 106–8, 123–4, 126–8.

[122] See Ackerknecht, 'Anticontagionism'; La Berge, *Mission and Method*, 90–4; Heaman, 'The Rise and Fall of Anticontagionism in France'; Stephan Girard to Jean Devèze, 30 August 1819, 17 December 1823, 26 January 1825; Devèze to Girard, 22 September 1821, Girard Papers, Library of the American Philosophical Society.

[123] O' Halloran, *Remarks*, xv.

or sought its liberalization. They opposed it on the grounds that it was medically unnecessary, that it was inhumane, and that it was irrational and unenlightened. They saw a close connection between tyranny and the arbitrary and, to them, unjustified use of such measures to pursue political ends. Although his subject was Spain, O'Halloran's remarks were clearly intended to resonate in Britain, where there was growing pressure for reform of quarantine from cotton merchants, humanitarians, and members of the medical profession, the most outspoken of which was Charles Maclean. It will be recalled that Maclean had been expelled from India for criticizing the Governor-General, Wellesley, and that he had set himself against all forms of what he perceived as tyranny. In the same year that O'Halloran's volume was published, Maclean completed a monograph entitled *Remarks on the British Quarantine Laws*, which was one of many books and pamphlets he wrote on this subject between 1817 and 1824. Maclean had also visited Spain, where he had witnessed outbreaks of yellow fever in the early 1820s. Like O'Halloran, he had developed close ties with reform-minded members of the Spanish medical profession, and both became members of the medical academies of Madrid and Barcelona.

Maclean was well known as a writer on 'contagious' diseases, on account of his military experience and his work in Levant, where he claimed to have contracted plague.[124] He saw the outbreak of yellow fever in Barcelona in 1821 as an opportunity to impress his controversial views upon the liberal government, sending a copy of one of his works on quarantine to the Spanish ambassador in London. Despite receiving no response, Maclean left for Madrid, where he was introduced to many physicians and learned societies. His voluminous writings were known to some of the more radical physicians in the city but had for some time been considered dangerous by the authorities. His book on epidemic diseases, for example, had to be smuggled into the country, and some physicians had been harshly treated for espousing similar ideas about contagion and quarantine. Since the liberal constitution had been established in 1820, there was rather more freedom of expression, but many physicians were still reluctant to voice their support for Maclean openly, fearing a return of the Bourbon regime which had been strongly committed to quarantine. Indeed, the country's physician elite, which was well represented in the Cortes, was still stridently contagionist in outlook.[125]

Once Maclean received permission to visit Barcelona, he proceeded to the city and there made common cause with a number of other liberal physicians who met regularly to discuss the outbreak of fever. Most were local doctors, but there were four other foreign physicians, including O'Halloran, two Frenchmen, and

[124] The fullest account of Maclean's experiences in the Levant are contained in his correspondence with Lord Grenville, in the Dropmore Papers, Add. MS 59265, BL. See also Maclean, *Remarks on the British Quarantine Laws*.

[125] Maclean, *Evils of Quarantine Laws*, 110–15.

an American.[126] In 1822, this group drafted a manifesto on the fever which disputed the commonly held view that it had arrived in Barcelona on board a Neapolitan naval vessel which had recently returned from Havana. Instead, they claimed that the fever had been produced by a miasma arising from filth and stagnant pools of water.[127] Maclean then proceeded to Madrid to lay the manifesto before the Cortes and gave a copy of the pamphlet to each of the 250 deputies sitting there. In return, he received what he described as 'an angry tirade from the pestilential contagionists', to which he responded by writing an additional pamphlet on the evils of sanitary laws which criticized a proposal by the Spanish Committee of Public Health for the introduction of a Sanitary Code.[128] Having been vexed by the activities of the medical commission sent by France to investigate the epidemic, many deputies were receptive to Maclean's views. The French commission included several prominent contagionists, the most influential of whom was Pariset, and it seemed likely that the commission would declare yellow fever a communicable disease. In anticipation of this, the French government erected a *cordon sanitaire* along the border with Spain; a move which was deeply resented, not only for disrupting commerce but because it harboured spies and afforded a refuge to traitors.[129] Thus, when the proposal was eventually debated in October 1822, the Code was rejected by the majority of deputies and sent back to the Committee of Public Health.[130]

Maclean saw this as a great victory for the opponents of contagion and quarantine. He thought that it was the first occasion on which the merits of quarantine laws had ever been debated in a political assembly and, while the Cortes had stopped short of wholly endorsing his position, he had at least delayed the introduction of a system of quarantine. He also believed that the progress made in Spain might have some impact upon debates over quarantine in Britain, in which he was then actively involved. However, he was pessimistic about the immediate future in Spain, for in 1823 troops comprising the French cordon were used to crush the constitutional government and restore the Bourbon monarchy.[131]

In Britain, the contributions made by Maclean and O'Halloran were overshadowed by an outbreak of yellow fever on Ascension Island. The fever broke out first amongst the crew of the naval sloop HMS *Bann*, which had sailed from Sierra Leone in March 1823. The crew were in good health until their arrival at Ascension, but shortly afterwards they began to fall ill. By 2 June, twenty of the crew were dead and the disease appeared to have spread to the island's garrison,

[126] Maclean, *Evils*, 122, 141.
[127] Ibid., 125, 130.
[128] Ibid., 170, 186.
[129] Mullett, 'Politics, Economics and Medicine', 233; Heaman, 'The Rise and Fall of Anticontagionism', 9.
[130] Maclean, *Evils*, 264–5, 295, 319, 343.
[131] Heaman, 'Anticontagionism', 9.

claiming a further sixteen lives. This outbreak was the subject of a report by Dr William Burnett, one of the commissioners in the medical department of the Royal Navy and formerly Inspector of Hospitals to the Mediterranean Fleet.[132] Burnett claimed that the fever was caused by a miasma emanating from the timbers of the ship, which became 'contagious' in the ill-ventilated conditions found below decks and in the island's barracks. The fever was not, however, contagious in the sense of being easily communicable from person to person.[133] It was a conclusion that appealed to many self-styled moderates within the medical profession, who inclined towards a belief in the atmospheric causes of such fevers but who did not rule out contagion under any circumstances. For this reason, Burnett's book was well reviewed in the *Medico-Chirurgical Review* edited by James Johnson, while the more 'extreme' views opposing contagion expressed in Charles Maclean's *Remarks* (1823) and *Evils of Quarantine Laws* (1824) were denounced. Although it urged the liberalization of quarantine, the *Review* concluded that Maclean's belligerence was damaging the case for reform.[134]

Perhaps because of its moderate tone, Burnett's report was regarded as more dangerous than the bilious outpourings of Maclean; it certainly prompted a vigorous defence by the pro-quarantine establishment. In a letter to the Lords of the Admiralty, which was published in *The Times*, no less a figure than Sir Gilbert Blane wrote that 'a great proportion of the medical officers of the navy ... disbelieve in the contagious nature of this fever'. This, according to Blane, was an irresponsible delusion:

Their Lordships will readily apprehend, from what has happened on this small scale, what must have been the effect of this opinion, if erroneous, held by those whose duty it is to suggest the requisite precautions in the case of the fleets, armies, garrisons, and great towns, which have been exposed to this malady for the last 30 years on the continent and islands of America, and for the last 23 years in the south of Europe; and what must in future be the effects of this singular delusion, should it continue to prevail and to be acted upon as heretofore in his Majesty's service by sea and land.[135]

132 Burnett studied at Edinburgh but left without taking a degree to serve as a surgeon's mate in the Navy. He was promoted to the rank of Surgeon in 1798 and served with distinction at the Nile and Trafalgar. He was appointed Physician and Inspector of Hospitals to the Mediterranean Fleet in 1810 and awarded an MD from the universities of St Andrews and Aberdeen in 1825. In 1814, he was placed in medical charge of the Russian fleet in the Medway, where he made observations on fevers among the crews. After the war, he settled at Chichester, where he became Physician to the Dispensary but was invited to become one of the commissioners of the Navy's Medical Board and eventually became Physician-General of the Navy. He was knighted in 1831 and appointed Physician-in-Ordinary to the king in 1835. See Bettany, *rev.* Herrick, 'Burnett, Sir William (1779–1861)'.

133 Burnett, *Official Report on the Fever which appeared on board H.M. Ship Bann, on the Coast of Africa.*

134 *Medico-Chirurgical Review*, series 2, 2 (1825), 9–10, 20–1.

135 Gilbert Blane to John Wilson Croker, Secretary to the Admiralty, *The Times*, 22 January 1824, 3.

Blane was referring to the Admiralty's resistance to the imposition of quarantine on its ships, fearing that it would hamper naval operations. During the French Wars, the Navy had often complained that its vessels were detained unnecessarily in foreign ports because of concerns that ships returning from the Caribbean might carry yellow fever.[136] Some years later, following an epidemic of yellow fever among British sailors in the Caribbean, the Admiralty also reacted negatively to a suggestion by William Pym that infected vessels be placed under quarantine. The Admiralty replied to Pym that 'The Lordships are of opinion that the regulations which you suggest in the nature of Quarantine restrictions, would not be attended with beneficial results, or are necessary, provided the usual precautions on board His Majesty's ships . . . are attended to.'[137] This presumably referred to the process of fumigation and cleansing.

Although Pym was out of step with opinion at the Admiralty, he was in tune with the thinking of successive governments about quarantine and the perceived threat from diseases such as yellow fever. Like Blane, he advised government to err on the side of caution and to bear in mind the diplomatic risks of unilateral liberalization or repeal. Britain's commercial and political rivals would portray any drastic moves in this direction as irresponsible, he warned, and would use them as a pretext to impose trade embargos or quarantines against British shipping. The damage caused by such measures would more than outweigh the advantages to be gained from unrestricted trade.[138] The government was faced with such a decision in 1824, the year in which Burnett's report was published. In response to pressure from cotton-manufacturing and mercantile interests, and their medical allies such as Maclean, the government considered the existing quarantine laws with respect to plague, the disease which most affected the booming trade in cotton with the eastern Mediterranean. It decided in favour of liberalization but against the repeal of the quarantine statute as demanded by the merchants and their supporters in Parliament.[139] That the government did not repeal the legislation was partly due to its conservative instincts and partly because it feared retaliation from countries that might see such a step as irresponsible.

On these matters, the opinions of government and those of its senior medical officials tended to be mutually reinforcing. The likes of Pym, Blane, and McGrigor were far from being reactionaries, but the opponents of quarantine

[136] e.g. letter from Office of Sick and Wounded Seamen to Admiralty Board, 19 August 1797, ADM/F/27, NMM.

[137] Quoted in Pym to Lords of the Privy Council, undated, Papers of the Sotherton-Estcourt family, F.549, GCRO.

[138] See Harrison, 'Disease, Diplomacy and International Commerce'; Booker, *Maritime Quarantine*, chap. 15.

[139] *Report of the Select Committee appointed to consider the Means of maintaining and improving the Foreign Trade of this Country, relative to Quarantine, 1824*; McDonald, 'The History of Quarantine in Britain during the 19th Century'; Pelling, *Cholera, Fever and English Medicine*, 27–30.

disliked it for the same reasons their senior officers defended it: they saw it as an instrument of state power and a bulwark of the established order. They also condemned quarantine as a crude and archaic method of disease prevention and argued that environmental management, based on the natural history of epidemic diseases, offered a more efficient and less onerous alternative.[140] In the first two decades of the nineteenth century, those who pressed for the liberalization or abolition of quarantine were unable to make much headway, but by the 1830s, they formed the clear majority in the medical establishments of the Army, Navy, and East India Company. As a book review in the *India Journal of Medical Science* put it: 'Yellow fever, Dysentery, Ophthalmia, were at one time supposed to be contagious, but who at the present day stands up for such a doctrine.'[141] The tide was beginning to turn in favour of the reform of quarantine, too. By the mid-1840s, colonial practitioners were beginning to exert considerable influence over government, their opinions being very much in tune with the sentiments of Robert Peel and the advocates of free trade. Although quarantine was not abolished in Great Britain, the middle decades of the century saw practitioners with colonial experience dominate discussions over yellow fever and cholera, nudging government ever further in the direction of liberalization.[142]

[140] This was true of sanitary measures on ships, as well as on land; see Foxhall, 'Disease at Sea'.
[141] Review of J. Hutchinson, *Observations on Cholera Asphyxia*, *India Journal of Medical Science*, 1 (1834), 129.
[142] Harrison, 'Disease, Diplomacy and International Commerce'.

Conclusion

In the Preface to the first volume of the *Transactions of the Medical and Physical Society of Bombay* (1838), Charles Morehead warned his readers that 'to be slavish imitators of the doctrines, and systems of the European schools, is to shew that we do not estimate our position here, at its true value to science'.[1] It was a statement that might have been made at any time in either India or the West Indies over the preceding century. It was not, as one might infer from the later history of the Indian medical services, a defensive statement, intended to bolster professional morale.[2] It was, rather, an expression of confidence grounded in empirical observation and personal experience. Practitioners who had worked for any length of time in India, the West Indies, or other overseas locations tended to emphasize the particularity of their diseases and the necessity of modifying therapeutics to suit their 'elusive and varying forms', as the naval surgeon Charles Curtis described them. Such ideas had been expressed with growing assertiveness in pamphlets, books, and journals from the late seventeenth century and, from about the middle of the eighteenth century, formed the core of a relatively distinct body of theory and practice. The peculiarities of colonial medicine were increasingly expressed in references to the diseases of 'warm', 'hot', and 'tropical' climates; terms that indicate not only their difference from diseases of temperate latitudes but a degree of similarity across what many contemporaries called the 'Torrid Zone'. The medicine of warm climates was also distinguished by the prominence that it gave to matters of 'race'. Racial ideas were by no means absent from medical writings on Britain, but in the medicine of warm climates the exploration and exposition of the relationship between climate and physical difference was often central.

There was, however, a degree of ambiguity in the way in which the diseases and medical practices of tropical lands were represented in Europe. When it suited them, practitioners who worked in warm climates stressed the singularity of their diseases and the need to modify European practice accordingly. Indeed, in some cases the teaching of European universities and hospitals appeared to be redundant. But most of these practitioners did not remain in the colonies all their professional lives. They sought ways to make their experience relevant to

[1] Morehead, 'Preface', *Transactions of the Medical and Physical Society of Bombay*, 1 (1838), ix.
[2] See Harrison, *Public Health in British India.*

medicine at home and often acknowledged similarities between the diseases of warm and temperate climates. This enabled them to claim that they could provide unique insights into the causes and prevention of diseases afflicting Britons who remained at home, and that the therapies they had learned during their time overseas could be used, with certain modifications, to treat them.

One of the reasons why they were able to do so was the perception that the British disease environment was changing. During the eighteenth century, there was increasing unease about outbreaks of 'crowd diseases' in jails, towns, factories, army barracks, and ships. Economic and social change, and the expansion of the armed services, gave rise to anxieties which often found their expression in fears about disease. Practitioners who had gained extensive experience of fevers overseas increasingly found employment in hospitals in Britain, including some newly created establishments such as fever hospitals and dispensaries for the sick poor. Indeed, they were sometimes instrumental in establishing them. In such institutions, they tended to use forms of treatment similar to those used in the colonies, John Clark's practice in Newcastle being a case in point. The expertise which colonial practitioners had gained in the treatment of chronic disorders also enabled them to occupy a niche in the treatment of invalids who had returned from the colonies. The same skills were useful in attracting patients afflicted with chronic ailments said to be characteristic of modern society: a range of nervous and dyspeptic disorders which many likened to the maladies of tropical invalids. Men with experience of working in the Indies were therefore among the most prominent practitioners in resorts such as Bath and Cheltenham, as well as being proprietors of some of the most fashionable spas.

Many practitioners who had never ventured overseas – Lyssons, Hamilton, and Beddoes, for example – also saw the potential relevance of colonial experience and began to employ colonial methods in the treatment of diseases in Britain. Others incorporated the findings of post-mortem dissections conducted in colonial hospitals, recognizing the great strides made in these institutions in the pathology of fevers, dysentery, and hepatitis. Among those who did so was the physician William Saunders, Britain's foremost authority on diseases of the liver. Saunders' work drew heavily on that of Indian surgeons who had elucidated the pathology of hepatic diseases and who suggested new forms of treatment based on their post-mortem observations. He was one of a growing number of practitioners and laypersons who became convinced of the therapeutic potential of mercurial drugs in diseases of the liver and the digestive system. Indeed, mercurial therapy represents one of the most striking examples of the 'circulation' of practices between the colonies and Europe. From small beginnings in south India, the use of mercury in a range of digestive disorders became common throughout the British Empire.

The history of mercurial therapy for hepatic and febrile disorders is significant because it was perhaps the first British remedy to derive its rationale largely from pathology. In this sense, it precedes developments normally associated with the infirmaries of revolutionary Paris. Indeed, all the characteristic elements of what have come to be known as 'hospital medicine' were present twenty or thirty years before in military and naval institutions in the colonies. Investigative autopsies were conducted as a matter of routine; symptoms in living patients were correlated with signs revealed post-mortem; pathological anatomy informed therapeutic practice; and trials of new drugs and therapies were made in a systematic manner among their patients. The results of these investigations had begun to percolate into medical knowledge and practice in Britain some years before the profession doffed its cap to Paris. It is no accident, either, that some of the champions of Paris medicine were reform-minded men with analogous experience in the colonies.

Amidst the upheavals of the French Wars, Britain also faced the very real possibility of the invasion of new diseases such as yellow fever and the return of old ones such as plague. Here, again, the experience of practitioners who had served overseas in a military or naval capacity seemed indispensable and, by the 1810s, the government began to turn to them for advice as well as to more established bodies like the Royal College of Physicians. Viewed in the wider context of the campaign for state recognition by surgeon-apothecaries, and the passage of the Apothecaries Act in 1815, this amounts to a significant dilution of traditional authority, in certain aspects of medicine at least. It also betokens a greater willingness on the part of government to involve itself in medical affairs. Government select committees on such matters as fumigation, the contagiousness of plague, and the utility of quarantine provide further indications of the same trend. In this public arena, colonial practitioners appealed to a wider public in an attempt to circumvent the authority wielded by the royal colleges.[3] It is important not to take this argument too far, however: the royal colleges retained considerable power and influence. And yet, these were signs of things to come, of an important shift in the balance of professional authority in which colonial practitioners had played an important part.

The impact made by medical practitioners who had worked in the colonies owed a good deal to their close ties with reformers in Britain, and to some extent in other countries. Some practitioners were attracted to work overseas by the promise of greater professional freedom and opportunities to observe diseases they could not see at home. Others were drawn by the prospect of discovering new remedies. Either way, most exhibited in their professional and private lives what Charles Maclean called a 'great independence of mind'. Their work in the tropics may thus be regarded as an extension or enlargement of investigations begun at home by medical practitioners and natural philosophers who tended to have a reformist agenda. There were extensive and close connections between practitioners working in India and the East Indies and like-minded individuals in

[3] See Kelly, '"Not from the College"'.

Dissenting circles in Britain and America, and also with colleagues in some of the Protestant nations of northern Europe. They were united not only by their desire for reform in medicine but by their earnest endeavours for the betterment of humanity. This entailed the provision of cheaper and more effective remedies, and the removal of restrictions on liberty and commerce, such as those represented by the old system of quarantine. Practitioners who had visited the West Indies as part of their military and naval service – men such as Gillespie, Trotter, and Blane – also tended to be strong in their condemnation of the slave trade and of conditions in plantations, although by no means uniformly so, while private practitioners who had gained employment in sugar plantations tended to support the status quo, for obvious reasons. In India, the improving spirit often lent itself uncritically to support of the East India Company as a kind of benevolent despotism that would sweep away oriental superstition and corruption. But there was also a degree of sympathy for and interest in local medical traditions which exhibited a strong sense of common humanity, and occasionally a kind of Romantic longing for an unsullied and uncomplicated existence. Indeed, some practitioners were ambivalent or even hostile to imperialism and commerce, believing that they corrupted all associated with them.

During and after the French Revolutionary and Napoleonic Wars, expressions of radical dissent among colonial practitioners were rare. But the patina of conservatism and respectability that now glossed the surgeons of the Army, Navy, and East India Company did not altogether stifle their reformist and cosmopolitan impulses. They continued to see themselves as being in the vanguard of medical progress and made common cause with like-minded individuals overseas, such as those in France, Spain, and America. They did not speak with one voice on matters such as contagion and quarantine, for example, but on the whole they tended to challenge accepted wisdom as represented by the Royal College of Physicians. They continued to stress the virtues of empirical observation over textual authority and of experience over tradition. By the 1820s, professional opinion had shifted substantially in their favour, with debates turning on the results of scientific trials. As the fate of Helenus Scott's controversial nitrous acid treatment shows, these did not always favour practitioners with overseas experience, but the case demonstrates that the fundamental principles long espoused by tropical practitioners had been accepted.

The cumulative effects of colonial expansion thus added substantial impetus to those who sought to reform British medicine during the eighteenth and early nineteenth centuries. In the main, these tended to be surgeons or surgeon-apothecaries rather than physicians, although many of the latter were also embracing what they regarded as scientific practice, grounded in the same empirical and experimental methods espoused by surgeons. The development of medicine in the British colonies must be seen as part of this process; indeed, the relationship between tropical and domestic practice is best seen in terms of reciprocity and critical engagement rather than a flow of ideas and practices in any particular direction. Recent work on 'networks' and on the 'circulation' of knowledge and practices captures the complexity of these interactions much better than the centralized and hierarchical models traditionally used to frame 'colonial science'.[4] But while acknowledging the existence of many overlapping (sometimes, transnational) networks, we ought not to lose sight of the power relationships which mediated all such transactions. The most important thing, perhaps, is to be specific about the terms of exchange. Medical knowledge was obtained and disseminated in many ways: it was sometimes purchased and sometimes freely given. On some occasions, it was shared among peers of roughly equal esteem or offered up in the hope of preferment or patronage. Medical practices were often emulated but also, not infrequently, imposed by military or naval authorities. The net effect of these transactions – however we choose to construe them – was to place medical knowledge obtained in the colonial tropics increasingly at the heart of British medicine. In this sense, medicine was no different from any other aspect of British private or public life, which was profoundly altered by the effects of colonial expansion.[5] Indeed, the last section of this book has attempted to show just how closely embroiled medical issues were with other concerns stemming directly or indirectly from international trade, war, and territorial acquisition. The emergence of what contemporaries celebrated as 'rational' or 'scientific' medicine was therefore intimately bound up with Britain's commercial and imperial interests, with the empire at home as well as overseas.

[4] e.g. Raj, *Relocating Modern Science*; Sivasundaram, 'Trading Knowledge'; Lester, 'Imperial Circuits and Networks'; Wade Chambers and Gillespie, 'Locality in the History of Science'.

[5] Colley, *Britons*; Hall, *Civilising Subjects*.

Bibliography

PRIMARY SOURCES

Archives and manuscripts

GREAT BRITAIN

Aberdeen Medico-Chirurgical Society, University of Aberdeen
Papers of Sir James McGrigor

Birmingham City Archives
Papers of James Watt

Bristol Record Office
Letters of George Clement
Papers of Rev. Thomas Morris

British Library
Asia, Pacific and African Collections:
Bengal Military Consultations
Bengal Public Proceedings
East India Company Marine
India Home Consultations
Madras Public Proceedings (Consultations)

European Manuscripts:
Manuscript of S. K. Bhuyan
Cruso papers
Papers of Sir Paul Jodrell
Papers of Col. John MacDonald
Letters from Dr Francis Maxwell
Diary of Kenneth Murchison
Raleigh papers
Papers of William Roxburgh
Spilsbury letters
Papers of J. C. Wade
Papers of H. H. Wilson

Add. MSS:
Correspondence of Sir Joseph Banks
Papers of Lord Dropmore

Derbyshire Record Office
Fitzherbert of Tissington Papers

Gloucestershire County Record Office
Papers of Capt. Richard Barlow
Correspondence of C. L. Davies
Dickinson family correspondence
Ducarel family papers
Memorandum of Mr Fortesque's Services in India
Returns of His Majesty's Forces, October 1767
Correspondence of the Huntley family
Papers of the Sotherton-Estcourt family

Hampshire County Record Office
Papers of the Earl of Malmesbury

Herefordshire Record Office
Correspondence of Henry Smith

Lincolnshire Archives
Papers collected by Sir Francis Hill

The National Archives
ADM 1/232
ADM 101
ADM 1/235

National Maritime Museum
ADM/F/27
F/7 CL

Natural History Museum
Papers of William Roxburgh

Plymouth and West Devon Record Office
Minutes and memoranda of Capt. Richard Creyke
John Glennys Papers

Robinson Library, Special Collections, University of Newcastle
Hospital Archives

Royal College of Physicians of Edinburgh
Anon, 'An Essay on the Hypochondriac Disease'
Papers of William Cullen
Papers of Sir John Pringle
Papers of William Roxburgh
Papers of Partick Russell
Lecture notes of Robert Whytt

Sheffield City Archives
Wentworth Woodhouse Muniments

University of Glasgow Library, Special Collections
MS Cullen

University of Nottingham
Bentinck Papers

Wellcome Library for the History and Understanding of Medicine
Western Manuscript Collection:
Papers of Sir George Ballingall
Collection of Nicolas Chervin
V. O. Gouraud, Memorandum on the French military hospital service
Papers of M. J. de Herrate
Papers of William Cuming
Papers of John Fothergill
Papers of Martin de Sesse y Lacasta
Letters of Lord George Macartney
Charles Middleton, Reports on Haslar Hospital
Journal of Surgeon Pigot
Commonplace book of Thomas Thomson

Royal Army Medical Corps Muniment Collection:
Alexander Allan Cormack (ed.), *The Mahratta Wars 1792–1805: Letters from the Front by Three Brothers – Nicholas, George and Thomas Carnegie of Charleton, Montrose*
William Fergusson, letters
William Fergusson, reports on hospitals in the West Indies

West Sussex Record Office
Goodwood MSS

Wiltshire and Swindon Record Office
Letters from Sir Paul Jodrell

INDIA

Maharashtra State Archives
Bombay, Hospital Board Diary
Public Department Diary

Tamil Nadu State Archives
Surgeon General's Records, Madras

West Bengal State Archives
Judicial (Criminal) Consultations

JAMAICA

National Library of Jamaica, Special Collections
Hospital records, 1739–48

UNITED STATES OF AMERICA

American Philosophical Society, Philadelphia
Girard papers

Green Library, Stanford University
Correspondence of Thomas de St Laurent

Lilly Library, University of Indiana, Bloomington
Wyndham MSS

Books and published reports

a Costa, Christaphori, *Aromatum & medicamentum in Orientali India nascentium* (Antwerp: Christophori Platini, 1582).

Ainslie, Whitelaw, *Observations on the Cholera Morbus of India: A Letter addressed to the Honourable Court of Directors of the East India Company* (London: Kingsbury, Parbury and Allen, 1825).

Alexander, William, *Experimental Essays on the following Subjects: I. On the external Application of Antiseptics in Putrid Diseases. II. On the Diseases and Effects of Medicines. III. On Diuretics and Sudorifics, Essay II* (London: s.n., 1790).

Allen, Colinus, *Dissertatio medica inauguralis, seu observations quaedem de febre remittente, quae grassabatur in insula Sancta Lucia, annis MDCCXCVI. MDCCXCVII* (Edinburgh: John Moir, 1818).

Alpini, Prosper, *De medicina Ægyptiorum. Libri quator. Iacobi Bontii, In Indiis archiatri, de medicina Indorum* (Paris: G. Pele & I. Duval, 1646).

Annesley, James, *Researches into the Causes, and Treatment of the more prevalent Diseases of India, and of Warm Climates more generally. Illustrated with Cases, Post-Mortem Examinations, and Numerous Coloured Engravings of Morbid Structures* (London: Longman, Rees, Orme, Browne and Green, 1828).

Anon., *Paracelsus his Aurora, & Treasure of the Philosophers. As also the Water-Stone of the Wise Men; Describing the Matter of, and Manner how to attain the universal Tincture* (London: J. H. Oxon., 1659).

Anon., *Traité de la Peste* (Paris: Guillaume Cavelier, 1722).

Anon., *Medicina Vindicata: Or, Reflections on Bleeding, Vomiting, and Purging, in the Beginning of Fevers, Small-Pox, Pleurises and other Acute Diseases, by a Fellow of the College of Physicians in Dublin* (London: James and John Knapton, 1728).

Armstrong, John, *Miscellanies* (London: T. Cadell, 1770).

Armstrong, Robert, *The Influence of Climate and other Agents on the Human Constitution, with reference to the Causes and Prevention of Disease among Seamen: with Observations on Fever in General, and an Account of the Epidemic Fever of Jamaica* (London: Longman, Brown, Green & Longman, 1843).

Arnott, Archibald, *Dissertatio medica inauguralis de febre remittente* (Edinburgh: C. Stewart, 1815).

Arthy, Elliot, *The Seaman's Medical Advocate: Or, An Attempt to shew that Five Thousand Seamen are, annually, during war, lost to the British Nation, in the West-India Merchant's*

Service, and on-board Ships of War on the West-India Station, through the Yellow Fever, And other Diseases and Means, from Causes which, it is conceived, are chiefly to be obviated, and unconnected with the Misfortunes of War or Dangers of the Seas (London: Richardson and Egerton, 1798).

Balfour, Francis, *Treatise on the Influence of the Moon in Fevers* (Calcutta: George Gordon, 1784).

Balfour, Francis, *A Treatise on Putrid Intestinal Remitting Fevers, in which the Laws of the febrile State and Sol-Lunar Influence being Investigated and Defined, are Applied to Explain the Nature of the Various Forms, Crises, and other Phenomena of these Fevers; and there is Deduced and Instituted an Improved Method of Curing Them* (Edinburgh: William Smellie, 1790).

Balfour, Francis, *A Treatise on the Action of Sol-Lunar Influence, in which it is inferred, from Observations on the Urine, etc, etc, that it occasions the Daily and Lunar Revolutions Observable in the State of Fevers, of other Diseases, and of Health, by producing coincident Changes in the Condition of the Constrictive Power and Balance of the Vascular System* (Edinburgh: William Smellie, 1791).

Balfour, Francis, *A Treatise on Sol-Lunar Influence in Fevers* (Calcutta: Company's Press, 1794).

Ballingall, George, *Practical Observations on Fever, Dysentery, and Liver Complaints; as they occur amongst the European Troops in India; with Introductory Remarks, on the Disadvantages of selecting Boys for Indian Military Service* (Edinburgh: David Browne and A. Constable & Co., 1818).

Bally, Victor, *Du typhus d'Amerique ou fièvre jaune* (Paris: Smith, 1814).

Baltimore City Health Department, *The First Thirty-Five Annual Reports, 1815–1849* (Baltimore: The Commissioner of Health of Baltimore, Maryland, 1853).

Bampfield, R. W., *A Practical Treatise on Tropical Dysentery, more particularly as it occurs in the East Indies; illustrated by Cases and Appearances on Dissection: to which is added a Practical Treatise on Scorbutic Dysentery, with some Facts and Observations relative to Scurvy* (London: Burgess & Hill, 1819).

Bancroft, Edward N., *Exposure of Misrepresentations by Dr McGrigor and Dr Jackson to the Commissioners of Military Enquiry* (London: T. Cadell & W. Davies, 1808).

Bancroft, Edward N., *A Letter to the Commissioners of Military Enquiry, containing some Animadversions on some Parts of their Fifth Report* (London: J. Murray, 1808).

Bancroft, Edward N., *An Essay on the Disease called Yellow Fever, with Observations concerning Febrile Contagion, Typhus Fever, Dysentery, and the Plague, partly delivered as the Gulstonian Lectures, before the College of Physicians, in the Years 1806 and 1807* (London: T. Cadell & W. Davies, 1811).

Bancroft, Edward N., *A Sequel to an Essay on the Yellow Fever; principally intended to prove, by incontestable Facts and important Documents, that the Fever, called Bulam, or Pestilential, has no Existence as a distinct, or a Contagious Disease* (London: J. Callow, 1817).

Barker, John, *An Inquiry into the Nature, Cause, and Cure of the present Epidemick Fever. Together with some general Observations concerning the Difference betwixt Nervous and Inflammatory Fevers, and the Method of treating each* (London: T. Astley, 1742).

Barker, John, *An Essay on the Agreement betwixt Ancient and Modern Physicians: or a Comparison between the Practice of Hippocrates, Galen, Sydenham, and Boerhaave, in Acute Diseases* (London: G. Hawkins, 1747).

Beddoes, Thomas (ed.), *Reports, principally concerning the Effects of the Nitrous Acid in the Venereal Disease, by Surgeons of the Royal Naval Hospital at Plymouth, and other Practitioners* (Bristol: J. Johnson, 1797).

Bellini, Laurentii, *Opuscula aliquot* (Lugduni Batavorum [Leiden]: Cornelium Boutesteyn, 1656).

Bernier, F., *Travels in the Mogul Empire A.D. 1656–1668*, tr. I. Brock, rev. A. Constable (New Delhi: S. Chand & Son, 1972).

Bichat, Xavier, *Anatomie Générale, appliqué a la Physiologie et a la Médecine*, 4 vols (Paris: Brosson, Gabon & Co., 1801).

Bichat, Xavier, *Physiological Researches on Life and Death*, tr. F. Gold (London: Longman, Hurst, Rees, Orme and Browne, 1815).

Blair, William, *Essays on the Venereal Disease, and its Concomitant Affections. Illustrated by a Variety of Cases: Essay I. Part I. On the Antivenereal Effects of the Nitric Acid, Oxygenated Muriate of Potash, and several analogous remedies, which have been lately proposed as substitutes for Mercury* (London: J. Johnson, 1798).

Bland, Humphry, *A Treatise of Military Discipline; in which is laid down and explained the Duty of the Officer and Soldier, thro' the several Branches of the Service* (London and Dublin, 1743).

Blane, Gilbert, *Observations on the Diseases Incident to Seamen* (London: Joseph Cooper, 1785).

Blane, Gilbert, *Observations on the Diseases Incident to Seamen*, 3rd edn. (London: Murray and Highley, 1799).

Blane, Gilbert, *Select Dissertations on Several Subjects of Medical Science* (London: Thomas and George Underwood, 1822).

Blicke, Charles, *An Essay on the Bilious or Yellow Fever of Jamaica, collected from the Manuscript of a late Surgeon* (London: T. Bechet & Co., 1772).

Boerhaave, W., *Boerhaave's Aphorisms: Concerning the Knowledge and Causes of Disease*, tr. J. Delacoste (London: W. & J. Innys, 1742).

Bolingbroke, Henry, *A Voyage to the Demerary: An Account of the Settlements there and on the Essequebo and Berbice* (Georgetown: The Daily Chronicle, 1941 [1807]).

Bontius, Jacobus, *De medicina Indorum* (Lugduni Batav. [Leiden]: Apud Franciscum Hackium, 1642).

Bontius, Jacobus, *An Account of the Diseases, Natural History, and Medicines of the East Indies*, tr. anon. (London: T. Noteman, 1769).

Boyle, Robert, *The General History of the Air, designed and begun by the Hon. Robert Boyle* (London: A. and J. Churchill, 1692).

Brande, W. T. and Parke, Samuel, *A Descriptive Account of Mr Thompson's Laboratory at Cheltenham for the Preparation of Cheltenham Salts, with a Chemical Analysis of the Waters whence they are produced* (Cheltenham: G. A. Williams, 1817).

Brett, F. H., *A Practical Essay on some of the Principal Diseases of India* (Calcutta: Thacker and Co., 1840).

Brocklesby, Richard, *Œconomical and Medical Observations, in Two Parts. From the Year 1758 to the Year 1763, inclusive. Tending to the Improvement of Military Hospitals, and to the Cure of Camp Diseases, incident to Soldiers. To which is subjoined, An Appendix, containing a curious Account of the Climate and Diseases in Africa, upon the Great River Senegal, and farther up than the Island of Senegal. In a Letter from Mr Boone,*

Practitioners in Physic to that Garrison for Three Years, to Dr Brocklesby (London: T. Beckett and P. A. De Hondt, 1764).

Brown, John, *The Works of Dr John Brown M.D. To which is prefixed a biographical Account of the Author by W. C. Brown*, 3 vols (London: J. Johnson, 1804).

Bryce, James, *An Account of the Yellow Fever, with a successful Method of Cure* (Edinburgh: W. Creech, 1796).

Buchan, William, *Domestic Medicine; or the Family Physician* (Philadelphia: John Dunlop, 1772).

Burke, Edmund, *A Philosophical Enquiry into the Origin of our Ideas of the Sublime and Beautiful* (Dublin: Graisberry & Campbell, 1771).

Burnett, William, *Official Report on the Fever which appeared on board H.M. Ship Bann, on the Coast of Africa; and amongst the Detachment of Royal Marines, forming the Garrison of the Island of Ascension, in the Year 1823* (London: Burgess and Hill, 1824).

Burt, Adam, *A Tract on the Biliary Complaints of Europeans in Hot Climates; founded on Observations in Bengal, and consequently designed to be particularly useful to those in that Country* (Calcutta: John Hay, 1785).

Burton, Richard, *Goa and the Blue Mountains; Or Six Months of Sick Leave* (London: R. Bentley, 1851).

Butterfield, L. H. (ed.), *The Letters of Benjamin Rush*, 2 vols (Princeton: Princeton University Press, 1951).

Campbell, Gulielmus, *Disputatio medica inauguralis de dysenteria complectens* (Edinburgh: Stevenson and Co., 1818).

Carter, Gulielmus Fransicus, *Tentamen medicum inaugurale de febre endemica occidentalium* (Edinburgh: D. Schaw and Son, 1818).

Cheyne, George, *The English Malady, or, A Treatise of Nervous Diseases of all Kinds, as Spleen, Vapours, Lowness of Spirits, Hypochondrial, and Hysterical Distempers, etc.* (London: G. Strahan, 1733).

Chisholm, Colin, *An Essay on the Malignant Pestilential Fever introduced into the West Indian Islands from Boullam, on the Coast of Guinea, as it appeared in 1793 and 1794* (London: C. Dilly, 1795).

Chisholm, Colin, *A Manual of the Climate and Diseases of Tropical Countries; in which a Practical View of the Statistical Pathology, and of the History and Treatment of the Diseases of those Countries, is attempted to be given: calculated chiefly as a Guide to the young medical Practitioner on his first resorting to those Countries* (London: Burgess and Hill, 1822).

Clark, John, *Observations on the Diseases of Long Voyages to Hot Countries, and particularly on those which prevail in the East Indies* (London: D. Wilson, 1773).

Clark, John, *A Collection of Papers intended to promote an Institution for the Cure and Prevention of Infectious Fevers in Newcastle and other populous Towns. Together with the Communications of the most eminent Physicians relative to the Safety and Importance of annexing Fever-Wards to the Newcastle and other Infirmaries* (Newcastle: S. Hodgson, 1802).

Clark, John, *Observations on the Diseases which prevail in Long Voyages to Hot Countries, particularly those in the East Indies; and in the same Diseases as they appear in Great Britain* (London: John Murray, 1809).

Clark, Thomas, *Observations on the Nature and Cure of Fevers, and of Diseases of the West and East Indies, and of America: with an Account of Dissections performed in those Climates and General Remarks on Diseases in the Army* (Edinburgh: Bell and Bradfute, 1801).

Clarke, James, *A Treatise on the Yellow Fever, as it appeared in the Island of Dominica in the Years 1793–4–5–6* (London: J. Murray and S. Highley, 1797).

Cleghorn, George, *Observations on the Epidemical Diseases in Minorca. From the Year 1744 to 1749. To which is prefixed, a short Account of the Climate, Productions, Inhabitants, and Endemical Distempers of that Island* (London: D. Wilson, 1751).

Cobbett, William, *Rural Rides*, 2 vols (London: Reeves & Turner, 1885).

Cockburn, Marcus, *Dissertatio medica inauguralis de dysenteria Indae orientalis* (Edinburgh: Stevenson and Co., 1818).

Cockburn, William, *The Present Uncertainty in the Knowledge of Medicines, in a Letter to the Physicians in the Commission for Sick and Wounded Seamen. With a Postscript to Physicians, shewing the Necessity of a True Theory of Diseases* (London: Benjamin Barker, 1703).

Cockburn, William, *Sea Diseases: Or, a Treatise of Their Nature, Causes and Cure* (2nd edn., London: George Strachan, 1706).

Colin, Anthoine (ed. and tr.), *Histoire des Drogues, Espiceries, et de Certains Medicamens Simples, qui naissent es Indes et en l'Amerique, divise en deux parties* (Lyon: Pillehotte, 1619).

Collett, Joseph, *The Private Letter Books of Joseph Collett, Sometime Governor of Fort St. George, Madras*, ed. H. H. Dodwell (London: Longmans, Green and Co., 1933).

Corner, B. C. and Booth, C. C. (eds.), *Chain of Friendship: Selected Letters of Dr John Fothergill of London, 1735–1780* (Cambridge, Mass.: Belknap Press, 1971).

Cruickshank, William, *The Results of the Trials of various Acids, and some other Substances, in the Treatment of Lues Venerea* (London: C. Dilly, 1797).

Currie, James, *Medical Reports on the Effects of Water, cold and warm, as a remedy in Fever and Febrile Diseases, whether applied to the surface of the Body, or used as a drink; with Observations on the nature of Fever, and on the Effects of Opium, Alcohol, and Inanition* (London: Cadell and Davies, 1797).

Currie, James, *Examination of the Prejudices commonly entertained against Mercury as beneficially applicable to most Hepatic Complaints* (London: J. M'Creery, 1809).

Curtin, Samuel, *Tentamen medicum inaugurale, de febre flava Indae Occidentalis* (Edinburgh: Balfour and Smellie, 1778).

Curtis, Charles, *An Account of the Diseases in India, as they appeared in the English Fleet, and in the Naval Hospital at Madras, in 1782 and 1783, with Observations on Ulcers, and the Hospital Sores of that Country* (Edinburgh: W. Laing, 1807).

da Orta, Garcia, *Coloquios dos Simples, e Drogas he cousas Mediçinais da India, & assi dalgûas fructas achadas nella onde se tratam algûas cousas tocantes amediçina, practica, & outras cousas boas, pera saber cópostos pello Doutor Garçia Dorta* (Goa: Ioannes de Endem, 1563).

da Silveira Caldiera, Joannes, *Disputatio medica inauguralis de febrius intermittentibus* (Edinburgh: Neill and Co., 1815).

Dancer, Thomas, *The Medical Assistant; or Jamaica Practice of Physic: designed chiefly for the use of Families and Plantations* (Kingston: Alexander Aikman, 1801).

Darwin, Erasmus, *Zoonomia: or, the Laws of Organic Life*, 2 vols (1st American edn.; Philadelphia: T. Dobson, 1797).

de Arejula, Don Juan Manuel, *Breve descripcion de la fiebre amarilla padecida en Cadiz y pueblos cornarcanos en 1800, en Medinasidonia en 1801, en Malaga en 1803, y en esta misma plaza y varias otras del reyno en 1804* (Madrid: Imprenta Real, 1806).

de Castenada, H. L., *The First Book of the Historie of the Discoverie and Conquest of the Portingales, in their dangerous Navigations, in the Time of King Don John, the Second of the Name*, tr. T. East (London: T. East, 1582).

de Faria y Sousa, Manuel, *The Portuguese Asia: Or, the History of the Discovery and Conquest of India by the Portuguese*, tr. J. Stevens (London: C. Brome, 1695).

de Jonnès, Moreau, *Monographie Historique et Médicale de la Fièvre Jaune des Antilles* (Paris: Migneret, Bechet & Crevot, 1820).

Delon, J., *A Voyage to the East Indies* (London: D. Browne, 1698).

Dickson, Samuel, *On the Prevalent Diseases of India. With New Physiological and Therapeutical Illustrations* (3rd edn.; Edinburgh: J. Anderson, 1833).

Dickson, Samuel, *The Fallacy of the Art of Physic, as taught in the Schools; with the development of new and important Principles of Practice* (Edinburgh: Adam & Charles Black, 1836).

Doughty, Edward, *Observations and Inquiries into the Nature and Treatment of the Yellow, or Bulam Fever, in Jamaica, and at Cadiz; particularly in what regards its primary Cause and assigned Contagious Powers: illustrated by Cases and Dissections* (London: Highley & Son, 1816).

Douglas, Robert, *The Genealogy of the Family of Lind and the Montgomeries of Smithton, written by Sir Robert Douglas, Baronet* (Windsor: s.n., 1795).

Edwards, W. F., *De l'influence des agens physiques sur la vie* (Paris: Crochard, 1824).

Falck, N. D., *A Treatise on the Medical Qualities of Mercury* (London: B. Law, 1776).

Falconer, William, *Remarks on the Influence of Climate, Situation, Nature of Country, Population, Nature of Food, and Way of Life, on the Disposition and Temper, Manners and Behaviours, Intellects, Laws and Customs, Forms of Government, and Religion, of Mankind* (London: C. Dilly, 1781).

Faria e Sousa, Manuel de, *The Portugues Asia: Or, The History of the Discovery and Conquest of India by the Portugues*, tr. J. Stevens (London: C. Brome, 1695 [1650]).

Fellowes, James, *Reports of the Pestilential Disorder of Andalusia, which appeared at Cadiz in the Years 1800, 1804, 1810, and 1813; with a Detailed Account of that Fatal Epidemic as it prevailed at Gibraltar, during the Autumnal Months of 1804; also Observations on the Remitting and Intermitting Fever, made in the Military Hospitals at Colchester, after the Return of the Troops from the Expedition to Zealand in 1809* (London: Longman, Hurst, Rees, Orme, and Brown, 1815).

Ferguson, Adam, *An Essay on the History of Civil Society* (Basel: J. J. Tourneisen, 1789).

Fisher, *Edward Tentamen medicum inaugurale, de febre flava, reionum calidarum* (Edinburgh: George Mudie, 1795).

Fogo, Thomas MacMillan, *Dissertatio medica inauguralis de febre flava Hispaniae* (Edinburgh: Abernethy and Walker, 1818).

Fontana, Niccola Fontana, *Osservazioni intorno alli Malattie che Attaccano gli Europeine' Clinici Caldi & nelle Lunghe Navigazioni di Niccola Fontana cremonese fatten el suo Viaggio alle Indie Orientali dall anno 1776 al 1781* (Livorno: Vincenzio Falorni, 1781).

Forbes, James, *Oriental Memoirs: Selected from a Series of Familiar Letters written during seventeen Years Residence in India*, 4 vols (New Delhi: Gian Publishing House, 1988 [1813]).

Fourcroy, A.-F., 'Preliminary Discourse', *Elements of Natural History, and of Chemistry*, tr. W. Nicholson (London: G. J. J. & J. Robinson, 1788).

Fryer, John, *A New Account of East India and Persia in Eight Letters being Nine Years Travels, begun 1672 and Finished 1681* (London: R. Chiswell, 1698).

Geddes, William, *Clinical Illustrations of the Diseases of India: As exhibited in the Medical History of a Body of European Soldiers for a Series of Years from their Arrival in that Country* (London: Smith, Elder & Co., 1846).

Gentleman of the Faculty [pseud.], *Anatomical Dialogues; or, a Breviary of Anatomy. Wherein all the Parts of the Human Body are concisely and accurately described, and their Uses explained; by which the Young Practitioner may attain a Right Method of Treating Diseases, as far as it depends on Anatomy. Chiefly compiled for the Use of the Young Gentlemen in the Navy and Army* (London: G. Robinson, 1778).

Gibney, William, *A Medical Guide to the Cheltenham Waters, containing Observations on their Nature and Properties; the Diseases in which they are beneficial or hurtful; with the Rules to be Observed during their Use* (Cheltenham: S. Bettison, 1824).

Gibson, John, *A Treatise on Bilious Diseases and Indigestion, with the Effects of Quassy and Natron in these Disorders* (London: Murray and Highley, 1799).

Gillespie, Leonard, *Observations on the Diseases which prevailed on Board a Part of His Majesty's Squadron, on the Leeward Island Station, between Nov. 1794 and April 1796* (London: J. Cuthell, 1800).

Gordon, Charles Alexander, *The Principal Diseases of India, briefly described: with Hints on the Duties of Medical Officers in that Country* (London: Trelawney William Saunders, 1847).

Gupta, P. C. (ed.), *Fort William – India House Correspondence and other Contemporary Papers relating thereto (Public Series)*, vol. XIII (Delhi: National Archives of India, 1959).

Halley, Edmund, 'An Historical Account of the Trade Winds, and Monsoons, observable in the Seas between and near the Tropicks, with an Attempt to assign the Physical cause of the said Winds', *Phil. Trans.*, 16 (1686), 153–68.

Halpin, W., *Fact versus Assertion, or Critical and Explanatory Observations on some Erroneous Statements, contained in Dr Adam Neale's Pamphlet on the Nature and Properties of the Cheltenham Waters* (London: s.n., 1820).

Herbert, Thomas, *Some Years Travels into Africa and Asia the Great, especially describing the famous Empires of Persia and Industant. As also divers other Kingdoms in the Orientall Indies, and Iles adjacent* (4th edn.; London: R. Everingham, 1677 [1638]).

Hillary, William, *A Rational and Mechanical Essay on the Smallpox* (London: G. Strahan, 1735).

Hillary, William, *An Inquiry into the Contents and Medicinal Virtues of Lincomb Spa Water, near Bath* (London: J. Leake & C. Hitch, 1742).

Hillary, William, *Observations on the Changes of the Air, and the Concomitant Epidemical Diseases in the Island of Barbadoes. To which is added, a Treatise on the Putrid Bilious Fever, commonly called the Yellow Fever; and such other Diseases as are indigenous or endemial in the West India Islands or in the Torrid Zone* (London: C. Hitch and L. Hawes, 1759).

Hoffman, Friedrich, *Fundamenta Medicinae*, tr. and ed. Lester S. King (London: MacDonald, 1971).

Houlston, Thomas, *Observations on Poisons; and on the use of Mercury in the Cure of obstinate Dysenteries* (London: H. Reynell, 1784).

House of Assembly, Jamaica, *Journals of the Assembly of Jamaica* (Kingston: House of Assembly Jamaica, 1821).

Howard, John, *An Account of the Principal Lazarettos in Europe; with various Papers relative to the Plague: together with further Observations on some foreign Prisons and Hospitals; and additional Remarks on the present State of those in Britain and Ireland* (Warrington: William Eyres, 1789).

Hunter, John, *Inaugural Disputation on the Varieties of Man*; dissertation to the Fellows of the Royal Society of Edinburgh (Edinburgh: Balfour and Smellie, 1775).

Hunter, John, *Observations on the Diseases of the Army in Jamaica and on the best Means of preserving the Health of Europeans in the Climate* (London: G. Nicol, 1788).

Huxham, John, *An Essay on Fevers and their various Kinds, as depending on different Constitutions of the Blood: with Dissertations on Slow Nervous Fevers; on Putrid, Pestilential, Spotted Fevers; on the Small-Pox; and on Pleurisies and Peripneumonies* (London: S. Austen, 1750).

Ingram, Dale, *An Historical Account of the several Plagues that have appeared in the World since the Year 1346 with an Enquiry into the present prevailing Opinion, that the Plague is a Contagious Distemper, capable of being transported in Merchandize, from one Country to another* (London: R. Baldwin, 1755).

Ingram, E. (ed.), *Two Views of British India: The Private Correspondence of Mr Dundas and Lord Wellesley: 1798–1801* (London: Adams and Dart, 1969).

Jackson, Robert, *A Treatise on the Fevers of Jamaica, with some Observations on the Intermitting Fever of America, and an Appendix, containing some Hints on the Means of Preserving the Health of Soldiers in Hot Climates* (London: J. Murray, 1791).

Jackson, Robert, *An Outline of the History and Cure of Fever, Endemic and Contagious* (Edinburgh: Mundell & Son, 1798).

Jackson, Robert, *A Sketch of the History and Cure of febrile Diseases; more particularly as they appear in the West Indies among the Soldiers of the British Army* (Stockton: T. & H. Eeles, 1817).

James, R., *The Modern Practice of Physic; as improv'd by the Celebrated Professors, H. Boerhaave, and F. Hoffman*, 2 vols (London: J. Hodges, 1746).

James, R., *A Dissertation on Fevers and Inflammatory Distempers, wherein an expeditious Method is proposed of Curing those dangerous Disorders* (London: J. Newberry, 1749).

Jameson, David, *Dissertatio medica inauguralis, de febris remmitentis curatione* (Edinburgh: C. Stewart, 1818).

Jameson, Thomas, *Essays on the Changes of the Human Body, at its Different Ages; the Diseases to which it is Predisposed in each Period of Life: and the Physiological Principles of its Longevity. The whole Illustrated by Analogies in Plants and Animals* (London: Longman, Hurst, Rees, Orme and Brown, 1811).

Jameson, Thomas, *A Treatise on Cheltenham Waters and Biliary Diseases, with Introductory Observations by John Fosbroke, Surgeon, Cheltenham* (2nd edn.; Cheltenham: S. C. Harper, 1825).

Johnson, James, *The Influence of Tropical Climates, more especially of the Climate of India, on European Constitutions; and the Principal Effects and Diseases thereby induced, their Prevention and Removal, and the Means of Preserving Health in Hot Climates rendered obvious to Europeans of every Capacity* (London: J. J. Callow, 1815).

Johnson, James, *A Practical Treatise on Derangements of the Liver, Digestive Organs, and Nervous System. To which is added an Essay on the Prolongation of Life, and Conservation of Health* (2nd edn.; London: for the author, 1818).

Johnson, James, *An Essay on Morbid Sensibility of the Stomach and Bowels, as the Proximate Cause, or Characteristic Condition of Indigestion, Nervous Irritability, Mental Despondency, Hypochondriasis, etc, to which are added Observations on the Diseases and Regimen of Invalids, on their Return from Hot and Unhealthy Climates* (2nd edn.; London: Thomas and George Unwin, 1827).

Johnson, James, *The Influence of Tropical Climates on European Constitutions* (London: Thomas and George Underwood, 1827).

Johnson, James, *Change of Air, or the Philosophy of Travelling; being Autumnal Excursions through France, Switzerland, Italy, Germany, and Belgium; with Observations and Reflections on the Moral, Physical, and Medicinal Influence of Travelling-Exercise, Change of Scene, Foreign Skies, and Voluntary Expatriations. To which is Prefixed, Wear and Tear of Modern Babylon* (London: S. Highley, 1831).

Johnson, James, *The Economy of Health or the Stream of Human Life from the Cradle to the Grave with Reflections Moral, Physical and Philosophical on the Successive Phases of Human Existence, the Maladies to which they are subjected and the Dangers that may be averted* (London: Highley, 1837).

Johnstone, James, *Some Account of the Medicinal Waters, near Tewkesbury; with Thoughts on the Use and Diseases of the Lymphatic Glands in a Letter to Edward Johnstone, M.D., A Physician to the General Hospital, Birmingham* (Tewkesbury: W. Dyde and Sons, 1790).

Jones, William, *Sir William Jones's Discourses*, 2 vols (London: W. H. Carpenter, 1821).

Kaye, J. W., *Peregrine Pulteney; Or, Life in India*, 2 vols (London: John Mortimer, 1846).

Khan, I., *The Shah Jahan Nama of 'Inyat Khan*, tr. A. R. Fuller, ed. W. E. Begley and Z. A. Desai (New Delhi: Oxford University Press, 1990).

King, Gulielmus J., *Disputatio medica quaedam de febre flava* (Edinburgh: Abernethy & Walker, 1819).

Knox, Robert, *The Races of Man: A Fragment* (London: Henry Renshaw, 1850).

Laitner, Christiano, *De Febrius et Morbis Acutis* (Venice: H. Albricium, 1721).

Lempriere, William, *A Tour from Gibraltar to Tangier, Sallee, Mogodore, Santa Cruz, Tarudant; and thence, over Mount Atlas, to Morocco: including a particular Account of the Royal Harem, etc.* (London: Walter, 1793).

Lempriere, William, *Practical Observations on the Diseases of the Army in Jamaica, as they occurred between the Years 1792 and 1797; on the Situation, Climate, and Diseases of that Island; and on the most probable Means of lessening Mortality among the Troops, and among Europeans in Tropical Climates*, 2 vols (London: T. N. Longman and O. Rees, 1799).

Lempriere, William, *Report on the Medicinal Effects of an Aluminous Chalybeate Spring, lately discovered at Sandrocks, in the Parish of Chale in the Isle of Wight, pointing out its Efficacy in the Walcheren and other Diseases incident to Soldiers who have served Abroad, and more particularly the Advantages to be derived from its Introduction into Private Practice* (Newport, Isle of Wight: Musson and Taylor, undated).

Lind, James, *An Essay on the Most Effectual Means of preserving the Health of Seamen, in the Royal Navy. Containing Directions proper for all those who undertake long Voyages at Sea, or reside in unhealthy Situations, with Cautions necessary for the Preservation of such Persons as attend the Sick in Fevers* (London: D. Wilson, 1762).

Lind, James, *An Essay on Diseases incidental to Europeans in Hot Climates with the Method of preventing their fatal Consequences* (London: T. Beckett & A. De Hondt, 1768).

Lind, James, *An Essay on Diseases incidental to Europeans in Hot Climates with the Method of preventing their fatal Consequences* (rev. edn.; London: J. & J. Richardson, 1808).

Lind, James, *A Treatise on the Putrid, and Remitting Marsh-Fever, which raged at Bengal in the year 1762* (Edinburgh: C. Elliot, 1776).

Lind, James, *Sketch for a Medical Education* (Windsor: s.n., 1800).

Lyssons, Daniel, *An Essay upon the Effects of Camphire and Calomel in Continual Fevers, illustrated by several Cases. To which is added, an occasional Observation upon the modern Practice of Inoculation. And from the whole is deduced an Argument in support of the Opinion, that the alimentary Canal is the principal Seat of a Fever* (London: E. Reeve, 1771).

M'Cabe, James, *Observations on the Cheltenham Waters, and the Diseases in which they are recommended. To which is annexed, An Analysis of the Salts and Waters, by several very eminent Chemists* (Cheltenham: G. A. Williams, 1820).

McCabe, James, *A Reply to Dr Neale's Pamphlet, respecting the Nature and Properties of the Mineral Waters of Cheltenham* (Cheltenham: G. A. Wiliams, 1820).

McCabe, James, *Directions for Drinking the Cheltenham Waters; with a Selection of Cases, illustrating their Effects in a great Variety* (Cheltenham: G. A. Williams, 1823).

McCabe, James, *Military Medical Reports; containing Pathological and Practical Observations illustrating the Diseases of Warm Climates* (Cheltenham: G. A. Williams, 1825).

M'Cann, F. A., *Dissertatio medica inauguralis de dysenteria tropica* (Edinburgh: D. Schaw and Son, 1818).

MacGregor, W. L., *Practical Observations on the Principal Diseases affecting the Health of the European and Native Soldiers in the North-Western Provinces of India; with a Supplement on Dysentery* (Calcutta: W. Thacker and Co., 1843).

M'Gregor [McGrigor], James, *Medical Sketches of the Expedition to Egypt* (London: John Murray, 1804).

McGrigor, James, *A Letter to the Commissioners of Military Enquiry, in reply to some Animadversions of Dr E. Nathaniel Bancroft on their Fifth Report* (London: John Murray, 1808).

McGrigor, James, *The Scalpel and the Sword: The Autobiography of the Father of Army Medicine*, ed. M. McGrigor (Dalkeith: Scottish Cultural Press, 2000).

M'Kinnal, Robertus, *Tentamen medicum inaugurale quaedam de dysenteria Indiae orientalis* (Edinburgh: Stevenson and Co., 1818).

Maclean, Charles, *A Treatise on the Action of Mercury, upon Living Bodies and its Application for the Cure of Diseases of Indirect Debility* (Philadelphia: William Young, 1797).

Maclean, Charles, *To the British Inhabitants of India* (Calcutta: s.n., 1798).

Maclean, Charles, *The Affairs of Asia considered in their Effects on the Liberties of Britain, in a Series of Letters, addressed to the Marquis of Wellesley, late Governor of India; including a Correspondence with the Government of Bengal, under that Nobleman, and a Narrative of Transactions involving the Annihilation of a personal Freedom of the Subject, and the Extinction of the Liberty of the Press in India* (London: s.n., 2nd edn., 1806).

Maclean, Charles, *On the State of Vaccination in 1810; in a Letter to the Rt. Hon. Richard Rider, H.M.'s Principal Secretary of State for the Home Department: with Remarks on the Report of the National Vaccine Establishment. Forming a Guide for Parents in deciding for the Safety of their Children* (London: s.n., 1810).

Maclean, Charles, *An Analytical View of the Medical Department of the British Army* (London: J. Stockdale, 1810).

Maclean, Charles, *A View of the Consequences of laying open the Trade to India, to Private Ships; with some Remarks on the Nature of the East India Company's Rights to their Territories, and the Trade depending on them; and on the Conduct and Issue of the late Negociation for a Renewal of their Exclusive Privileges* (London: A. J. Valpy, 1813).

Maclean, Charles, *Remarks on the Evidence delivered before both Houses of Parliament, on the East-India Company's Affairs* (London: Black, Parry & Co., 1813).

Maclean, Charles, *Results of an Investigation respecting Epidemic and Pestilential Diseases: including Researches in the Levant concerning the Plague*, 2 vols (London: Thomas & George Underwood, 1817).

Maclean, Charles, *Suggestions for the Prevention and Mitigation of Epidemic and Pestilential Diseases, comprehending the Abolition of Quarantines and Lazarettos: with some opportune Remarks upon the Danger of Pestilence from Scarcity* (London: s.n., 1817).

Maclean, Charles, *Practical Illustrations of the Progress of Medical Improvement, for the last Thirty Years: Or, Histories of Cases of Acute Diseases, as Fevers, Dysentery, Hepatitis and Plague, treated according to the Principles of the Doctrine of Excitation, by Himself and other Practitioners, chiefly in the East and West Indies* (London: s.n., 1818).

Maclean, Charles, *The Triumph of Public Opinion: Being a Standing Lesson to the Throne, the Parliament, and the People: with proposed Articles of Impeachment against the Ministries of the Crown, in the Case of Her Majesty, Caroline, Queen of England* (London: T. & J. Allman, 1820).

Maclean, Charles, *Specimens of Systematic Misrule; or Immense Sums annually expended in upholding a single Imposture; Discoveries of the highest importance to all Mankind smothered; and Injustice perpetrated, for Reasons of State; from Official Proceedings and Correspondence of the Ministries of the Crown, the Privy Council, the Board of Trade, the Levant Company, etc, etc, etc and Reports of Committees of the House of Commons, and of the College of Physicians, during an Investigation for a Period of nearly Four Years: Illustrative of the real Remote Cause of all the Distresses of the Nation, and of their sole efficient Remedy* (London: H. Hay, 1820).

Maclean, Charles, *Remarks on the British Quarantine Laws, and the so-called Sanitary Laws of the Continental Nations of Europe, especially those of Spain* (London: Black, Perry & Co., 1823).

Maclean, Charles, *Evils of Quarantine Laws, and Non-Existence of Pestilential Contagion; deduced from the Phenomena of the Plague of the Levant, the Yellow Fever of Spain, and the Cholera Morbus of Asia* (London: T. G. Underwood, 1824).

M'Lean, Hector, *An Enquiry into the Nature, and Causes of the Great Mortality among the Troops at St. Domingo: with Practical Remarks on the Fever of that Island, and Directions, for the Conduct of Europeans on their first Arrival in Warm Climates* (London: T. Cadell, 1797).

Mabit, J., *Essai sur les Maladies de l'Armée de St.-Domingue en l'anXI, et principalement sur la Fièvre Jaune* (Paris: École de Médicine, 1804).

Madras Government, Medical Board, *Medical Reports* (Madras: Government Press, 1831).

Makittrick, Jacob, *Dissertatio medica inauguralis de febre indiae occidentalis maligna flava* (Edinburgh: A. Donaldson, 1764).

Manningham, Richard, *A Discourse concerning the Plague and Pestilential Fevers* (London: Robinson, 1758).

Martin, François, *Mémoirs: Travels to Africa, Persia and India 1664–1670*, tr. A. Ray (Calcutta: Subarnarekha, 1990).

Martin, James Ranald, *The Influence of Tropical Climates on European Constitutions, including Practical Observations on the Nature and Treatment of the Diseases of Europeans on their Return from Tropical Climates* (London: J. Churchill, 1856).

Martin, Montgomery, *The History, Antiquities, Topography, and Statistics of Eastern India; Comprising the Districts of Behar, Shahabad, Bhagulpoor, Goruckpoor, Dinajpoor, Puraniya, Ronggopoor, and Assam, in relation to their Geology, Mineralogy, Botany, Agriculture, Commerce, Manufactures, Fine Arts, Population, Religion, Education, Statistics, etc. Surveyed under the Orders of the Supreme Government, and collated from the original Documents at the E.I. House*, 6 vols (New Delhi: Cosmo Publications, 1976 [1838]).

Matthews, Henry, *The Diary of an Invalid: Being the Journal of a Tour in Pursuit of Health in Portugal, Italy, Switzerland and France in the Years 1817, 1818, and 1819* (London: John Murray, 1820).

Mead, Richard, *Medical Precepts and Cautions* (London: J. Brindley, 1751).

Meade, Joannes, *Disputatio medica inauguralis quaedem de fibre flava* (Edinburgh: P. Neill, 1819).

Millar, John, *Observations on Antimony, read before the Medical Society of London, and published at their Request* (London: J. Johnson, 1774).

Milman, Francis, *An Enquiry into the Source from whence the Symptoms of the Scurvy, and of putrid Fevers arise; and into the Seat which those Affections occupy in the Animal Œconomy; with a View of ascertaining a more just Idea of putrid Diseases than has generally been formed of them* (London: J. Dodsley, 1782).

Monro, Donald, *An Account of the Diseases which were most frequent in the British Military Hospitals in Germany, from January 1761 to the Return of the Troops to England in March 1763. To which is added An Essay on the Means of Preserving the Health of Soldiers, and conducting Military Hospitals* (London: A. Millar, D. Wilson and T. Durham, 1764).

Morison, James, *Origin of Life and Cause of Diseases, clearly explained, demonstrated, and put in a new Light, accounting for our Senses and Feelings: A Physical Treatise, dedicated to the Council and Professors of the London University* (London: s.n., 1828).

Morison, James, *Morisonia; or Family Adviser of the British College of Health. Being a Collection of the Works of Mr Morison, the Hygeist* (London: College of Health, 1831).

Morison, James, *The Practical Proofs of the Soundness of the Hygeian System of Physiology, giving Incontrovertible Testimony to the Afflicted of the inestimable Value of Morison's Vegetable Universal Medicines* (London: M. Shepheard Moat, 1832).

Morton, Richard, *Pyretologia: seu exercitationes de morbis universalibus acutis* . . . (London: S. Smith, 1692).

Moseley, Benjamin, *A Treatise on Tropical Diseases; on Military Operations; and on the Climate of the West Indies* (1st edn.; London: T. Cadell, 1789).

Moseley, Benjamin, *A Treatise on Tropical Diseases; on Military Operations; and on the Climate of the West Indies* (3rd edn.; London: T. Cadell, 1792).

Moseley, Benjamin, *On Hydrophobia, its Prevention and Cure. With a Description of the Different Stages of Canine Madness* (London: Longman & Co., 1808).

Narvaez, O., et al., *Memoire pour Chévalier Chirurgien-major, au Régiment de la Martinique, et Apothicaire en la Ville du Fort Royal* . . . *contre M. Bagour, ecrivian principal des Colonies faisant fo[n]tion de Contrôleur* (St Pierre: s.n., 1788).

Newell, T., *A Letter to the Editor of the City Gazette upon the Misrepresentations contained in a Pamphlet recently Published by Dr Neale, upon the Subject of the Cheltenham Waters by Thomas Newell, M.D., Surgeon Extraordinary to the King* (London: s.n., 1820).

Norford, Gulielmo, *Concise et practicae observations de intermittentibus febribus curandis* (London: S. Crowder, T. Cadell and H. Payne, 1780).

Norton, G., *On the Prevalent Diseases of India. With New Physiological and Therapeutical Illustrations* (Edinburgh: J. Anderson, 1833).

O'Halloran, Thomas, *Remarks on the Yellow Fever of the South and East Coasts of Spain* (London: Callow & Wilson, 1823).

Oliver, William, *A Practical Essay on Fevers containing Remarks on the Hot and Cool Methods of their Cure* (London: T. Goodwin, 1704).

Orme, Robert, *Historical Fragments of the Mogul Empire, of the Morattoes, and of the English concerns in Indostan; from the Year M.D.C.LIX. Origin of the English Establishment, and of the Company's Trade, at Broach and Surat; and a General Idea of the Government and People of Indostan* (London: F. Wingrave, 1805).

Orton, Reginald, *An Essay on the Epidemic Cholera of India* (London: Burgess and Hill, 1831; first published, Madras, 1820).

Pariset, Étienne, *Observations sur la Fièvre Jaune, faites a Cadix, en 1819* (Paris: Audot, 1820).

Parkes, E. A., *Researches into the Pathology and Treatment of the Asiatic or Algide Cholera* (London: Churchill, 1847).

Pearson, John, *Observations on the Effects of Various Articles of the Materia Medica in the Cure of Lues Venerea: Illustrated with Cases* (London: J. Callow, 1800).

Philadelphia Academy of Medicine, *Proof of the Origin of the Yellow Fever, in Philadelphia and Kensington, in the Year 1797, from Domestic Exhalation* (Philadelphia: T. & S. F. Bradford, 1798).

Philadelphian, A [pseud.], *Occasional Essays on the Yellow Fever* (Philadelphia: John Ormerod, 1800).

Pinckard, George, *Notes on the West Indies: Written during the Expedition under the Command of the Late General Sir Ralph Abercomby: Including Observations on the Island of Barbadoes, and the Settlements captured by the British Troops, upon the Coast of Guiana, likewise Remarks relating to the Creoles and Slaves of the Western Colonies, and the Indians of South America: with occasional Hints, regarding the Seasoning, or Yellow Fever of Hot Climates*, 3 vols (London: Longman, Hurst, Rees, and Orme, 1806).

Piso, Willem, *De Indiae utriusque re naturali et medica libri quatuordecim* (Amsterdam: Elzevir, 1658).

Playfair, George, *Tentamen medicum inaugurale de febre flava calpensi* (Edinburgh: P. Neill, 1819).

Playfair, George, *The Taleef Shereef, or Indian Materia Medica. Translated from the Original* (Calcutta: Baptist Mission Press, 1833).

Powell, Charles, *A Treatise on the Nature, Causes, and Cure, of the Endemic, or Yellow Fever of Tropical Climates, as it occurs in the West Indies; to which Europeans are more particularly liable on their first Arrival* (London: J. Callow, 1814).

Priestley, Robert, *A Few Interesting Remarks on Bilious Disorders, particularly the Jaundice and Yellow Fever, etc, highly important to Persons of Fashion, the Sedentary, and those who inhabit or frequent Tropical Climates; recommending the Anti-Bilious Powder, a Certain and Experimental Remedy* (Leeds: Thomas Gill, 1798).

Pringle, John, *Observations on the Diseases of the Army* (London: A. Miller et al., 1768 [1752]).

Pym, William, *Observations upon the Bulam Fever, which has of late Years prevailed in the West Indies, on the coast of South America, at Gibraltar, Cadiz, and other parts of Spain: with a Collection of Facts proving it to be a highly contagious Disease* (London: J. Callow, 1815).

Quier, John, et al., *Letters and Essays on the Smallpox and Inoculation* (London and Edinburgh: J. Murray and C. Elliot, 1778).

Raleigh, Walter, *Observations on Idiopathic Dysentery, as it occurs in Europeans in Bengal, particularly in Reference to the Anatomy of that Disease* (Calcutta: W. Thacker & Co., 1842).

Ramazzini, Bernardino, *Health Preserved* (London: John Whiston, 1751).

Raynal, Abbé, *A Philosophical and Political History of the Settlement and Trade of the Europeans in the East and West Indies*, tr. J. O. Justamond, 2 vols (London: W. Strahan and T. Cadell, 1783).

Renny, Robert, *An History of Jamaica. With Observations on the Climate, Scenery, Trade, Productions, Negroes, Slave Trade, Diseases of Europeans, Customs, Manners, and Dispositions of the Inhabitants. To which is added, an Illustration of the Advantages, which are likely to result, from the Abolition of the Slave Trade* (London: J. Cawthorn, 1807).

Report from the Committee on Dr C. Smyth's Petition, respecting his Discovery of Nitrous Fumigation (1802), House of Commons Parliamentary Papers Online.

Report of the Select Committee appointed to consider the Means of maintaining and improving the Foreign Trade of this Country, relative to Quarantine, 1824 (London: J. M. Richardson, 1824).

Robertson, Robert, *An Essay on Fevers; wherein their theoretic Genera, Species, and various Denominations, are, from Observation and Experience, for Thirty Years, in Europe, Africa, and in the intermediate Seas, reduced to their characteristic Genus, Febrile Infection; and the Cure established on Philosophical Induction* (London: G. G. and J. J. Robertson, 1790).

Robertson, Robert, *Observations on Fevers and other Diseases, which occur on Voyages to Africa and the West Indies* (London: John Murray, 1791).

Robertson, Robert, *Directions for Administering Peruvian Bark, in a fermented State, in Fever, and other Diseases* (London: March & Teape, 1799).

Rouppé, Louis Ludovicus, *De morbis navigantium. Accedit observation de effectu extracti cicutae Storkiano in cancro* (Leiden: T. Haak, 1764).

Rowe, George, *Illustrated Cheltenham Guide* (Wakefield: S. R. Publishers, 1969 [1845]).

Roxburgh, William, *Plants of the Coast of Coromandel* (Serampore: Baptist Mission Press, 1820).

Royle, J. F., *An Essay on the Antiquity of Hindoo Medicine, including an introductory Lecture to the Course of Materia Medica and Therapeutics, delivered at King's College* (London: William H. Allen & J. Churchill, 1837).

Rush, Benjamin, *An Account of the Bilious Remitting Fever* (Philadelphia: Thomas Dobson, 1794).

Russell, Alexander, *The Natural History of Aleppo, and Parts Adjacent, containing a Description of the City, and the Principal Natural Productions in its Neighbourhood, together with an Account of the Climate, Inhabitants, and Diseases; particularly of the*

PLAGUE, with the Methods used by the Europeans for their Prevention (London: A. Millar, 1756).

Russell, Patrick, *A Treatise of the Plague: Containing an Historical Journal, and Medical Account, of the Plague, at Aleppo, in the Years 1760, 1761, and 1762. Also, Remarks on Quarantines, Lazarettoes, and the Administration of Police in Times of Pestilence* (London: G. G. J. and J. Robinson, 1791).

Rutherford, G. S., *Dissertatio medica inauguralis de dysenteria Bataviae orientalis* (Edinburgh: s.n., 1818).

Saletore, B. A. (ed.), *Fort William–India House Correspondence*, vol. IX, *Public Series, 1782–5* (New Delhi: National Archives of India, 1959).

Saunders, William, *A Treatise on the Structure, Economy, and Diseases of the Liver; together with An Inquiry into the Properties and Component Parts of the Bile and Biliary Concretions* (2nd edn.; London: J. Philips, 1795).

Saunders, William, *A Treatise on the Structure, Economy, and Diseases of the Liver* (4th edn.; London: s.n., 1809).

Scott, Helenus, *The Adventures of a Rupee. Wherein are interspersed Various Anecdotes Asiatic and European. A new Edition to which is prefixed Memoirs of the Life of the Author and to which there are annexed, His Remarks concerning the Inhabitants of Africa* (London: J. Murray, 1783 [1782]).

Sinclair, John, *The Plough, Joint Stock Farming Society, for Ascertaining the Principles of Agricultural Improvement; Submitted to the Consideration of the Friends to Agricultural and other Public Improvements* (London: W. Bulmer, 1800).

Slare, Frederick, *Experiments and Observations upon Oriental and other Bezoar Stones, which Prove them to be of no Use in Physick* (London: T. Goodwin, 1715).

Sloane, Hans, *A Voyage to the Islands Madera, Barbadoes, Nieves, St. Christophers, and Jamaica with the Natural History of the Herbs and Trees, four-footed Beasts, Fishes, Birds, Insects, Reptiles, etc, of the last of these Islands, to which is prefixed, an Introduction, wherein there is an Account of the Inhabitants, Air, Waters, Diseases, Trade, &c of the Place*, 2 vols (London: s.n., 1707–25).

Stanhope Smith, Samuel, *An Essay on the Causes of the Variety of Complexion and Figure in the Human Species: To which are added, Strictures on Lord Kames's Discourse on the Original Diversity of Mankind* (Edinburgh: C. Elliot & T. Kay, 1788).

Steel, Galterus (Walter), *Dissertatio medica inauguralis de febre insularum Indae Occidentalis* (Edinburgh: Stevenson & Co., 1818).

Strotter, Edward, *Criticon Febrium: Or, A Critical Essay on Fevers; with the Diagnosticks and Methods of Cure, in all the different Species of them. To which is prefix'd a large Introduction concerning the Use and Abuse of Mathematicks in Physick, and the Basis on which Indications are founded: Where also the Euodia Medicorum is annex'd* (London: Charles Rivington, 1716).

Sydenham, Thomas, *The Whole Works of that Excellent Practical Physician, Dr Thomas Sydenham*, tr. J. Pechey (London: R. Wellington, 1705).

Tavernier, J. B., *Les Six Voyages de Jean Baptiste Tavernier, Ecuyer Baron D'Aubonne, Qu'il a fait en Turque, en Perse, et aux Indies* (Paris: Clouzier & Barbin, 1676).

Taylor, John, *Travels from England to India, in the Year 1789, by way of the Tyrol, Venice, Scandaroon, Aleppo, and over the Great Desert to Bussora: with Instructions for Travellers; and an Account of the Expence of Travelling*, 2 vols (London: S. Low, 1799).

Terry, Edward, *The Travels of Pietro della Valle, a noble Roman, into East-India and Arabia Deserta. In which, the several Countries, together with the Customs, Manners, Traffique, and Rites both Religious and Civil, of those Oriental Princes and Nations, are faithfully described: In familiar Letters to his Friend Signor Mario Schipano whereunto is added a Relation of Sir Thomas Roe's Voyage into the East-Indies* (London: Herringham, 1665).

Thompson, Frederick, *An Essay on the Scurvy: Shewing Effectual and Practicable Means for Its Prevention at Sea* (London: J. Robinson, 1790).

Thomson, James, *A Treatise on the Diseases of Negroes as they occur in the Island of Jamaica, with Observations on the Country Remedies* (Kingston: Alexander Aikman, 1820).

Tissot, S., *A Dissertation on the Sensible and Irritable Parts of Animals* (London: J. Nurse, 1755).

Tommasini, J., *Reserches pathologiques sur la fièvre de Livourne de 1804, sur la fièvre jaune d'Amérique, et sur les maladies qui leur sont analogues* (Paris: Arthus-Bertrand, 1812).

Towne, Richard, *A Treatise of the Diseases most frequent in the West-Indies, and herein more particularly of those which occur in Barbadoes* (London: John Clarke, 1726).

Trapham, Thomas, *A Discourse of the State of Health in the Island of Jamaica. With a provision therefore calculated from the Air, the Place, and the Water: The Customs and Manners of Living, etc* (London: R. Boulter, 1679).

Trotter, Thomas, *Observations on the Scurvy; with a Review of the Opinions lately advanced on that Disease, and a new Therapy defended, on the approved Method of Cure, and the Induction of Pneumatic Chemistry* (2nd edn.; London: T. Longman, 1792 [1785]).

Trotter, Thomas, *Medicina Nautica: An Essay on the Diseases of Seamen: Comprehending the History of Health in His Majesty's Fleet, under the Command of Richard Earl Howe* (London: T. Cadell & W. Davies, 1797).

Trotter, Thomas, *An Essay, Medical, Philosophical, and Chemical, on Drunkenness, and Its Effects on the Human Body* (London: Longman et al., 1804).

Trotter, Thomas, *A View of the Nervous Temperament; Being a Practical Enquiry into the Increasing Prevalence, Prevention, and Treatment of those Diseases commonly called Nervous, Bilious, Stomach and Liver Complaints; Indigestion; Low Spirits; Gout, etc.* (London: Longman, Hurst, Rees and Orme, 1807).

Trotter, Thomas, *A Practicable Plan for Manning the Royal Navy, and Preserving our Maritime Ascendancy, without Impressment: Addressed to Admiral Lord Viscount Exmouth, K.G.B.* (Newcastle and London: Longman, Hurst, Rees, Orme and Brown, 1819).

Twining, William, *Clinical Illustrations of the More Important Diseases of Bengal, with the Result of an Inquiry into their Pathology and Treatment* (Calcutta: Baptist Mission Press, 1832).

Twining, William, *A Practical Account of the Epidemic Cholera, and of the Treatment requisite in the Various Modifications of that Disease* (London: Parbury Allen and Co., 1833).

Urquhart, Thomas, *Substance of a Letter to Lord Viscount Melville, written in May 1815, with the Outlines of a Plan to Raise British Seamen, and to form their Minds to Volunteer the Naval Service when Required; to do away with the Evil of Impressment, and Man our Ships effectually with Mercantile Seamen* (London: W. Philips, 1815).

Valentin, Louis, *Traité de la fièvre jaune d'Amerique* (Paris: Mequignon, 1803).

Veitch, Jacob, *Disputatio medica inauguralis de methodo tratandi, et praevendi, febrem flavam Indarium Occidentalium* (Edinburgh: Adam Neill, 1808).

von Troil, Uno, *Letters on Iceland, containing Observations on the Civil, Literary, Ecclesiastical, and Natural History; Antiquities, Volcanos, Basaltes, Hot Springs, Customs, Dress, Manners of the Inhabitants, &c., &c.* (London: W. Richardson, 1780).

Wade, John P., *Select Evidences of a Successful Method of Treating Fever and Dysentery in Bengal*, 2 vols (London: John Murray, 1791).

Wade, John P., *Nature and Effects of Emetics, Purgatives, Mercurials, and Low Diet, in Disorders of Bengal and Similar Latitudes* (London: John Murray, 1792).

Wade, John P., *A Paper on the Prevention and Treatment of the Disorders of Seamen and Soldiers in Bengal* (London: John Murray, 1793).

Ward, William, *A View of the History, Literature, and Mythology, of the Hindoos: Including a minute Description of their Manners and Customs, and Translations from their Principal Works*, 2 vols (Serampore: Mission Press, 1818).

Warren, Henry, *A Treatise concerning the Malignant Fever in Barbados, and the neighbouring Islands: with an Account of the Seasons there, from the Year 1734 to 1738, in a Letter to Dr Mead* (London: Fletcher Gyles, 1740).

Watson, Alexander, *Dissertatio medica inauguralis quaedem de febre Bataviae* (Edinburgh: A. Smellie, 1819).

Watt, Jacob T. B., *Dissertatio medica inauguralis, quaedam de dysenteria complectens* (Edinburgh: G. Creech, 1809).

White, Gulielmus, *Dissertation medica inauguralis de febre remittente* (Batavia: S. J. Luchtmans, 1775).

Willis, Thomas, *Diatribe duae Medico-Philosophicae: Quarum prior agit de Fermentione, sive de motu intestine particularum in quovis corpore; altera de Febrius, sive de motu earundem in sanguine Animalium. His accessit Dissertatio Epistolica de Urinis* (Amsterdam: Gerbrandus Schaghen, 1663).

Wilson Philip, A. P., *An Experimental Inquiry into the Laws of the Vital Functions, with some Observations on the Nature and Treatment of Internal Diseases* (London: Thomas and George Underwood, 1818).

Woodall, John, *The Surgion's Mate or Military and Domestique Surgery, discovering faithfully and plainly ye Method and Order of ye Surgeons Chest, ye Uses of the Instruments, the Vertues and Operations of ye Medicines, ye exact Cures of Wounds made by Gunshott and otherwise . . . with a Treatise of ye Cure of ye Plague* (London: R. Young, 1617).

Woodcock, Samuel, *Dissertatio medica inauguralis quaedem de febre flava Indarium Occidentalium* (Edinburgh: Abernethy & Walker, 1809).

Yates, William and Maclean, Charles, *A View of the Science of Life; on the Principles established in the Elements of Medicine of the late celebrated John Brown M.D., with an Attempt to Correct some of the Errors of that Work* (Dover, N H: Samuel Bragg, 1801).

Articles and book chapters

Addison, Thomas, 'The Pleasures of the Imagination', in A. Ross (ed.), *Selections from* The Tatler *and* The Spectator *of Steele and Addison* (London: Penguin, 1982), 364–406.

Annesley, James, 'Medical Observations', in H. Murray et al. (eds.), *Histories and Descriptive Statements of British India* (Edinburgh: Oliver and Boyd, 1832), 353–67.

Anon., 'An Account of the Success of Inoculation for the Small-Pox at Jamaica', in John Quier, Thomas Fraser, John Hume, George Monro, Ambrose Dawson, and Dr Dodsell, *Letters and Essays on the Small-Pox and Inoculation, the Measles, the Dry Bell-Ache, the Yellow, and Remitting, and Intermitting Fevers of the West Indies.... By Different Practitioners* (London: John Murray, 1778).

Anon., 'The Process suggested by James Charmichael Smyth, M.D., F.R.S., for determining the Effect of the Nitric Acid in destroying Contagion. Extracted from an Account of the Experiment made by the Desire of the Lords Commissioners of the Admiralty on Board the Union Hospital Ship, 1796', *Philosophical Magazine*, 2 (1798), 68–73.

Anon., 'Review of William Fowle's Practical Treatise on the Different Fevers of the West Indies (1800)', in *Medical and Physical Journal*, 4 (1800), 354.

Arnott, F. S., 'Report on the Health of the 1st Bombay European Regiment (Fusiliers), from 1st April 1846 to 31st March 1854', *Transactions of the Medical and Physical Society of Bombay*, 2nd series, 2 (1854–5), 102–211.

Atkinson, J., 'Popular Notions on Health and Disease Examined', *India Journal of Medical Science*, 1 (1834), 113–15.

Balfour, Francis, 'Observations respecting the remarkable Effects of Sol-Lunar Influence in the Fevers of India; with the Scheme of an Astronomical Ephemeris for the Purposes of Medicine and Meteorology', *Asiatick Researches*, 8 (1808), 21–2.

Bell, J., 'Special Report upon the Sulphate of Quina', in Madras Government, *Madras Medical Reports*, 257–8.

Blane, Gilbert, 'On the Comparative Health of the British Navy, from the Year 1779 to the Year 1814, with Proposals for its farther Improvement', in idem, *Select Dissertations*, 1–64.

Blane, Gilbert, 'On the Medical Service of the Fleet in the West Indies in the Year 1782', in idem, *Select Dissertations*, 65–86.

Blane, Gilbert, 'Warning to the British Public against the Alarming Approach of the Indian Cholera', in *Cholera Morbus: Its Causes, Prevention, and Cure: with Disquisitions on the Contagious or Non-Contagious Nature of this dreadful Malady, by Sir Henry Holford, Sir Gilbert Blane, and eminent Birmingham Physicians, and the Lancet, and Medical Gazette, together with ample Directions regarding it, by the College of Physicians and Board of Health* (Glasgow: W. R. M'Phan, 1831), 9–21.

Blumenbach, J., 'On the Possibility of Casual Mutilations in the Bodies of Animals becoming in the Course of Time hereditary Marks of Distinction', *Philosophical Magazine*, 4 (1799), 1–2.

Caveri, Gernelli, 'A Voyage round the World by Dr John Francis Gernelli Caveri, containing the most remarkable Things he saw in Indostan', in J. P. Guha (ed.), *India in the Seventeenth Century. Being an Account of the two Voyages to India by Ovington and Thevenot. To which is added the Indian Travels of Caveri* (New Delhi: Associated Publishing House, 1976), vol. 2, 189–335.

Cawley, Thomas, 'An Account of the Dysentery, as it appeared among His Majesty's Troops in Jamaica during the late War; with Dissections explaining the proximate Cause of that Disease; and a more simple and efficacious Method of Treatment thence resulting described', *London Medical Journal*, 7 (1786), 337–71.

Chisholm, Colin, 'An Account of the Cachexia Africana', *Medical and Physical Journal*, 2 (1799), 172–3.

Clark, John, 'Observations on the Hepatitis', *Medical and Philosophical Commentaries*, 5 (1777–8), 423–8.

Clayton, John, 'A letter from Mr John Clayton, Rector of Crofton at Wakefield in Yorkshire, to the Royal Society, 12 May 1688, giving "An Account of several Observables in Virginia, and in his Voyage thither, more particularly concerning the Air"', *Phil. Trans.*, 17 (1693), 781–95.

Coleman, J. G., 'Cases of Dysentery, treated in the Hospital of the B Troop, of the 1st Brigade of Horse Artillery, with Observations', in Madras Government, *Madras Medical Reports*, 181–97.

Comstock, Joseph, 'Remarks on the Bilous, or Yellow Fever, with some Hints for the more free and frequent use of Mercurial Medicines therein', *Medical Repository*, 4 (1807), 21–7.

Currie, William, 'An Enquiry into the Causes of the Insalubrity of flat and marshy Situations; and Directions for preventing or correcting the Effects thereof', *Medical and Physical Journal*, 6 (1801), 493–501.

da Cunha, J. G., 'Notes on the Treatment of Cholera and on the Opium Question, with Antiquarian and Historical References to Bombay', *Transactions of the Medical and Physical Society of Bombay*, new series 1 (1882), 77–88.

Dancer, Thomas, 'Observations on the Contagiousness and Importation of Yellow Fever', *Medical Repository*, 1, 2nd series (1804), 247–54.

Davidson, George, 'Experiments with the Eudiometer, made at Martinique', *Medical and Physical Journal*, 2 (1799), 386–7.

Davidson, George, 'Practical and Diagnostic Observations on Yellow Fever, as it occurs in Martinque, and on the remedial Effects of Calomel and Opium in the same; together with some Remarks on the Glandular Disease of Barbadoes', in *Medical Repository*, 2 (1805), 244–52.

Dick, William, 'Observations on Dropsies prevailing among the Troops in the East Indies', *Medical and Philosophical Commentaries*, 6 (1778), 212–13.

Eckard, J. F., 'Correction of Chisholm's Misstatement respecting the Prevalence of the Malignant Fever at St. Thomas's's', *Medical Repository*, 2nd series, 1 (1804), 336–8.

Ffrith, S., 'Practical Remarks on the Similarity of American and Asiatic Fevers, and on the Efficacy of Black Henbane and White Vitriol in curing Intermittent Fevers and Dysentery', *Medical Repository*, 4 (1807), 145–8.

Fisher, Miers, 'Account of a remarkable Change of Colour in a Negro', *Memoirs of the Manchester Literary and Philosophical Society*, 5 (1708), 314–18.

Geddes, William, 'Observations on Dysentery, extracted from the Quarterly Medical Reports of the Right Wing of the Madras European Regiment, with details of Cases of that Disease', in Madras Government, *Madras Medical Reports*, 143–80.

Geddes, William, 'Report on the Sulphate of Quinine', in Medical Board, Madras Government, *Medical Reports*, 201–39.

Gillespie, Leonard, 'An Account of the Means employed on board His Majesty's Sloop *Weasel* to preserve the Health of the Crew during a Voyage to Africa and the West Indies; with a Reply to some Remarks lately published by M. Chausser, Surgeon at Dijon. Communicated in a Letter to Dr Simmons by Mr Leonard Gillespie, Surgeon in the Navy, and late Assistant Surgeon to His Majesty's Naval Hospital at St. Lucia', *Gentleman's Magazine*, 57 (1788), 709–10.

Goodeve, H. H., 'Sketch of Medical Progress in the East', *Quarterly Journal of the Calcutta Medical and Physical Society* (1837), 124–56.

Hamilton, Robert, 'An Account of a successful Method of treating Inflammatory Diseases, by Mercury and Opium', *Medical Commentaries*, 9 (1783–4), 191–205.

Henderson, Stewart, 'An Inquiry into the Causes which produce Disease among the Troops at the Cape of Good Hope, with a view to discover the most effectual Means of Prevention; – to which is added, the Outline of a Plan of Military Hospitals, on a principle and construction tending to introduce a more successful treatment of the Sick', *Medical and Physical Journal*, 1 (1799), 455–62.

Jackson, Robert, 'Some Observations on the Connexion of the new and full Moon with the Invasion and Relapse of Fevers', *London Medical Journal*, 8 (1787), 25–33.

Jackson, Robert, 'Additional Remarks on the supposed Influence of the Moon in Fevers', *London Medical Journal*, 8 (1787), 300–4.

Jephson, J., 'Statistical Report of Sukkur', *Transactions of the Medical and Physical Society of Bombay*, 5 (1842), 80–2.

Johnson, Henry J., 'A Sketch of the Life, and some Account of the Works, of the late Dr James Johnson', *Medico-Chirurgical Review and Journal of Practical Medicine*, n.s. 3 (1846), 1–48.

Jones, William, 'Botanical Observations on Select Indian Plants', *Asiatick Researches*, 4 (1793–4), 231–303.

Lawrence, J., 'Cases of Cholera with Observations', in Medical Board, Madras Government, *Medical Reports: Containing Observations on Cholera, Dysentery, the Effects of Sulphate of Quinine as a Remedy of Fever, and on Inflammation of Veins, with the Cases of these Diseases; and Notices relative to the Treatment of Syphilis without Mercury, and the Utility of an Indian Remedy in Ophthalmia* (Madras: Government Press, 1831), 64–79.

Lind, James, 'An Account of the Efficacy of Mercury in the Cure of Inflammatory Diseases, and the Dysentery', *London Medical Journal*, 8 (1787), 43–56.

Lind, James, 'Some Remarks on the supposed Influence of the Moon on Fevers', *London Medical Journal*, 8 (1787), 145–7.

Lining, John, 'Extracts of Two Letters from Dr John Lining, Physician at Charles-Town in South Carolina to James Jurin, M.D., F.R.S. Giving an Account of Statical Experiments made several Times in a Day upon Himself, for one whole Year, accompanied with Meteorological Observations; to which are subjoined Six General Tables, deduced from the whole Year's Course', *Phil. Trans.*, 42 (1742–3), 491–509.

Lister, S. W., 'Report of Cholera Epidemica in the Right Wing of H.M.'s 46th Regiment, Bellary, May 1824', in Medical Board, Madras, *Medical Reports* (Madras: Government Press, 1831), 5–9.

Lister, S. W. and Evans, T., 'Report of Cholera in the 45th Regiment N.I., during the March from Bellary to Hyderabad, etc., in October and November, 1824', in Madras Medical Board, *Medical Reports* (Madras: Government Press, 1831), 13–27.

Maclarty, Dr, 'History of a Case of the Epidemic Fever of Jamaica terminating successfully; in which a very large quantity of Mercury was employed, without any obvious Operation during the Fever', *Annals of Medicine*, 1 (1796), 328–33.

Malcolmson, J. G., 'Report on the Use of Quinine in Fever, in the "A" Troop 1st Horse Brigade, and 1st Battalion of Artillery', in *Madras Medical Reports,* (1831), 240–6.

Martin, William, 'Letter to Mr Dacosta, Librarian, &c., to the Royal Society, from Mr William Martin, containing an Extract of a Letter from his Son at Bengal, on the Heat of the Climate', *Phil. Trans.*, 57 (1767), 217–18.

Mason, Abraham, 'Extract of a Letter to the Reverend Thomas Birch, D.D., Secretary to the Royal Society, from Mr Abraham Mason of Barbadoes, relating to an extraordinary agitation of the Sea there, 31st of March 1761, and an epidemical Disorder in that Island', *Phil. Trans.*, 52 (1762), 477–8.

Mitchill, Dr, 'Thoughts on Quarantines and Lazarettos: addressed to Richard Bayley, Esq., Health Officer of the Port of New York', *Medical Repository,* 1st series, 5 (1805), 243–54.

Moore, W., 'Is the habitual use of Opium in Moderation Injurious?', *Transactions of the Medical and Physical Society of Bombay,* new series 1 (1882), 14–27.

Morehead, C., 'Notes on the Treatment and Pathology of Intermittent and Remittent Fever as observed in the European General Hospital at Bombay, during the five Years, from July 1838 to July 1843', *Transactions of the Medical and Physical Society of Bombay,* 6 (1843), 170–209.

Mortimer, W., 'Observations on the Treatment of Dysentery; more especially in reference to the use of Ipecacuan in this Disease, as employed in the General Hospital of Fort St. George, from February 1828, to July 1829', in Medical Board, Madras Government, *Medical Reports,* 89–142.

Mouat, J., 'On the Climate of Bangalore, and the Prevalence of Hepatitis at that Station', *Transactions of the Medical and Physical Society of Calcutta,* 6 (1833), 1–32.

Murray, J., 'Observations on the good and bad Effects of Calomel in some of the Diseases of India', *Transactions of the Medical and Physical Society of Bombay,* 5 (1842), 145–54.

Neale, Adam, 'A Letter to a Professor of Medicine in the University of Edinburgh respecting the Nature and Properties of the Mineral Waters of Cheltenham', in *A Collection of all the Papers, relative to the Alleged Adulteration of the Cheltenham Waters, without Comment or Observation, leaving it entirely to the Dispassionate Reader to Make his Observations thereon . . . to which is added, A Reply by James M'Cabe, M.D.* (Cheltenham: G. A. Williams, 1820), unpaginated.

Norton, G., 'Intermittent Fever', *Madras Journal of Medicine,* 1 (1852), 3–8.

O'Shaughnessy, W. B., et al., 'First Report of the Committee for the Preparation of a Pharmacopoeia for Bengal', *Quarterly Journal of the Medical and Physical Society of Calcutta,* 6 (1838), 153–65.

Ovington, John, 'A Voyage to Suratt in the Year 1689', in J. P. Guha (ed.), *India in the Seventeenth Century. Being an Account of the Two Voyages to India by Ovington and Thevenot. To which is added the Indian Travels of Caveri* (New Delhi: Associated Publishing House, 1976), vol. 1 (entire volume).

Priestley, Joseph, 'Observations on different Kinds of Air', *Phil. Trans.*, 62 (1772), 147–264.

Priestley, Joseph, 'On the noxious Quality of the Effluvia of Putrid Marshes', a letter from Priestley to Pringle, *Phil. Trans.*, 64 (1774), 90–4.

Pringle, John, 'Some Experiments on Substances resisting Putrefaction', *Phil. Trans.*, 46 (1750), 480–8, 525–34, 550–8.

Rule, John, 'Considerations on the Origin, Causes and Character of Yellow Fever, as it appears in the United States and West-Indies', *Medical Repository*, 6 (1809), 323–30.

Rush, Benjamin, 'Facts intended to prove the Yellow Fever not to be Contagious, and Instances of its supposed Contagion explained upon other Principles', *Medical Repository*, 6 (1803), 155–70.

Ryan, Dennis, 'Farther Remarks on the Method of treating the Remittent Fevers of the West Indies; with Observations on the best Means of preserving Health in Jamaica', *London Medical Journal*, 2 (1782), 63–80.

Scarman, J., 'Observations on Cholera', in Madras Government, *Madras Medical Reports*, 80–6.

Stubbe, Henry, 'An Enlargement of the Observations, formerly publish'd [on the Caribe Islands], made and generously imparted by that Learn'd and Inquisitive Physitian, Dr Stubbes', *Phil. Trans.*, 3 (1668), 699–709.

Timoni, Dr, 'An Account of the Plague at Constantinople', in S. Miles (ed.), *Medical Essays and Observations relating to the Practice of Physic and Surgery* (London: S. Birt, 1745), vol. 2, 69–76.

Trotter, Thomas, 'On the Means of Destroying Contagion,' *Medical and Physical Journal*, 3 (1800), 245–7.

Vage, T., 'Criticism on the Treatment of the Venereal Disease', *Medical and Physical Journal*, 3 (May 1800), 465.

van Linschoten, J. H., 'Observations of the East Indies' (1583), in J. T. Wheeler (ed.), *Early Travels in India (16th and 17th Centuries). Reprints of Rare and Curious Narratives of Old Travellers in India, in the Sixteenth and Seventeenth Centuries* (New Delhi: Deep Publications, 1964), 161–228.

Vernati, Philberto, 'Of the Nature of a certain Stone, found in the Indies, in the Head of a Serpent', *Phil. Trans.*, 57 (1767), 102–3.

Watson, John, 'Some Observations on the Diseases that occurred on Board the Ship Europa, in the Service of the Hon. East India Company, during a Voyage from England to and from Madras and Bengal', *Medical Facts and Observations*, 5 (1794), 20–43.

Whytt, Robert, 'Observations on the Nature, Causes, and Cure of those Disorders which are commonly called Nervous, Hypochondriac, or Hysteric', in *Works* (Edinburgh: T. Becket and P. A. De Hondt, 1768), 646–7.

Wise, T. A., 'Observations on the Vitality of the Blood', *India Journal of Medical Science*, 1 (1834), 154–8.

Wright, William, 'Description of the Jesuit's Bark Tree of Jamaica and the Caribbees', *Phil. Trans.*, 67 (1777), 504–12.

Wright, William, 'Practical Observations on the Treatment of Acute Diseases; particularly those of the West Indies', *Medical Facts and Observations*, 7 (1797), 1–25.

Newspapers and periodicals

Annals of Medicine
Asiatick Researches
Bath and Cheltenham Gazette

Bombay Courier
Cheltenham Chronicle
Gentleman's Magazine
India Journal of Medical Science
Jamaica Physical Journal
Journal of Practical Medicine
Journals of the Assembly of Jamaica
The Lancet
London Medical Journal
London Medical Repository
Madras Journal of Medicine
Madras Quarterly Medical Journal, Medical Commentaries
Medical and Philosophical Commentaries
Medical and Physical Journal
Medical Facts and Observations
Medical Museum
Medical Repository
Medico-Chirurgical Review
Memoirs of the Manchester Literary and Philosophical Society
Philosophical Magazine
Philosophical Transactions of the Royal Society
The Times
Transactions of the Medical and Physical Society of Calcutta
Transactions of the Medical and Physical Society of Bombay
Transactions of the Royal Society of Edinburgh

SECONDARY SOURCES

Books

Ackerknecht, Erwin H., *Medicine at the Paris Hospital, 1794–1848* (Baltimore: Johns Hopkins University Press, 1967).

Ackerknecht, Erwin H., *Therapeutics: From the Primitives to the 20th Century* (New York: Hafner Press, 1973).

Ackroyd, Marcus, Brockliss, Laurence, Moss, Michael, Retford, Kate, and Stevenson, John, *Advancing with the Army: Medicine, the Professions, and Social Mobility in the British Isles 1790–1850* (Oxford: Oxford University Press, 2006).

Alavi, Seema, *Islam and Healing: Loss and Recovery of an Indo-Muslim Medical Tradition, 1600–1900* (Basingstoke: Palgrave, 2008).

Alavi, Seema (ed.), *The Eighteenth Century in India* (New Delhi: Oxford University Press, 1992).

Anderson, M. S., *War and Society in Europe of the Old Regime 1618–1789* (Stroud: Sutton, 1998).

Anderson, R. G. W. and Lawrence, Christopher (eds.), *Science, Medicine and Dissent: Joseph Priestley (1733–1804)* (London: The Wellcome Institute/Science Museum, 1987).

Anderson, Warwick, *The Cultivation of Whiteness: Science, Health and Racial Destiny in Australia* (Melbourne: Melbourne University Press, 2002).
Anderson, Warwick, *Colonial Pathologies: American Tropical Medicine, Race, and Hygiene in the Philippines* (Durham and London: Duke University Press, 2006).
Arasaratnam, Sinnappah, *Maritime India in the Seventeenth Century* (Delhi: Oxford University Press, 1994).
Arnold, David, *Colonizing the Body: State Medicine and Epidemic Disease in Nineteenth-Century India* (Berkeley: University of California Press, 1993).
Arnold, David, *Science, Technology and Medicine in Colonial India* (Cambridge: Cambridge University Press, 2000).
Arnold, David (ed.), *Warm Climates and Western Medicine* (Amsterdam and Atlanta: Rodopi, 1996).
Bala, Poonam, *Imperialism and Medicine in Bengal: A Socio-Historical Perspective* (New Delhi: Sage, 1991).
Bala, Poonam (ed.), *Biomedicine as a Contested Site: Some Revelations in Imperial Contexts* (Lanham: Lexington, 2009).
Baldwin, Peter, *Contagion and the State in Europe 1830–1930* (Cambridge: Cambridge University Press, 1999).
Banton, Michael, *Racial Theories* (Cambridge: Cambridge University Press, 1987).
Barrell, John, *The Infection of Thomas De Quincey: A Psychopathology of Imperialism* (New Haven and London: Yale, 1991).
Barrett, Frank A., *Disease and Geography: The History of an Idea* (Toronto: Geographical Monographs, 2000).
Bayly, C. A., *Indian Society and the Making of the British Empire* (Cambridge: Cambridge University Press, 1987).
Bayly, C. A., *Empire and Information: Intelligence Gathering and Social Communication in India, 1780–1870* (Cambridge: Cambridge University Press, 1996).
Bayly, C. A., *The Birth of the Modern World, 1780–1914* (Oxford: Blackwell, 2004).
Berman, Morris, *Social Change and Scientific Organization: The Royal Institution 1799–1844* (London: Heinemann, 1978).
Bewell, Alan, *Romanticism and Colonial Disease* (Baltimore: Johns Hopkins University Press, 1999).
Bhattacharya, Sanjoy, Harrison, Mark, and Worboys, Michael, *Fractured States: Smallpox, Public Health and Vaccination Policy in British India 1800–1947* (Hyderabad: Orient Longman, 2005).
Black, Jeremy, *A Military Revolution? Military Change and European Society 1550–1800* (Basingstoke: Macmillan, 1991).
Black, Jeremy, *European Warfare 1660–1815* (London and New Haven: Yale University Press, 1994).
Black, Jeremy, *The British Seaborne Empire* (New Haven: Yale University Press, 2004).
Bonner, Thomas Neville, *Becoming a Physician: Medical Education in Britain, France, Germany, and the United States, 1750–1945* (Baltimore: Johns Hopkins University Press, 1995).
Booker, John, *Maritime Quarantine: The British Experience c. 1650–1900* (Aldershot: Ashgate, 2007).

Boxer, C. R., *Portuguese Society in the Tropics: The Municipal Councils of Goa, Macao, Bahia, and Luanda, 1510–1800* (Madison and Milwaukee: University of Wisconsin Press, 1965).

Brain, Peter, *Galen on Bloodletting: A Study of the Origins, Development and Validity of His Opinions, with a Translation of the Three Works* (Cambridge: Cambridge University Press, 1985).

Brewer, John, *The Sinews of Power: War, Money and the English State, 1688–1783* (London: Routledge, 1994).

Brockliss, Laurence, *Calvet's Web: Enlightenment and the Republic of Letters in Eighteenth-Century France* (Oxford: Oxford University Press, 2002).

Brockliss, Laurence and Jones, Colin, *The Medical World of Early Modern France* (Oxford: Clarendon Press, 1997).

Brockliss, Laurence, Cardwell, John, and Moss, Michael, *Nelson's Surgeon: William Beatty, Naval Medicine and Trafalgar* (Oxford: Oxford University Press, 2005).

Brockway, Lucille H., *Science and Colonial Expansion: The Role of the British Royal Botanical Gardens* (New Haven and London: Yale University Press, 1979).

Bruijn, Iris, *Ship's Surgeons of the Dutch East India Company: Commerce and the Progress of Medicine in the Eighteenth Century* (Leiden: Leiden University Press, 2009).

Bryant, Arthur, *Years of Victory, 1802–1812* (London: Collins, 1944).

Buckley, Roger N., *The British Army in the West Indies: Society and the Military in the Revolutionary Age* (Gainesville: University Press of Florida, 1998).

Bynum, W. F., *Science and the Practice of Medicine in the Nineteenth Century* (Cambridge: Cambridge University Press, 1994).

Bynum, W. F. and Porter, R. (eds.), *Medical Fringe and Medical Orthodoxy 1750–1850* (London: Croom Helm, 1987).

Cannon, John, *Parliamentary Reform, 1640–1832* (Cambridge: Cambridge University Press, 1994).

Cantlie, Neil, *A History of the Army Medical Department*, 2 vols (Edinburgh: Churchill Livingstone, 1974).

Carpenter, Kenneth J., *The History of Scurvy and Vitamin C* (Cambridge: Cambridge University Press, 1986).

Chang, Hsiu-Jung, Farrington, Anthony, Huang Fu-San, Ts'ao Yung-Ho, Wu Mi-Tsa, *The English Factory in Taiwan 1670–1685* (Taipei: National Taiwan University Press, 1995).

Christie, Ian R., *Wilkes, Wyvil and Reform: The Parliamentary Movement in British Politics 1760–1785* (Aldershot: Ashgate, 1994).

Coleman, William, *Yellow Fever in the North: The Methods of Early Epidemiology* (Madison: University of Wisconsin Press, 1987).

Colley, Linda, *Britons: Forging the Nation 1707–1837* (New Haven: Yale University Press, 1992).

Collingham, E. M., *Imperial Bodies: The Physical Experience of the Raj, c. 1800–1947* (Cambridge: Polity, 2001).

Cook, Harold J., *The Decline of the Old Medical Regime in Stuart London* (Ithaca, NY: Cornell University Press, 1986).

Cook, Harold J., *Matters of Exchange: Commerce, Medicine, and Science in the Dutch Golden Age* (New Haven: Yale University Press, 2007).

Cooper, Frederick and Stoler, Ann Laura (eds.), *Tensions of Empire: Colonial Cultures in a Bourgeois World* (Berkeley: University of California Press, 1991).
Corbin, Alain, *The Foul and the Fragrant: Odor and the French Social Imagination* (Cambridge, Mass.: Harvard University Press, 1986).
Corfield, Penelope J., *Power and the Professions in Britain 1700–1850* (London: Routledge, 1995).
Crawford, D. G., *Roll of the Indian Medical Service* (London: Thacker, 1930).
Crewe, Duncan, *Yellow Jack and the Worm: British Naval Administration in the West Indies, 1739–1748* (Liverpool: Liverpool University Press, 1993).
Crosby, Alfred W., *The Columbian Exchange: Biological and Cultural Consequences of 1492* (Westport, Conn.: Greenwood Press, 1972).
Cunningham, A. and Jardine, N. (eds.), *Romanticism and the Sciences* (Cambridge: Cambridge University Press, 1990).
Curtin, Philip D., *The Image of Africa* (Madison: University of Wisconsin Press, 1964).
Curtin, Philip D., *The Atlantic Slave Trade: A Census* (Madison: University of Wisconsin Press, 1969).
Curtin, Philip D., *Death By Migration: Europe's Encounter with the Tropical World in the Nineteenth Century* (Cambridge and New York: Cambridge University Press, 1989).
Dalrymple, William, *The Last Mughal: The Fall of a Dynasty, Delhi, 1857* (London: Bloomsbury, 2006).
Debus, Allen G., *The English Paracelsians* (London: Oldbourne, 1965).
Desmond, Adrian, *The Politics of Evolution: Morphology, Medicine, and Reform in Radical London* (Chicago and London: University of Chicago Press, 1989).
Desmond, Ray, *The European Discovery of the Indian Flora* (Oxford: Oxford University Press, 1992).
Dictionary of National Biography, <http://www.ox.oxforddnb.com>
Digby, Anne, *Making a Medical Living: Doctors and Patients in the English Market for Medicine, 1720–1911* (Cambridge: Cambridge University Press, 1994).
Douglas, Robert, *The Genealogy of the Family of Lind, and the Montgomeries of Smithton* (Windsor: Private Press of James Lind, 1795).
Drayton, Richard, *Nature's Government: Science, Imperial Britain, and the 'Improvement' of the World* (New Haven: Yale University Press, 2000).
Drew, John, *India and the Romantic Imagination* (New Delhi and Oxford: Oxford University Press, 1987).
Drew, Robert, Peterkin, A., and Johnston, W., *Commissioned Officers in the Medical Services of the British Army 1660–1960* [a.k.a. *Drew's Roll*] (London: The Wellcome Institute, 1968).
Driver, F. and Martins, L. (eds.), *Tropical Visions in an Age of Empire* (Chicago and London: University of Chicago Press, 2005).
Duffy, C., *The Military Experience in the Age of Reason* (London and New York: Routledge & Kegan Paul, 1987).
Duffy, John, *A History of Public Health in New York City 1625–1866* (New York: Russell Sage Foundation, 1968).
Dunn, Richard, *Sugar and Slaves: The Rise of the Planter Class in the English West Indies, 1624–1713* (Chapel Hill and London: University of North Carolina Press, 2000).
Durey, Michael, *The Return of the Plague: British Society and the Cholera 1831–2* (Dublin: Gill and Macmillan, 1979).

Edmond, Rod, *Leprosy and Empire: A Medical and Cultural History* (Cambridge: Cambridge University Press, 2006).

Ernst, Waltraud, *Mad Tales from the Raj: The European Insane in British India, 1800–1858* (London: Routledge, 1991).

Ernst, Waltraud and Harris, Bernard, *Race, Science and Medicine, 1700–1960* (London: Routledge, 1999).

Fara, Patricia, *Sympathetic Attractions: Magnetic Practices, Beliefs, and Symbolism in Eighteenth-Century England* (Princeton: Princeton University Press, 1996).

Feldback, Ole, *India Trade under the Danish Flag, 1772–1808* (Copenhagen: Studentlitteratur, 1969).

Fisher, Michael (ed.), *The Politics of the British Annexation of India, 1757–1857* (Delhi: Oxford University Press, 1993).

Fissell, Mary E., *Patients, Power, and the Poor in Eighteenth-Century Bristol* (Cambridge: Cambridge University Press, 1991).

Floyd-Wilson, Mary, *English Ethnicity and Race in Early Modern Drama* (Cambridge: Cambridge University Press, 2003).

Foucault, Michel, *Madness and Civilization*, tr. Richard Howard (London: Random House, 1965).

Foucault, Michel, *Discipline and Punish: The Birth of the Prison*, tr. A. Sheridan (Harmondsworth: Penguin, 1979).

Foucault, Michel, *The History of Sexuality*, vol. i, tr. R. Hurley (New York: Vintage, 1980).

Foucault, Michel, *The Birth of the Clinic: An Archaeology of Medical Perception* (London: Routledge, 1997).

Frank, R., *Harvey and the Oxford Physiologists* (Berkeley: University of California Press, 1980).

French, R. K., *Robert Whytt, The Soul, and Medicine* (London: Wellcome Institute for the History of Medicine, 1969).

French, R. K., *Medicine before Science: The Rational and Learned Doctor from the Middle Ages to the Enlightenment* (Cambridge: Cambridge University Press, 2003).

Furber, Holden, *Rival Empires of Trade in the Orient, 1600–1800* (Minneapolis: University of Minnesota Press, 1976).

Gascoigne, John, *Joseph Banks and the English Enlightenment: Useful Knowledge and Polite Culture* (Cambridge: Cambridge University Press, 1994).

Gascoigne, John, *Science in the Service of Empire: Joseph Banks, the British State, the British State and the Uses of Science in the Age of Revolution* (Cambridge: Cambridge University Press, 1998).

Geggus, David, *Slavery, War, and Revolution: The British Occupation of Saint Domingue 1793–1798* (Oxford: Clarendon Press, 1982).

Gelfand, Toby, *Professionalizing Modern Medicine: Paris Surgeons and Medical Science and Institutions in the Eighteenth Century* (Westport, Conn.: Greenwood Press, 1980).

Glacken, Clarence, *Traces on the Rhodian Shore: Nature and Culture in Western Thought from Ancient Times to the End of the Eighteenth Century* (Berkeley: University of California Press, 1990 [1973]).

Goldgar, Anne, *Impolite Learning: Conduct and Community in the Republic of Letters, 1680–1750* (New Haven: Yale University Press, 1995).

Goldwater, J., *Mercury: A History of Quicksilver* (Baltimore: York Press, 1972).
Golinski, Jan, *Science as Public Culture: Chemistry and Enlightenment in Britain, 1760–1820* (Cambridge: Cambridge University Press, 1999 [1992]).
Gradish, S., *The Manning of the British Navy during the Seven Years' War* (London: Royal Historical Society, 1980).
Grafton, Anthony (with Shelford, April and Sirasi, Nancy), *New Worlds, Ancient Texts: The Power of Tradition and the Shock of Discovery* (Cambridge, Mass.: Belknap/ Harvard University Press, 1992).
Grove, Richard H., *Green Imperialism: Colonial Expansion, Tropical Island Edens and the Origins of Environmentalism, 1600–1860* (Cambridge: Cambridge University Press, 1995).
Guy, Alan J., *Œconomy and Discipline: Officership and Administration in the British Army 1714–63* (Manchester: Manchester University Press, 1985).
Haakonssen, Lisabeth, *Medicine and Morals in the Enlightenment: John Gregory, Thomas Percival and Benjamin Rush* (Amsterdam and Atlanta: Rodopi Press, 1997).
Haigh, Elizabeth, *Xavier Bichat and the Medical Thought of the Eighteenth Century* (Medical History, Supplement No.4, 1984).
Halévy, Elie, *The Growth of Philosophical Radicalism* (Boston: The Beacon Press, 1955).
Hall, Catherine, *Civilizing Subjects: Metropole and Colony in the English Imagination, 1830–1867* (Cambridge: Polity, 2002).
Hamilton, Douglas J., *Scotland, the Caribbean and the Atlantic World, 1750–1820* (Manchester: Manchester University Press, 2005).
Hamlin, Christopher, *Public Health and Social Justice in the Age of Chadwick: Britain, 1800–1854* (Cambridge: Cambridge University Press, 1998).
Hammond, J. L. and Hammond, B., *The Village Labourer 1760–1832* (Gloucester: Sutton, 1987).
Hannaford, Ivan, *Race: The History of an Idea in the West* (Baltimore and London: Johns Hopkins University Press, 1996).
Hannaway, C. and La Berge, A. (eds.), *Constructing Paris Medicine* (Amsterdam: Rodopi, 1998).
Harrison, Mark, *Public Health in British India: Anglo-Indian Preventive Medicine, 1859–1914* (Cambridge: Cambridge University Press, 1994).
Harrison, Mark, *Climates and Constitutions: Health, Race, Environment and British Imperialism in India, 1600–1859* (Delhi: Oxford University Press, 1999).
Hart, Gwen, *A History of Cheltenham* (Leicester: Leicester University Press, 1965).
Haynes, Douglas M., *Imperial Medicine: Patrick Manson and the Conquest of Tropical Disease* (Philadelphia: University of Pennsylvania Press, 2001).
Hemby, Phyliss M., *The English Spa, 1560–1815: A Social History* (London: Athlone, 1989).
Higston Fox, R., *Dr John Fothergill and His Friends: Chapters in Eighteenth Century Life* (London: Macmillan, 1919).
Honigsbaum, Mark, *The Fever Trail: The Hunt for a Cure for Malaria* (London: Macmillan, 2001).
Hudson, Geoffrey L., *British Military and Naval Medicine, 1600–1830* (Amsterdam and New York: Rodopi, 2007).

Hunter, Michael, *The Royal Society and its Fellows, 1660–1700: The Morphology of an Early Scientific Institution* (Chalfont St Giles: British Society for the History of Science, 1985).

Jacob, James R., *Henry Stubbe, Radical Protestantism and the Early Enlightenment* (Cambridge: Cambridge University Press, 2002).

Jacob, Margaret C., *The Newtonians and the English Revolution, 1689–1720* (Hassock: Harvester, 1976).

Jacyna, L. S., *Philosophic Whigs: Medicine, Science and Citizenship in Edinburgh, 1789–1848* (London: Routledge, 1994).

Janković, Vladimir, *Reading the Skies: A Cultural History of English Weather, 1650–1820* (Manchester: Manchester University Press, 2000).

Jenner, Mark and Wallis, Patrick, *Medicine and the Market in England and its Colonies, c. 1450–c. 1850* (Basingstoke: Palgrave, 2007).

Jennings, Eric T., *Curing the Colonisers: Hydrotherapy, Climatology and French Colonial Spas* (Durham, NC: Duke University Press, 2006).

Jones, Colin, *The Charitable Imperative: Hospitals and Nursing in Ancien Regime and Revolutionary France* (London: Routledge, 1989).

Jones, J. R., *The Anglo-Dutch Wars of the Seventeenth Century* (New York: Longman, 1996).

Jordanova, Ludmilla, *Sexual Visions: Images of Gender and Medicine between the Eighteenth and Twentieth Centuries* (London: Harvester Wheatsheaf, 1989).

Kaufmann, Matthew H., *The Regius Chair of Military Surgery in the University of Edinburgh, 1806–55* (Amsterdam and New York: Rodopi, 2003).

Keel, Othmar, *L'Avenement de la Médicine Clinique Moderne en Europe: 1750–1815: Politiques, Institutions et Savoirs* (Montreal: Presses de l'Université de Montreal, 2001).

Kejariwal, O. P., *The Asiatic Society of Bengal and the Discovery of India's Past* (New Delhi: Oxford University Press, 1988).

Keller, Richard C., *Colonial Madness: Psychiatry in French North Africa* (Chicago: University of Chicago Press, 2007).

Kennedy, Dane, *Magic Mountains: Hill Stations and the British Raj* (Berkeley: University of California Press, 1996).

King, Lester S., *The Road to Medical Enlightenment, 1650–1695* (London: MacDonald, 1970).

King, Lester S., *The Philosophy of Medicine in the Early Eighteenth Century* (Cambridge, Mass.: Harvard University Press, 1978).

King-Hele, Desmond, *Erasmus Darwin: A Life of Unequalled Achievement* (London: Macmillan, 1963).

Kiple, Kenneth F., *The Caribbean Slave: A Biological History* (Cambridge: Cambridge University Press, 1984).

Kiple, Kenneth F. (ed.), *The African Exchange: Towards a Biological History of Black People* (Durham, NC: Duke University Press, 1987).

Knoeff, Rina, *Herman Boerhaave (1668–1738): Calvinist Chemist and Physician* (Amsterdam: Royal Netherlands Academy of Arts and Sciences, 2002).

Kopf, David, *British Orientalism and the Bengal Renaissance: The Dynamics of Indian Modernization 1773–1835* (Berkeley and Los Angeles: University of California Press, 1969).

Kumar, Anil, *Medicine and the Raj: British Medical Policy in India 1835–1911* (New Delhi: Sage, 1998).
Kumar, Deepak, *Science and the Raj 1857–1905* (Delhi: Oxford University Press, 1995).
La Berge, Ann F., *Mission and Method: The Early Nineteenth-Century French Public Health Movement* (Cambridge: Cambridge University Press, 1992).
Lane Furdell, Elizabeth, *The Royal Doctors 1485–1714: Medical Personnel at the Tudor and Stuart Courts* (Rochester, NY: University of Rochester Press, 2001).
Langford, Paul, *A Polite and Commercial People: England, 1727–1783* (Oxford: Clarendon Press, 1989).
Langford, Paul, *Public Life and the Propertied Englishman, 1689–1798* (Oxford: Clarendon Press, 1991).
Laquer, Thomas, *Making Sex: Body and Gender from the Greeks to Freud* (Cambridge, Mass. and London: Harvard University Press, 1990).
Lawrence, Christopher, *Medicine and the Making of Modern Britain 1700–1920* (London: Routledge, 1994).
Lawrence, Susan, *Charitable Knowledge: Hospital Pupils and Practitioners in Eighteenth-Century London* (Cambridge: Cambridge University Press, 1996).
Leach, Douglas, *Roots of Conflict: British Armed Forces and Colonial Americans, 1677–1763* (Chapel Hill: University of North Carolina Press, 1986).
Lindeboom, G. A., *Hermann Boerhaave: The Man and His Work* (London: Methuen, 1968).
Lindeboom, G. A., *Boerhaave and Great Britain: Three Lectures on Boerhaave with Particular Reference to His Relations with Great Britain* (Leiden: Brill, 1974).
Livingstone, David N., *Putting Science in its Place: Geographies of Scientific Knowledge* (Chicago: Chicago University Press, 2003).
Lloyd, C. and Coulter, J. L. S., *Medicine and the Navy 1200–1900, vol. iii: 1714–1815* (Edinburgh and London: E. and S. Livingstone, 1961).
Lloyd, G. E. R. (ed.), *Hippocratic Writings* (London: Penguin, 1983).
Lorimer, Douglas A., *Colour, Class and the Victorians: English Attitudes to the Negro in the Mid-Nineteenth Century* (Leicester: Leicester University Press, 1978).
Loudon, Irvine, *Medical Care and the General Practitioner, 1750–1850* (Oxford: Clarendon Press, 1986).
MacKenzie, John M., *Orientalism: History, Theory and the Arts* (Manchester: Manchester University Press, 1995).
Maclean, Ian, *Logic, Signs and Nature in the Renaissance: The Case of Learned Medicine* (Cambridge: Cambridge University Press, 2002).
Maehle, A.-H., *Drugs on Trial: Experimental Pharmacology and Therapeutic Innovation in the Eighteenth Century* (Amsterdam and Atlanta: Rodopi, 1999).
Markovits, C., Pouchepadass, J., and Subrahmanyam, S. (eds.), *Society and Circulation: Mobile People and Itinerant Cultures in South Asia, 1750–1950* (Delhi: Permanent Black, 2003).
Marshall, Peter J., *Bengal: The British Bridgehead, Eastern India, 1740–1828* (Cambridge: Cambridge University Press, 1987).
Marshall, Peter J. (ed.), *The Eighteenth Century in Indian History: Evolution or Revolution?* (New Delhi: Oxford University Press, 2003).
Marshall, Peter J. and Williams, G., *The Great Map of Mankind: Perceptions of New Worlds in the Age of Enlightenment* (London: Dent, 1982).

Maultiz, Russell, *Morbid Appearances: The Anatomy of Pathology in the Early Nineteenth Century* (Cambridge: Cambridge University Press, 1987).

Metcalf, Thomas R., *Ideologies of the Raj*, The New Cambridge History of India, III.4 (Cambridge: Cambridge University Press, 1994).

Mohanavelu, C. S., *German Tamilology: German Contributions to Tamil Language, Literature and Culture during the Period 1706–1945* (Madras: South India Saiva Siddhanta Works Publishing Society, 1993).

Morris, R. J., *Cholera, 1832* (New York: Holmes and Meier, 1976).

Mukherjee, S. N., *Sir William Jones: A Study in Eighteenth-Century British Attitudes to India* (London: Sangam Books, 1987).

Parker, Geoffrey, *The Military Revolution: Military Innovation and the Rise of the West, 1500–1800* (Cambridge: Cambridge University Press, 1996).

Parker, Geoffrey, *The Army of Flanders and the Spanish Road 1567–1659* (2nd edn.; Oxford: Oxford University Press, 2004).

Pelling, Margaret, *Cholera, Fever and English Medicine, 1825–1865* (Oxford: Oxford University Press, 1978).

Pelling, Margaret, *Medical Conflicts in Early Modern London: Patronage, Physicians and Irregular Practitioners, 1550–1640* (Oxford: Clarendon Press, 2003).

Pernick, Martin, *A Calculus of Suffering: Pain, Professionalism and Anesthesia in Nineteenth Century America* (New York: Columbia University Press, 1985).

Philip, Mark (ed.), *The French Revolution in British Popular Politics* (Cambridge: Cambridge University Press, 1991).

Philip, Mark (ed.), *Resisting Napoleon: The British Response to the Threat of Invasion, 1797–1815* (Aldershot: Ashgate, 2006).

Pickstone, John V., *Ways of Knowing: A New History of Science, Technology and Medicine* (Manchester: Manchester University Press, 2000).

Porter, Roy, *Doctor of Society: Thomas Beddoes and the Sick Trade in Late-Enlightenment England* (London and New York: Routledge, 1992).

Powell, J. H., *Bring Out Your Dead: The Great Plague of Yellow Fever in Philadelphia in 1793* (Philadelphia: University of Pennsylvania Press, 1949).

Prakash, Om, *European Commercial Enterprise in Pre-Colonial India*, The New Cambridge History of India, II.5 (Cambridge: Cambridge University Press, 1998).

Raistrick, Arthur, *Quakers in Science and Industry* (Newton Abbott: David and Charles, 1968).

Raj, Kapil, *Relocating Modern Science: Circulation and the Construction of Knowledge in South Asia and Europe, 1650–1900* (Basingstoke: Palgrave, 2007).

Ranger, T. and Slack, P. (eds.), *Epidemics and Ideas: Essays on the Historical Persception of Pestilence* (Cambridge: Cambridge University Press, 1992).

Richardson, Ruth, *Death, Dissection and the Destitute* (London: Routledge and Kegan Paul, 1987).

Riley, James C., *The Eighteenth Century Campaign to Avoid Disease* (New York: St Martin's Press, 1987).

Risse, Guenther, *Hospital Life in Enlightenment Scotland: Care and Teaching at the Royal Infirmary of Edinburgh* (Cambridge: Cambridge University Press, 1986).

Roberts, Michael, *The Military Revolution, 1560–1660* (Belfast: M. Boyd, 1956).

Rodger, N. A. M., *The Wooden World: An Anatomy of the Georgian Navy* (London: Fontana, 1986).

Rosner, Lisa, *Medical Education in the Age of Improvement: Edinburgh Students and Apprentices, 1760–1826* (Edinburgh: Edinburgh University Press, 1991).

Rousseau, George S., *Nervous Acts: Essays on Literature, Culture and Sensibility* (Basingstoke: Palgrave, 2004).

Rusnock, Andrea, *Vital Accounts: Quantifying Health and Population in Eighteenth-Century England and France* (Cambridge: Cambridge University Press, 2002).

Said, Edward W., *Culture and Imperialism* (London: Chatto & Windus, 1993).

Schiebinger, L., *Plants and Empire: Colonial Bioprospecting in the Atlantic World* (Cambridge, Mass.: Harvard University Press, 2004).

Schiebinger, L. and Swan, C. (eds.), *Colonial Botany: Science, Commerce, and Politics in the Early Modern World* (Philadelphia: University of Philadelphia Press, 2005).

Schofield, Robert E., *The Enlightenment of Joseph Priestley: A Study of His Life and Works from 1733 to 1773* (Philadelphia: Pennsylvania University Press, 1996).

Semmelink, J., *Geschiedenis der Cholera in Oost-Indie voor 1817* (Utrecht: C. H. E. Breijer, 1885).

Shapin, Steven *A Social History of Truth: Civility and Science in Seventeenth-Century England* (Chicago: Chicago University Press, 1994).

Shapin, Steven and Schaffer, Simon, *Leviathan and the Air Pump: Hobbes, Boyle, and the Experimental Life* (Princeton: Princeton University Press, 1985).

Sheridan, Richard B., *Doctors and Slaves: A Medical and Demographic History of Slavery in the British West Indies, 1680–1834* (Cambridge: Cambridge University Press, 1985).

Siraisi, Nancy G., *The Clock and the Mirror: Girolamo Cardano and Renaissance Medicine* (Princeton: Princeton University Press, 1997).

Sivasundaram, Sujit, *Nature and the Godly Empire: Science and Evangelical Mission in the Pacific, 1795–1850* (Cambridge: Cambridge University Press, 2005).

Slack, Paul, *The Impact of Plague in Tudor and Stuart England* (Oxford: Clarendon Press, 1985).

Spary, Emma, *Utopia's Garden: French Natural History from the Old Regime to Revolution* (Chicago: University of Chicago Press, 2000).

Stansfield, Dorothy A., *Thomas Beddoes M.D., 1760–1808* (Dordrecht: D. Reidel, 1984).

Stepan, Nancy L., *The Idea of Race in Science: Great Britain 1800–1960* (London: Macmillan, 1982).

Stepan, Nancy L., *Picturing Tropical Nature* (London: Reaktion Books, 2001).

Subrahmanyam, Sanjay, *Explorations in Connected History: Mughals and Franks* (Delhi: Oxford University Press, 2005).

Thomas, Peter D. G., *John Wilkes: A Friend to Liberty* (Oxford: Oxford University Press, 1996).

Thompson, Andrew S., *Imperial Britain: The Empire in British Politics, c. 1880–1932* (Harlow: Routledge, 2000).

Thomson, E. P., *The Making of the English Working Class* (London: Penguin, 1991).

Travis Howard, Jr, William, *Public Health Administration and the Natural History of Disease in Baltimore, Maryland 1797–1920* (Washington, DC: Carnegie Institution of Washington, 1924).

Uglow, Jenny, *The Lunar Men: The Friends Who Made the Future* (London: Faber & Faber, 2002).
Vaughan, Alden T., *The Roots of American Racism: Essays on the Colonial Experience* (New York: Oxford University Press, 1995).
Vess, David M., *Medical Revolution in France, 1789–1796* (Gainesville: University Press of Florida, 1975).
Von Arni, Eric Gruber, *Hospital Care and the British Standing Army, 1660–1714* (Aldershot: Ashgate, 2006).
Wahrman, Dror, *The Making of the Modern Self: Identity and Culture in Eighteenth-Century England* (London and New Haven: Yale University Press, 2004).
Ward, J. R., *British West Indian Slavery 1750–1834: The Process of Amelioration* (Oxford: Clarendon Press, 1988).
Warner, John Harley, *The Therapeutic Perspective: Medical Practice, Knowledge, and Identity in America, 1820–1885* (Princeton: Princeton University Press, 1986).
Warner, John Harley, *Against the Spirit of System: The French Impulse in Nineteenth-Century American Medicine* (Princeton: Princeton University Press, 1998).
Wear, Andrew, *Knowledge and Practice in English Medicine, 1550–1680* (Cambridge: Cambridge University Press, 2000).
Webster, Charles, *The Great Instauration: Science, Medicine and Reform, 1626–1660* (London: Duckworth, 1975).
Wheeler, Roxann, *The Complexion of Race: Categories of Difference in Eighteenth-Century British Culture* (Philadelphia: University of Pennsylvania Press, 2000).
Williams, Glyn, *The Prize of All the Oceans: The Triumph and the Tragedy of Anson's Voyage Around the World* (London: Harper Collins, 1999).
Wilson, Kathleen (ed.), *A New Imperial History: Culture, Identity and Modernity in Britain and the Empire, 1660–1840* (Cambridge: Cambridge University Press, 2004).
Winther, Paul C., *Anglo-European Science and the Rhetoric of Empire: Malaria, Opium, and British Rule in India, 1756–1895* (Lanham: Lexington Books, 2003).
Wood, P. (ed.), *Science and Dissent in England 1688–1945* (Aldershot: Ashgate, 2004).

Articles and book chapters

Ackerknecht, Erwin H., 'Anticontagionism between 1821 and 1867', *Bulletin of the History of Medicine*, 22 (1948), 562–93.
Alsop, J. D., 'Warfare and the Creation of British Imperial Medicine, 1600–1800', in Hudson (ed.), *British Military and Naval Medicine*, 23–50.
Arnold, David, 'India's Place in the Tropical World, 1770–1930', *Journal of Imperial and Commonwealth History*, 26 (1998), 1–21.
Austin, P. B., rev. Herrick, Claire, 'Barker, John (1708–1749), *physician*', *DNB*.
Bailey, Eva, 'Cheltenham and the Indian Connection', *Cheltenham Local History Society Journal*, 14 (1998), 48–51.
Barfoot, Michael, 'Brunonianism under the Bed: An Alternative to University Medicine in Edinburgh in the 1780s', in Bynum and Porter (eds.), *Brunonianism*, 22–43.
Bartholemew, Michael, 'Lind, James (1716–1794)', *DNB*.
Bates, Don G., 'Thomas Willis and the Fevers Literature of the Seventeenth Century', in Bynum and Nutton (eds.), *Theories of Fever*, 45–70.

Bettany, G. T., rev. Herrick, Claire E. J., 'Burnett, Sir William (1779–1861)', *DNB.*

Birken, William, 'The Dissenting Tradition in English Medicine of the Seventeenth and Eighteenth Centuries', *Medical History*, 39 (1995), 197–218.

Blair, J. S. G., 'Pringle, Sir John (1707–1782)', *DNB.*

Boomgaard, Peter, 'Dutch Medicine in Asia, 1600–1900', in D. Arnold (ed.), *Warm Climates and Western Medicine* (Amsterdam and Atlanta: Rodopi, 1996), 42–64.

Booth, Christopher C., 'William Hillary, Pupil of Boerhaave', *Medical History*, 7 (1963), 297–315.

Booth, Christopher C., 'Hillary, William (1697–1763)', *DNB.*

Boulger, G. S., rev. Patrick Wallis, 'Russell, Alexander (1714–1768)', *DNB.*

Boxer, C. R., 'Two Pioneers of Tropical Medicine: Garcia d'Orta and Nicolas Monardes', *Diamante*, 14 (1963), 1–36.

Brockliss, Laurence, 'Before the Clinic: French Medical Teaching in the Eighteenth Century', in La Berge and Hannaway (eds.), *Constructing Paris Medicine*, 71–115.

Brod, Manfred, 'Thomas Trapham, surgeon (?–1683)', *Abingdon Area Archaeological and Historical Society*, Newsletter, Spring 2005, <http://www.AAAHS.org.uk>.

Brown, Michael, 'Making Sense of Modernity's Maladies: Health and Disease in the Industrial Revolution', *Endeavour*, 30 (2006), 108–12.

Brown, Michael, 'Medicine, Quackery and the Free Market: The "War" against Morison's Pills and the Construction of the Medical Profession, c. 1830–c. 1850', in M. S. R. Jenner and P. Wallis (eds.), *Medicine and the Market in England and its Colonies* (Basingstoke: Palgrave, 2007).

Brown, Michael, 'From Foetid Air to Filth: The Cultural Transformation of British Epidemiological Thought, ca. 1780–1848', *Bulletin of the History of Medicine*, 82 (2008), 515–44.

Brown, Theodore M., 'The College of Physicians and the Acceptance of Iatromechanism in England, 1665–1695', *Bulletin of the History of Medicine*, 44 (1970), 12–30.

Brunton, Deborah, 'Moseley, James (1742–1819)', *DNB.*

Bynum, W. F., 'Cullen and the Study of Fevers in Britain, 1760–1820', in W. F. Bynum and V. Nutton (eds.), *Theories of Fever from Antiquity to the Enlightenment, Medical History Supplement*, No.1 (London: Wellcome Institute for the History of Medicine, 1981), 135–48.

Bynum, W. F., 'Treating the Wages of Sin: Venereal Disease and Specialism in Eighteenth-Century Britain', in W. F. Bynum and Roy Porter (eds.), *Medical Fringe and Medical Orthodoxy 1750–1850* (London: Croom Helm, 1987), 5–28.

Bynum, W. F., 'Cullen, William (1710–1790)', *DNB.*

Carey, Daniel, 'Compiling Nature's History: Travellers and Travel Narratives in the Early Royal Society', *Annals of Science*, 54 (1997), 269–92.

Chakrabarti, Pratik, '"Neither of meate nor drinke, but what the Doctor alloweth": Medicine amidst War and Commerce in Eighteenth-Century Madras', *Bulletin of the History of Medicine*, 80 (2006), 1–38.

Chitnis, A. C., 'Medical Education in Edinburgh, 1790–1826, and Some Victorian Social Consequences', *Medical History*, 17 (1973), 173–85.

Christie, J. R. R., 'The Origins and Development of the Scottish Scientific Community, 1680–1760', *History of Science*, 12 (1974), 122–41.

Cleruzio, Antonio, 'From Van Helmont to Boyle: A Study of the Transmission of Helmontian Chemical and Medical Theories in Seventeenth-Century England', *British Journal for the History of Science*, 26 (1993), 303–34.

Cook, Harold J., 'Practical Medicine in the British Armed Forces after the "Glorious Revolution"', *Medical History*, 34 (1979), 1–26.

Cook, Harold J., 'Physicians and the New Philosophy: Henry Stubbe and the Virtuosi-Physicians', in French and Cunningham (eds.), *Medical Revolution*, 246–71.

Cook, Harold J., 'The Society of Chemical Physicians, the New Philosophy, and the Restoration Court', *Bulletin of the History of Medicine*, 61 (1987), 61–77.

Cook, Harold J., 'Sydenham, Thomas (*bap.* 1624, *d.* 1689), *physician*', *DNB*.

Cook, Harold J., 'Global Economies and Local Knowledge in the East Indies: Jacobus Bontius Learns the Facts of Nature', in L. Schiebinger and C. Swan (eds.), *Colonial Botany: Science, Commerce, and Politics in the Early Modern World* (Philadelphia: University of Pennsylvania Press, 2005), 100–18.

Cooter, Roger, 'Anticontagionism and History's Medical Record', in P. Wright and A. Treacher (eds.), *The Problem of Medical Knowledge: Examining the Social Construction of Medicine* (Edinburgh: Edinburgh University Press, 1982), 87–108.

Copper, Thompson, rev. Wallis, Patrick, 'Lind, James (1736–1812)', *DNB*.

Cosgrove, Denis, 'Tropic and Tropicality', in F. Driver and L. Martins (eds.), *Tropical Visions in an Age of Empire* (Chicago and London: University of Chicago Press, 2005), 197–216.

Craton, Michael, 'Dr John Quier', *Jamaica Journal*, 8 (1974), 44–7.

Creighton, Charles, rev. Reznick, Jeffery S., 'Bancroft, Edward Nathaniel (1772–1842)', *DNB*.

Crimmin, P. K., 'The Sick and Hurt Board and the Health of Seamen, c. 1770–1806', *Journal of Maritime Research*, 4 (1999), 83–115.

Cunningham, Andrew, 'Sydenham versus Newton: The Edinburgh Fever Dispute of the 1690s between Andrew Brown and Archibald Pitcairne', in W. F. Bynum and V. Nutton, *Theories of Fever from Antiquity to the Enlightenment*: *Medical History*, Supplement No.1 (London: Wellcome Institute for the History of Medicine, 1981), 71–98.

Cunningham, Andrew, 'Thomas Sydenham and the "Good Old Cause"', in R. French and A. Wear (eds.), *The Medical Revolution of the Seventeenth Century* (Cambridge: Cambridge University Press, 1989), 164–90.

Cunningham, Andrew, 'The Transformation of Hippocrates in Seventeenth-Century Britain', in D. Cantor (ed.), *Reinventing Hippocrates* (Aldershot: Ashgate, 2002), 91–115.

Cunningham, Andrew, 'Medicine to Calm the Mind: Boerhaave's Medical System, and Why It Was Adopted in Edinburgh', in Andrew Cunningham and R. French (eds.), *The Medical Enlightenment of the Eighteenth Century* (Cambridge: Cambridge University Press, 1990), 40–66.

Curtin, Philip D., 'The White Man's Grave: Image and Reality, 1780–1850', *Journal of British Studies*, 1 (1961), 64–110.

Daston, Lorrain, 'The Ideal and Reality of the Republic of Letters in the Enlightenment', *Science in Context*, 4 (1991), 367–86.

De Lacy, Margaret, 'Currie, James (1756–1805)', *DNB*.

De Lacy, Margaret, 'Fothergill, John (1712–1780)', *DNB*.

Deacon, Harriet, 'The Politics of Medical Topography: Seeking Healthiness at the Cape during the Nineteenth Century', in R. Wrigley and G. Revill (eds.), *Pathologies of Travel* (Amsterdam and Atlanta: Rodopi, 2000), 279–98.

Dettlebach, Michael, 'The Stimulations of Travel: Humboldt's Physiological Construction of the Tropics', in F. Driver and L. Martins (eds.), *Tropical Visions in an Age of Empire* (Chicago and London: Chicago University Press, 2005), 43–58.

Drayton, Richard, 'Maritime Networks and the Making of Knowledge', in D. Cannadine (ed.), *Empire, the Sea and Global History: Britain's Maritime World, c. 1763–c. 1840* (Basingstoke: Palgrave, 2007), 72–82.

Drescher, Seymour, 'The Ending of the Slave Trade and the Evolution of European Racism', *Social Science History*, 14 (1990), 415–50.

Endersby, Jim, 'A Garden Enclosed: Botanical Barter in Sydney, 1818–39', *British Journal for the History of Science*, 33 (2000), 313–34.

Ernst, Waltraud, 'Colonial Policies, Racial Politics and the Development of Psychiatric Institutions in Early Nineteenth-Century British India', in W. Ernst and B. Harris (eds.), *Race, Science and Medicine, 1700–1960* (London: Routledge, 1999), 80–100.

Feingold, Mordechai, 'Stubbe [Stubbes, Stubb], Henry (1632–1676), *author and physician*', *DNB*.

Figlio, Karl, 'Theories of Perception and the Physiology of Mind in the Late Eighteenth Century', *History of Science*, 13 (1975), 177–212.

Fitzpatrick, Martin, 'Latitudinarianism at the Parting of the Ways: A Suggestion', in John Walsh, Colin Haydon, and Stephen Taylor (eds.), *The Church of England, c. 1689–c. 1833: From Toleration to Tractarianism* (Cambridge: Cambridge University Press, 1993), 209–27.

Foucault, Michel, 'The Politics of Health in the Eighteenth Century', in C. Gordon (ed.), *Michel Foucault: Power/Knowledge. Selected Interviews and Other Writings 1972–1977*, (Brighton: Harvester Press, 1980), 166–82.

Friesen, John, 'Archibald Pitcairne, David Gregory and the Scottish Origins of English Tory Newtonianism, 1688–1715', *History of Science*, 61 (2003), 163–91.

Frost, Alan, 'The Antipodean Exchange: European Horticulture and Imperial Designs', in D. P. Miller and P. H. Reil (eds.), *Visions of Empire: Voyages, Botany and Representations of Nature* (Cambridge: Cambridge University Press, 1996), 58–79.

Gascoigne, John, 'Anglican Latitudinarianism, Rational Dissent and Political Radicalism in the Late Eighteenth Century', in Knud Haakonssen (ed.), *Enlightenment and Religion: Rational Dissent in Eighteenth-Century England* (Cambridge: Cambridge University Press, 1996), 219–40.

Geggus, David, 'Yellow Fever in the 1790s: The British Army in Occupied St Domingue', *Medical History*, 23 (1979), 38–58.

Goldenberg, David M., 'The Development of the Idea of Race: Classical Paradigms and Medieval Elaborations', *International Journal of the Classical Tradition*, 5 (1999), 561–70.

Goodwin, Gordon, rev. Reznick, Jeffrey S., 'Chisholm, Colin (c. 1747–1825)', *DNB*.

Goodwin, Gordon, rev. Carter, Philip, 'Fryer, John (*d.* 1733), *traveller and writer*', *DNB*.

Goulding, Christopher, 'The Real Doctor Frankenstein?', *Journal of the Royal Society of Medicine*, 95 (2002), 257–9.

Grout, Andrew, 'Geology and India, 1775–1805: An Episode in Colonial Science', *South Asia Research*, 10 (1990), 1–19.

Guerrini, Anita, 'Archibald Pitcairne and Newtonian Medicine', *Medical History*, 31 (1987), 70–83.

Guerrini, Anita, 'Isaac Newton, George Cheyne and the "Principia Medicinae"', in Roger French and Andrew Wear (eds.), *The Medical Revolution of the Seventeenth Century* (Cambridge: Cambridge University Press, 1989), 222–45.

Harris, Steven J., 'Long-Distance Corporations, Big Sciences, and the Geography of Knowledge', *Configurations* (Spring 1998), 6, 269–304.

Harrison, Mark, 'Medicine and the Management of Modern Warfare', *History of Science*, 34 (1996), 379–410.

Harrison, Mark, '"The Tender Frame of Man": Disease, Climate and Racial Difference in India and the West Indies, 1760–1860', *Bulletin of the History of Medicine*, 70 (1996), 68–93.

Harrison, Mark, 'From Medical Astrology to Medical Astronomy: Sol-Lunar and Planetary Theories of Disease in British Medicine, c. 1700–1850', *British Journal for the History of Science*, 33 (2000), 25–48.

Harrison, Mark, 'Was There an Oriental Renaissance in Medicine? The Evidence of the Nineteenth-Century Medical Press', in D. Finklestein and D. M. Peers (eds.), *Negotiating India in the Nineteenth-Century Media* (London: Macmillan, 2000), 233–53.

Harrison, Mark, 'Medicine and Orientalism: Perspectives on Europe's Encounter with Indian Medical Systems', in Harrison and Pati (eds.), *Health, Medicine and Empire*, 37–87.

Harrison, Mark, 'Science and the British Empire', *Isis*, 96 (2005), 56–63.

Harrison, Mark, 'Disease, Diplomacy and International Commerce: The Origins of International Sanitary Regulation in the Nineteenth Century', *Journal of Global History*, 1 (2006), 197–217.

Harrison, Mark, 'Disease and Medicine in the Armies of British India, 1750–1830: The Treatment of Fevers and the Emergence of Tropical Therapeutics', in Hudson (ed.), *British Military and Naval Medicine*, 87–120.

Harrison, Mark, 'Racial Pathologies: Morbid Anatomy in British India, 1770–1850', in B. Pati and M. Harrison (eds.), *The Social History of Health and Medicine in Colonial India* (Hyderabad: Orient Longman, 2008), 173–94.

Harrison, Mark, 'Medical Experimentation in British India: The Case of Dr Helenus Scott', in H. Ebrahimnejad (ed.), *The Development of Modern Medicine in Non-Western Countries: Historical Perspectives* (London: Routledge, 2009), 23–41.

Harrison, Mark, 'Introduction', in M. Harrison, M. Jones, and H. Sweet (eds.), *From Western Medicine to Global Medicine: The Hospital Beyond the West* (Hyderabad: Orient Blackswan, 2009), 1–32.

Heaman, E. A., 'The Rise and Fall of Anticontagionism in France', *Canadian Bulletin of the History of Medicine*, 12 (1995), 3–25.

Holoway, S. W. F., 'The Apothecaries Act 1815', Parts I and II, *Medical History*, 10 (1966), 107–29, 221–36.

Hudson, Geoffrey L., 'Disabled Veterans and the State in Early Modern England', in D. A. Gerber (ed.), *Disabled Veterans in History* (Ann Arbor: University of Michigan Press, 2000), 117–44.

Inkster, Ian, 'Marginal Men: Aspects of the Social Role of the Medical Community in Sheffield, 1790–1850', in J. Woodward and D. Richards (eds.), *Health Care and Popular Medicine in Nineteenth-Century England* (London: Croom Helm, 1977), 128–63.

Jacob, Margaret C., 'The Anglican Origins of Modern Science: The Metaphysical Foundation of a Whig Constitution', *Isis*, 71 (1980), 251–67.

Jacob, Margaret C., 'Scientific Culture in the Early English Enlightenment: Mechanisms, Industry and Gentlemanly Facts', in A. Kors and P. Korshin (eds.), *Anticipations of the Enlightenment* (Philadelphia: University of Pennsylvania Press, 1987), 134–64.

Jacyna, Stephen, 'Immanence or Transcendence: Theories of Life and Organization in Britain, 1790–1835', *Isis*, 74 (1983), 310–29.

Jensen, Niklas Thode, 'The Medical Skills of the Malabar Doctors in Tranquebar, India: As Recorded by Surgeon T. L. F. Folly', *Medical History*, 49 (2005), 489–515.

Jewson, N. D., 'Medical Knowledge and the Patronage System in Eighteenth-Century England', *Sociology*, 8 (1974), 369–85.

Jewson, N. D., 'The Disappearance of the Sick Man from Medical Cosmology', *Sociology*, 10 (1976), 225–44.

Keel, Othmar, 'The Politics of Health and the Institutionalisation of Clinical Practices in Europe in the Second Half of the Eighteenth Century', in W. F. Bynum and Roy Porter, *William Hunter and the Eighteenth-Century Medical World* (Cambridge: Cambridge University Press, 1985), 207–58.

Keel, Othmar, 'Was Anatomical and Tissue Pathology a Product of the Paris Clinical School or Not?', in La Berge and Hannaway (eds.), *Constructing Paris Medicine*, 117–83.

Kelly, Catherine, '"Not From the College, but Through the Public and the Legislature": Charles Maclean and the Relocation of Medical Debate in the Early Nineteenth Century', *Bulletin of the History of Medicine*, 82 (2008), 545–69.

Kennedy, Dane, 'Guardians of Edenic Sanctuaries: Paharis, Lepchas, and Todas in the British Mind', *South Asia*, 14 (1991), 118–40.

King, L. S., 'The Blood-Letting Controversy: A Study in the Scientific Method', *Bulletin of the History of Medicine*, 35 (1961), 1–13.

Kiple, Kenneth F., 'Deficiency Diseases in the Caribbean', in Rotberg (ed.), *Disease in Human History*, 231–48.

Kiple, Kenneth F., 'Race, War and Tropical Medicine in the Eighteenth-Century Caribbean', in D. Arnold (ed.), *Warm Climates and Western Medicine* (Amsterdam: Rodopi, 1996), 65–79.

Klein, H. S. and Engermann, S. L., 'A Note on Mortality in the French Slave Trade in the Eighteenth Century', in H. A. Gemery and J. S. Hogendorn (eds.), *The Uncommon Market: Essays on the Economic History of the Atlantic Slave Trade* (New York: Academic Press, 1979), 261–72.

Kniz, Kay D., 'Curiosities, Commodities and Transplanted Bodies in Hans Sloane's "Natural History of Jamaica"', *William and Mary Quarterly*, 3rd series, 57 (2000).

Kopperman, Paul E., 'The British Army in North America and the West Indies, 1755–83: A Medical Perspective', in Hudson (ed.), *British Military and Naval Medicine*, 51–86.

Kupperman, Karen Ordahl, 'Fear of Hot Climates in the Anglo-American Colonial Experience', *William and Mary Quarterly*, 3rd series, 41 (1984), 214–40.

La Berge, Ann and Hannaway, Caroline, 'Paris Medicine: Perspectives Past and Present', in La Berge and Hannaway (eds.), *Constructing Paris Medicine*, 1–69.

Lawrence, Christopher, 'The Nervous System and Society in the Scottish Enlightenment', in B. Barnes and S. Shapin (eds.), *Natural Order: Historical Studies of Scientific Culture* (London: Sage, 1979), 19–40.

Lawrence, Christopher, 'Priestley in Tahiti: The Medical Interests of a Dissenting Chemist', in Anderson and Lawrence (eds.), *Science, Medicine and Dissent*, 11–28.

Lawrence, Christopher, 'Cullen, Brown and the Poverty of Essentialism', in W. F. Bynum and R. Porter (eds.), *Brunonianism in Britain and Europe* (London: Wellcome Institute for the History of Medicine, 1988), 1–21.

Lawrence, Christopher, 'Ornate Physicians and Learned Artisans: Edinburgh Medical Men, 1726–1776', in Bynum and Porter (eds.), *William Hunter and the Eighteenth-Century Medical World*, 153–76.

Lawrence, Christopher, 'The Power and the Glory: Humphry Davy and Romanticism', in Cunningham and Jardine (eds.), *Romanticism and the Sciences*, 213–27.

Lawrence, Christopher, 'Disciplining Disease: Scurvy, the Navy, and Imperial Expansion, 1750–1825', in D. P. Miller and P. H. Reill (eds.), *Visions of Empire: Voyages, Botany, and the Representation of Nature* (Cambridge: Cambridge University Press, 1996), 80–106.

Lesch, John E., 'Science and Medicine in France: The Emergence of Experimental Physiology, 1790–1855' (Cambridge, Mass. and London: Harvard University Press, 1984).

Lester, Adam, 'Imperial Circuits and Networks: Geographies of the British Empire', *History Compass*, 4 (2006), 124–41.

Levere, Trevor H., 'Dr Thomas Beddoes (1750–1808): Science and Medicine in Politics and Society', *British Journal for the History of Science*, 17 (1984), 187–204.

Levere, Trevor H., 'Dr Thomas Beddoes (1760–1808) and the Lunar Society of Birmingham: Collaborations in Medicine and Science', *British Journal for Eighteenth-Century Studies*, 30 (2007), 209–66.

Levere, Trevor H., 'Natural Philosophers in a Coffee House: Dissent, Radical Reform and Pneumatic Chemistry', in P. Wood (ed.), *Science and Dissent in England 1688–1945* (Aldershot: Ashgate, 2004), 131–46.

Lindeboom, G. A., 'Boerhaave's Debt to British Science and British Medicine's Debt to Boerhaave', in G. A. Lindeboom, *Boerhaave and Great Britain: Three Lectures on Boerhaave with Particular Reference to His Relations with Great Britain* (Leiden: Brill, 1974), 1–21.

Lonie, Iain M., 'Fever Pathology in the Sixteenth Century: Tradition and Innovation', in Bynum and Nutton (eds.), *Theories of Fever*, 19–44.

McDonald, J. C., 'The History of Quarantine in Britain during the 19th Century', *Bulletin of the History of Medicine*, 25 (1951), 22–44.

Macleod, Emma V., 'British Attitudes to the French Revolution', *Historical Journal*, 50 (2007), 689–709.

MacLeod, Roy, 'On Visiting the "Moving Metropolis": Reflections on the Architecture of Imperial Science', in N. Reingold and M. Rothenberg (eds.), *Scientific Colonialism:*

A Cross-Cultural Comparison (Washington, DC: Smithsonian Institution Press, 1987), 217–49.

MacLeod, Roy, 'Introduction', in R. MacLeod (ed.), *Nature and Empire: Science and the Colonial Enterprise, Osiris* (2000), 15, 1–13.

McNeill, J. R., 'The Ecological Basis of Warfare in the Caribbean, 1700–1804', in M. Utlee (ed.), *Adapting to Conditions* (Tuscaloosa: University of Alabama Press, 1986), 26–42.

Maehle, A.-H., 'Clark, John (*bap.* 1744, *d.* 1805)', *DNB.*

Martensen, Robert L., 'Hippocrates and the Politics of Medical Knowledge in Early Modern England', in D. Cantor (ed.), *Reinventing Hippocrates* (Aldershot: Ashgate, 2002), 116–35.

Mathias, Peter, 'Swords and Ploughshares: The Armed Forces, Medicine and Public Health in the Late Eighteenth Century', in J. M. Winter (ed.), *War and Economic Development* (Cambridge: Cambridge University Press, 1975), 91–102.

Maulitz, Russell C., 'Channel Crossing: The Lure of French Pathology for English Medical Students, 1816–36', *Bulletin of the History of Medicine*, 55 (1981), 475–96.

Meier, R. Y., '"Sympathy" in the Neurophysiology of Thomas Willis', *Clio Medica*, 17 (1982), 95–111.

Mitchison, Rosalind, 'Sir John Sinclair (1683–1750)', *DNB.*

Moore, Norman, rev. Herrick, Claire 'George Cleghorn (1716–1789)', *DNB.*

Moore, Norman, rev. Herrick, Claire E. J., 'Fellowes, Sir James (c. 1771–1857)', *DNB.*

Moore, Norman, rev. Hankins, Richard, 'Huxham, John (c. 1692–1768)', *DNB.*

Mullett, Charles F., 'Politics, Economic and Medicine: Charles Maclean and Anti-contagion in England,' *Osiris*, 10 (1952), 224–51.

Munk, W., *Roll of the Royal College of Physicians of London*, 3 vols (London: Royal College of Physicians, 1878).

Nicholson, Malcolm, 'Alexander von Humboldt and the Geography of Vegetation', in Cunningham and Jardine (eds.), *Romanticism and the Sciences*, 169–88.

Nicholson, Malcolm, 'Giovanni Battista Morgagni and Eighteenth-Century Physical Examination', in C. Lawrence (ed.), *Medical Theory, Surgical Practice* (London: Routledge, 1992), 101–34.

Niebyl, P. H., 'The Non-Naturals', *Bulletin of the History of Medicine*, 45 (1971), 486–92.

Orange, Derek, 'Rational Dissent and Provincial Science: William Turner and the Newcastle Literary and Philosophical Society', in I. Inkster and J. Morrell (eds.), *Metropolis and Province: Science in British Culture 1780–1850* (London: Hutchinson, 1983), 205–30.

Pearson, M. N., 'First Contacts between Indian and European Medical Systems: Goa in the Sixteenth Century', in D. Arnold (ed.), *Warm Climates and Western Medicine* (Amsterdam and Atlanta: Rodopi, 1996), 20–41.

Pernick, Martin, 'Politics, Parties and Pestilence: Epidemic Yellow Fever in Philadelphia and the Rise of the First Party System', in J. W. Leavitt and R. L. Numbers (eds.), *Sickness and Health in America: Readings in the History of Medicine and Public Health* (Madison: University of Wisconsin Press, 1985), 356–71.

Pickstone, John V., 'Bureaucracy, Liberalism and the Body in Post-Revolutionary France: Bichat's Physiology and the Paris School of Medicine', *History of Science*, 19 (1981), 115–42.

Pickstone, John V., 'Ferriars's Fever to Kay's Cholera: Disease and Social Structure in Cottonopolis', *History of Science*, 22 (1984), 401–19.

Pickstone, John V., 'Dearth, Dirt and Fever Epidemics: Rewriting the History of British "Public Health", 1780–1850', in T. Ranger and P. Slack (eds.), *Epidemics and Ideas: Essays on the Historical Perception of Pestilence* (Cambridge: Cambridge University Press, 1992), 125–48.

Pickstone, John V., 'Ways of Knowing: Towards a Historical Sociology of Science, Technology and Medicine', *British Journal of the History of Science*, 26 (1993), 433–58.

Porter, Roy, 'Health Care in Enlightenment England: Knowledge, Power and the Market', in H. Binneveld and R. Dekker (eds.), *Curing and Insuring: Essays on Illness in Past Times, The Netherlands, Belgium, England and Italy, Sixteenth to Twentieth Centuries* (Hilversum: Verloren, 1993), 95–111.

Porter, Roy, 'Introduction' to Thomas Trotter's *An Essay, Medical, Philosophical, and Chemical, on Drunkenness, and its Effects on the Human Body* (London: Routledge, 1988).

Porter, Roy, 'Consumption: Disease of the Consumer Society?', in J. Brewer and R. Porter (eds.), *Consumption and the World of Goods* (London: Routledge, 1993), 58–84.

Porter, Roy, 'Diseases of Civilization', in W. F. Bynum and R. Porter (eds.), *Companion Encyclopedia of the History of Medicine* (London: Routledge, 1994), 585–600.

Porter, Roy, 'The Eighteenth Century', in L. I. Conrad, M. Neve, V. Nutton, R. Porter, and A. Wear, *The Western Medical Tradition: 800 BC to AD 1800* (Cambridge: Cambridge University Press, 1995), 371–476.

Power, D'A., rev. Herrick, Claire E. J., 'Pym, Sir William (1772–1861)', *DNB*.

Power, D'A., rev. McConnell, Anita, 'John Thomson (1765–1846)', *DNB*.

Rather, L. J., '"The Six Things Non-Natural": A Note on the Origin and Fate of a Doctrine and Phrase', *Clio Medica*, 3 (1968), 337–47.

Rattansi, P. M., 'The Helmontian-Galenist Controversy in Restoration England', *Ambix*, 12 (1964), 1–23.

Risse, Guenter B., 'The Brownian System of Medicine: Its Theoretical and Practical Implications', *Clio Medica*, 5 (1970), 45–51.

Risse, Guenter B., 'Brunonian Therapeutics: New Wine in Old Bottles?', in W. F. Bynum and R. Porter (eds.), *Brunonianism in Britain and Europe, Medical History*, Supplement No. 8 (1988), 46–62.

Risse, Guenter B., 'Hysteria at the Edinburgh Infirmary: The Construction and Treatment of a Disease, 1770–1800', *Medical History*, 32 (1988), 1–22.

Risse, Guenter B., 'The History of Therapeutics', in W. F. Bynum and V. Nutton (eds.), *Essays in the History of Therapeutics* (Amsterdam and Atlanta: Rodopi, 1991), 3–12.

Rodger, N. A. M., 'Phipps, Constantine John, second Baron Mulgrave in the peerage of Ireland and Baron Mulgrave in the peerage of Great Britain (1744–1792)', *DNB*.

Ross, Angus, 'Arbuthnot, John (*bap.* 1667, *d.* 1735)', *DNB*.

Rupke, Nicolaas A. and Wonders, Karen, 'Humboldtian Representations in Medical Cartography', in N. A. Rupke (ed.), *Medical Geography in Historical Perspective* (*Medical History*, Supplement No. 20, 2000), 163–75.

Rusnock, Andrea, 'Hippocrates, Bacon, and Medical Meteorology at the Royal Society, 1700–1750', in D. Cantor (ed.), *Reinventing Hippocrates* (Aldershot: Ashgate, 2002), 135–53.

Rusnock, Andrea, 'Jurin, James (*bap.* 1684, *d.* 1750), *physician and natural philosopher*', *DNB.*

Saakwa-Mante, Norris, 'Western Medicine and Racial Constitutions: Surgeon John Atkins' Theory of Polygenism and Sleepy Distemper in the 1790s', in W. Ernst and B. Harris (eds.), *Science, Race and Medicine, 1700–1960* (London: Routledge, 1999), 29–57.

Schaffer, Simon, 'Priestley's Questions: A Historiographic Survey', *History of Science,* 22 (1984), 151–82.

Schaffer, Simon, 'Measuring Virtue: Eudiometry, Enlightenment and Pneumatic Medicine', in Clark, Golinski, and Schaffer (eds.), *The Medical Enlightenment of the Eighteenth Century,* 281–318.

Schaffer, Simon, 'The Consuming Flame: Electrical Showmen and Tory Mystics in the World of Goods', in J. Brewer and R. Porter (eds.), *Consumption and the World of Goods* (London: Routledge, 1994), 489–526.

Schofield, Robert E., 'Priestley, Joseph (1733–1804)', *DNB.*

Sheridan, Richard B., 'The Guinea Surgeons on the Middle Passage: The Provision of Medical Services in the British Slave Trade', *International Journal of African Historical Studies,* 14 (1987), 601–25.

Sivasundaram, Sujit, 'Trading Knowledge: The East India Company's Elephants in India and Britain', *Historical Journal,* 48 (2005), 27–63.

Sivasundaram, Sujit, '"A Christian Benares": Orientalism, Science and the Serampore Mission of Bengal', *Indian Economic and Social History Review,* 44 (2007), 111–45.

Smith, Dale C., 'Medical Science, Medical Practice, and the Emerging Concept of Typhus in Mid-Eighteenth-Century Britain', in Bynum and Nutton (eds.), *Theories of Fever,* 121–34.

Stepan, Nancy, 'Biology and Degeneration: Races and Proper Places', in S. L. Gilman and J. E. Chamberlain (eds.), *Degeneration: The Dark Side of Progress* (New York: Columbia University Press, 1985), 97–120.

Stevenson, Lloyd, 'The Siege of Warwick Lane: Together with a Brief History of the Society of the Collegiate Physicians', *Journal of the History of Medicine,* 7 (1952), 105–21.

Stewart, Larry, 'The Edge of Utility: Slaves and Smallpox in the Early Eighteenth Century', *Medical History,* 29 (1985), 54–70.

Stuchtey, Benedikt, 'Introduction: Towards a Comparative History of Science and Tropical Medicine in Imperial Cultures since 1800', in B. Stutchtey (ed.), *Science Across the European Empires 1800–1950* (Oxford: Oxford University Press, 2005), 1–46.

Styles, J., 'Product Innovation in Early Modern London', *Past and Present,* 168 (2000), 124–69.

Thackray, Arthur, 'Natural Knowledge in Cultural Context: The Manchester Model', *American Historical Review,* 79 (1974), 672–709.

Thomas, Stephen W., 'Doctoring Ideology: James Grainger's *The Sugar Cane* and the Bodies of Empire', *Early American Studies,* 4 (2006), 78–111.

Valle, Ellen, '"The Pleasure of Receiving your Favour": The Colonial Exchange in Eighteenth-Century Natural History', *Journal of Historical Pragmatics,* 5 (2004), 313–36.

Vaughan, Megan, 'Slavery, Smallpox and Revolution: 1792 in Île de France (Mauritius)', *Social History of Medicine*, 13 (2000), 1–28.

Waddington, Ivan, 'The Struggle to Reform the Royal College of Physicians, 1761–1771: A Sociological Analysis', *Medical History*, 17 (1975), 107–26.

Wade Chambers, David and Gillespie, Richard, 'Locality in the History of Science: Colonial Science, Technoscience, and Indigenous Knowledge', in MacLeod (ed.), *Nature and Empire*, 221–40.

Wallace, J., 'Thomas Trotter (1760–1832)', *DNB*.

Wallace, J., 'Sir Gilbert Blane (1749–1834)', *DNB*.

Warner, John Harley, 'The Idea of Science in English Medical Education: The "Decline of Science and the Rhetoric of Reform", 1815–45', in R. French and A. Wear (eds.), *British Medicine in an Age of Reform* (London: Routledge, 1991), 136–64.

Weber, Gay, 'Science and Society in Nineteenth-Century Anthropology', *History of Science*, 12 (1974), 260–83.

Webster, Charles, 'English Medical Reformers of the Puritan Revolution: A Background to the "Society of Chemical Physitians"', *Ambix*, 14 (1967), 16–41.

Wilson, Leonard, 'Fevers and Science in Early Nineteenth-Century Medicine', *Journal of the History of Medicine and Allied Sciences*, 3 (1978), 386–407.

Wujastyk, Dominick, 'Change and Creativity in Early Modern Indian Medical Thought', *Journal of Indian Philosophy*, 33 (2005), 95–118.

Zuckerman, Arnold, 'Plague and Contagionism in Eighteenth-Century England: The Role of Richard Mead', *Bulletin of the History of Medicine*, 78 (2004), 273–308.

Zupanov, Ines, 'Drugs, Health, Bodies and Souls in the Tropics: Medical Experiments in Sixteenth-Century Portuguese India', *Indian Economic and Social History Review*, 39 (2002), 1–43.

Unpublished theses

Bateson, Jonathan, '"Open up a few corpses: you will dissipate at once the darkness": Morbid Anatomy in England from Harvey to Morgagni', University of Oxford D.Phil. thesis (2007).

Charters, Erica M., 'Disease, War and the Imperial State: The Health of the British Armed Forces during the Seven Years War, 1756–63', University of Oxford D.Phil. thesis (2007).

Foxhall, Katherine, 'Disease at Sea: Convicts, Emigrants, Ships and the Ocean in the Voyage to Australia, c. 1830–1860', University of Warwick Ph.D. thesis (2008).

Kelly, Catherine, '"Not Surgeons Alone, but Medical Officers": The Effects of the French Revolutionary and Napoleonic Wars on British Military Medicine', University of Oxford D.Phil. thesis (2008).

Lawrence, Christopher J., 'Medicine as Culture: Edinburgh and the Scottish Enlightenment', University of London Ph.D. thesis (1984).

Tröhler, Ulrich, 'Quantification in British Medicine and Surgery, 1750–1830, with Special Reference to its Introduction in Therapeutics', University of London Ph.D. thesis (1978).

Vaughan, Louella K., '"Improvements in the Art of Healing": William Heberden (1710–1801) and the Emergence of Modern Medicine in Eighteenth-Century England', University of Oxford D.Phil. thesis (2004).

Index

Aberdeen University 158, 168, 169, 263, 264, 283 n.132
acids 131, 134, 158–71 197, 202, 214, 220, 241, 274
A Costa, Christophori 34
Admiralty, the 10, 17, 72, 144, 238, 241, 243 n.20, 265, 283, 284
aetiology 25–120, 47–63, 64–88, 89–115, 119
Africa 4, 12–16, 37, 39, 43, 45, 49, 60, 72, 106, 127, 132, 133, 186, 191, 208, 248, 252, 263, 26–67, 271–2, 276, 282
Africans 41, 45, 49, 50, 94, 108, 110, 111–12, 268, *see also* slaves
African medical practitioners 14
ague 44, 51, *see also* fevers
air 30, 31, 33, 36, 37, 38–40, 41, 43, 44, 45, 52, 55–6, 59–62, 66–72, 74–7, 83, 85–7, 93, 95, 98, 102, 114, 135, 141, 158–60, 165, 171, 172, 173, 174, 181, 215, 219, 227, 229, 230, 235–6, 240–1, 243, 249, 251, 257, 267, 271, 272–3
Albermarle, duke of 46
Aleppo 57, 131
Alexander, William 141
Alpinus (Prosper Alpini) 36–7, 48
America, Central 15, 64, 274; *see also* Caribbean
America, North 2, 7, 9, 11, 12, 13, 14, 20, 27, 45, 53, 57, 60, 64, 80, 81 n.84, 84, 94 n.17, 109, 111, 132, 155, 157, 158, 171, 179, 187, 194, 203, 208, 233, 238, 245, 251, 256, 257, 262–4, 269, 271, 273, 280, 282–3
America, South 15, 48, 90, 134, 136
Amie, Dr 188
Amsterdam 35
anatomy 2, 6, 9, 27, 32, 52 n.23, 62, 65, 68, 70, 90, 92, 94, 95, 97, 112, 190, *see also* pathological anatomy
Andaman Islands 91
Anderson, Dr 161
Anglicans 48, 58, 59, 61, 78, 261
Annals of Medicine, The 162, 164, 165
Annesley, James 95–100, 195, 199, 225
Antigua 19, 21, 107, 215, 218
antimonial drugs 132, 139, 142–5, 172, 179, 180, 184, 193
antiphlogistics 121, 147, 149, 181, 202
antiseptics 66, 67, 77, 131–3, 149, 198
anxiety, *see* fear
apothecaries 13, 22, 28, 31, 53, 54, 80, 86, 89, 90, 95, 121, 142, 158, 163
Arabic medicine 29, 34
Arbuthnot, John 59–61, 63, 74
Arcot, nawab of 135, 150
Aristotelianism 28, 29
Armstrong, Robert 112
Army 1, 3, 5–7, 10, 14, 16, 18, 19, 20–2, 31, 33, 50–2, 54, 62 n.65, 65, 66, 69, 74, 80, 81, 83–5, 87, 94, 95, 100, 101, 103–7, 113, 119, 120, 127, 133, 142–5, 148, 150–7, 162, 164, 166, 168–9, 172–3, 175, 178–80, 182–6, 188, 189, 190, 191, 195, 198, 202, 212–14, 216–18, 220, 222, 224–6, 234, 245
  35th Regiment 275
  46th Regiment 100
  56th Regiment 183
  67th Regiment 183
  70th Regiment 275
  77th Regiment 161
  88th Regiment 168
  Royal Artillery 164, 262
  Royal Regiment 102, 189, 226
  West India Regiment 286
  York Rangers 224

Arthy, Elliot 18, 258–9
Atlantic Ocean 7, 13, 115, 238
atmosphere, *see* air
Avicenna 29
Ayurveda 97, 123, 124, 147, 200

Bacon, Francis 29, 30, 59, 81
Baillie, Mathew 52, 166, 168
Balfour, Francis 132, 149
Ballantyne, Mr 126, 144 n.81
Ballingall, George 189–91, 194–5
Bally, Victor 111–12, 188
Baltimore 263
Bampfield, R. W. 194
Bancroft, Edward 105–6, 272–9
Bandar Abass 38
Banks, Sir Joseph 11, 70, 136, 159–60, 162, 165–6, 171, 186, 250
Bann, HMS 282–3
Barbados 13, 14, 19, 46, 48–50, 55–6, 70, 110, 125–6, 129 n.48, 136
barbiers 36, 40
Barclay, James 190
Barfleur, The 238
bark (Peruvian, Jesuits), *see* cinchona
Barker, Sir George 81
Barker, John 33, 61–2
Busbridge, The 153, 177
Batavia 35–7, 76, 176
Bath 55, 140, 211, 225, 288
Bathurst 208
bathing 109, 121, 165, 166, 167–9, 171, 180–4, 186–8, 192, 194, 196, 201, 213–17, 220–1, 223, 231
Bayly, C. A. 135
bazaars 4, 8, 12, 22, 137, 147
Beddoes, Thomas 71, 79, 160, 163–4, 166–9, 173, 245, 288
Belfast 90
Bellini, Lorenzo 144
Bengal 69, 70, 76, 90, 91, 92, 93, 100, 127, 132, 148, 149 n.14, 150–1, 152 175–7, 179, 192, 199–200, 236
  Bengal Medical Service 70, 76 n.54, 95 n.26, 101 n.51, 175, 179
Bencoolen 127
Bentinck, William 97
Berlin 137
Berwick, HMS 238
Bewell, Alan 253
bezoar stone 137–9
Bible, The 140, 246
Bichat, Xavier 2, 89, 93, 228
bile 32, 44, 49, 52, 56, 85, 92–6, 98, 102, 105–7, 114, 124, 125, 127–8, 133, 141, 144, 145, 147–54, 156, 157, 160–1, 166, 172–6, 180–1, 183–4, 188, 203 211–13, 215–16, 218–25, 228–9
biliary theory, *see* bile
bilious diseases, *see* bile
Black, Joseph 158, 166, 240
Blackmantle, Bernard 225
Blair, William 165
Bland, general 18
Blane, Sir Gilbert 17–18, 90, 157, 241, 243, 250, 259, 260–1, 265, 270, 283, 284, 290
Blicke, Charles 128
blood 29, 30, 38, 45, 47–8, 49, 50, 52, 56, 62, 83, 84 n.100, 85, 121–5, 128, 134, 139, 140, 181, 184, 186, 190, 196, 213, 223, 248, 257, 268
  blood-letting, 38, 41, 121–9, 130–1, 153, 172, 179–203, *see also* humours
Blumenbach, J. F. 94, 112
Boards of Health 261, 275, 277
Boerhaave, Herman 31–3, 47, 48, 52, 54, 56, 59, 62–3, 124–5, 128, 146–7, 181
Bogue, Mr 126, 131
Bombay 21, 22, 39, 77, 158, 241, 243, 250
Bombay Courier, The 160, 162
Bontius (Jacob de Bondt) 35–8, 40, 44, 48, 52, 54, 56, 59, 62, 63, 124–6, 128, 146–7, 181
botany 30, 34 n.34, 48 n.5, 121, 129, 134 n.29, 135–7
Boyle, Robert 31, 40, 44
Bradford 53–4

brain, the 102, 106–7, 199, 219, *see also* nervous system
Brazil 48 n.5, 90
Bristol 163–5, 167, 173, 263
British Empire, the 3, 6, 28, 115, 158, 168, 209, 227, 234, 236, 254, 287–91
Brocklesby, Richard 16–17
Brookes, The 238
Broussais, F. J. V. 97, 98, 102, 195
Brown, John 62, 97, 101–2, 104–7, 109, 172–80, 242, 244–5
Brunonianism, *see* Brown, John
Bryce, James 153–4, 258
Buffon, comte de 83, 112
Burke, Edmund 70

Cadiz 103, 254, 273, 279
Calcutta 21–3, 76, 95–6, 100–1, 126, 131, 136–7, 149, 175–7, 183
General Hospital 100–1, 174, 198
Medical College 23 n.107, 95–7, 100
Medical and Physical Society 23 n.107, 95, 97, 100
calomel, *see* mercurial drugs
Cambridge, University of 5, 6, 39, 47, 59, 124, 264, 272, 275
camphire 67, 139–42, 156
Cape of Good Hope, the 90, 231
Carnatic, the 135
Caroline, The 90–1
Caribbean, the 4–5, 12, 13 n.48, 14–15, 18, 20, 29, 41, 48, 50, 80, 81 n.84, 108, 110, 144, 155 n.45, 184, 186, 188, 191, 207, 240, 254, 257–8, 263, 266, 271, 273, 275–6, 280, 284, *see also* West Indies
Cartegena 15
Cartesians 47, *see also* mechanical medicine, mathematics
castor oil 148, 150
Caventou, J. 197
Caveri, J. F. G. 123
Cawley, Thomas 84
Celsus 59
Ceylon 35
Chadwick, Edwin 249
Chamberlain, Mr 155
Charlestown 264
Chatham, Lord 260
Cheltenham 211–26, 234, 288
Cheltenham Chronicle 225
chemistry 28–9, 31–2, 55–6, 59, 62, 66–7, 70–1, 97, 113, 121, 126, 129, 133–5, 142, 145–71, 172, 197, 212, 215–16, 223, 238, 240–1, 246, 267, 274, *see also* airs, antimonial drugs, mercurial drugs, nitric acid
Chervin, Nicolas 109, 280
Cheyne, George 124, 235, 237, 244–5, 248
China 70, 91
Chingleput 22
Chisholm, Colin 105–6, 111, 153–4, 157, 168, 171, 214, 262–4, 267, 270–2, 276
cholera 92, 95–102, 132, 196, 200, 208, 213, 221, 254–5, 261, 285
cinchona 13, 58, 67, 125–7, 130, 133–4, 136, 144–5, 149 n.14, 150–1, 179, 184, 187, 192, 195, 197, *see also* quinine
circulation, of the blood 29, 48, 96, 107, 121, 141, 190, *see also* blood, physiology, vascular system
circulation, concept of 12, 14, 186, 213, 291
Clark, James 153–5, 267
Clark, John 74–80, 83–4, 127, 131–3, 144, 148–9, 156, 165, 192, 240, 247, 271, 288
Clark, Thomas 152
Cleghorn, George 51–4, 57–8, 62–3, 70, 75, 79, 81, 86, 131–2, 191
climate 4, 8, 12, 16, 17, 19, 27, 29–46, 48–52, 55–7, 60–3, 64–88, 91–4, 98–100, 105, 107–12, 113–15, 119, 122, 123, 125–8, 131, 132, 133, 134, 140, 142, 143, 144–5, 149, 151, 154, 156, 159, 171, 172, 173, 175–6, 178, 181, 183, 185–6, 190–7, 199, 201–3, 208, 220,

227–32, 235–6, 238, 245, 255–7, 259, 264, 266, 268, 270, 272, 276, 287–91, *see also* cold, damp, heat, humidity, rainfall, seasons, tropics
clinical trials, *see* trials
Clarence, duke of 91, 261
classification of disease, *see* nosography
Cobbett, William 183, 225
Cockburn, William 124, 130
cold 49, 74, 85, 93, 125, 149, 151, 171, 173, 175, 180–4, 186–8, 192, 196, 213–14, 216, 218–19, 229–31, 243, 251, 266, 272
Colebrook, Sir George 148
Columbo 35
commerce 3, 6 n.18, 8, 9, 11, 12, 13, 16, 17, 21, 35, 36, 37, 39, 44, 61, 111, 115, 137, 143, 158, 178, 186, 209, 227, 234–6, 237, 238, 245, 246, 247, 251, 254–5, 258, 261–3, 273, 280, 282, 284, 285, 290–1
Constantinople 222
constitutions 30, 33, 38, 41, 46, 49, 55, 69, 74, 83, 87–8, 91, 93, 97–102, 108–9, 111–15, 127–8, 167, 191, 193, 199, 201, 208, 220, 228–30, 235–6, 246, 249–50, 257, 259, 266–7, 272, 281, *see also* race
consumerism 9, 115, 209, 211–25, 277, 234–5, 237, 245, 247, 248
consumption 228, 230, *see also* diet, digestive system, diseases of civilization
contagion 30, 57, 67, 69, 77, 79, 85–6, 103, 106, 109, 159, 174, 183, 191, 208, 241–3, 247–8, 250–1, 254–85, 290, *see also* cholera, crowd diseases, epidemics, plague, typhus, yellow fever
Cook, Captain James 241
Cooper, Sir Astley 91
Copenhagen, University of 137
Corbyn, Frederick 97
Cormack, George 152
Coromandel coast 76, 91, 135 n.34, 147, *see also* Madras, Tranquebar, Vizagapatam
corpuscular theories, *see* particulate theories
Cossens, J. 224
crowd diseases 61, 65, 77, 242, 247–8, 251, 267, 270, 288, *see also* contagion, epidemics, typhus, ventilation
Cruickshank, William 164
Cullen, William 8, 32, 62, 75, 85–6, 97, 172–3, 179, 180, 258, 261
cultivation 49, 68, 76–7, 248, *see also* agriculture, improvement
Cumberland, duke of 66
Cunningham, Andrew 32
Currie, James 78–9, 165, 186–7, 192
Curtis, Charles 287
Cuvier, Georges 94

D'Aguillar, Benjamin 177
Daman, raja of 123
damp 48, 49, 55–6, 61, 64, 69, 72, 87, 93, 98, 229, 245, 247, *see also* humidity, rain
Dancer, Thomas 166, 187, 270
Danish settlements 134–7
Da Orta, Garcia 33–6, 38
Darwin, Erasmus 62, 69, 94, 97, 173, 180, 193–4, 233, 236 n.38, 242, 248
Davidson, George 186
Davy, Humphry 167
De Arejula, Don Juan Manuel 188, 274
De Faria y Sousa, Manuel 35
De Jonnès, Moreau 188
De Thevenot, M. 138, 139
debility 172, 174–5, 180–1, 184, 190, 193, 197, 199, 219, 234, 246
degeneration 83, 93, 98, 101, 111, 159, 244, 248–9, 253, 266 n.51, *see also* constitutions, race
Delon, J. 123
Demerera 104, 187, 263
Devonshire, duke of 260
Dickinson, Colonel 196 n.132, 213

Dickson, Samuel 101–2, 212–13, 226
diet 34, 35–6, 38, 41, 49, 66, 74, 77, 110, 114, 121, 150, 162, 173, 199 n.154, 213, 221, 229–30, 233–4, 246, 268
digestive system, diseases of 227–8, 231, 233–4, 236, *see also* diseases of civilization, dysentery, nervous diseases
discipline 3, 18, 20, 23, 61, 152, 238, 243–4, 250, 259, 268, 278
diseases of civilization 211–26, 227–36, 237–53
dissection, *see* pathological anatomy
Dissent 5–7, 33, 42, 53, 58–9, 63, 66, 69, 71, 75–8, 113, 171, 240, 261, 265, 290, *see also* radicalism, reform
Diu 138
Dominica, *see* St Domingue
Doughty, Edward 103, 183–4
drainage 49, 77, 271
Drescher, Seymour 111
dropsy 40, 45, 49, 219
drugs, *see* medicines
Drummond, Dr 133
drunkenness 238, 246–7
Dublin 52
Dublin, The 179
Ducarel, Gustavus 148
Dundee 158
Dury, Andrew 56
Dutch East India Company 35–7, 48 n.5, 176
Dutch West Indies 83, 263
dysentery 3, 5, 23, 34, 35, 36, 39, 40, 49, 51, 66, 68, 72, 76, 84, 85, 88, 91, 92, 101, 102, 106, 110, 122, 126, 132 n.13, 146, 149–52, 154, 156–7, 168, 212, 218, 221, 230, 233, 285, 288

East India Company 1, 3, 5–6, 8, 10, 13, 16, 21–3, 33, 39, 50, 65, 69, 71, 74–8, 80, 85, 105, 113, 119, 127–8, 132, 145–6, 148, 150–2, 156, 158, 165, 169, 171–2, 174, 176, 178, 207, 216–18, 220, 225, 234, 240, 247, 269, 271, 279, 285, 290, *see also* Dutch East India Company
  Marine 74, 77–8, 132, 144, 153, 174, 240, 258
East Indies, the 1, 8, 21, 33–40, 41, 43–5, 48, 64, 76, 81, 90–1, 105, 122, 127–8, 131, 139–40, 149, 151, 156, 164, 172, 174, 183, 191, 197, 219, 248, 287–91
economy 16–20, 74, 78, 97, 115, 195, 223
Edinburgh, *see also* Royal College of Physicians of
  Infirmary 2, 85, 141, 185
  Philosophical and Medical Society 71
  Royal Society of 71, 268
  University 6, 8, 10–11, 17, 31–2, 52–4, 57, 65, 68–72, 74, 85, 95 n.26, 104, 124, 135, 136, 150, 158, 165–6, 169, 172–3, 184–6, 188, 190–1, 216, 220, 222–4, 228, 238, 257, 261–2, 268, 271, 275, 283 n.132
Edwards, W. F. 112, 114
effeminacy, *see* masculinity
Egypt 36, 37, 49, 94, 142, 155, 166, 248, 254, 260–1, 272–3
electricity 95, 102, 180
elephantiasis 14, 49, 102
emetics 121–2, 127–8, 130, 133, 140, 143, 145, 149–50, 173, 184, 193–5, 218
empirical medicine 1, 2, 9, 10, 27, 30–1, 33, 50, 56, 59–60, 75 n.50, 76, 113–14, 120, 129, 130, 139–41, 150–1, 172, 203, 274
eudiometry 271
England 29, 31, 41–3, 44, 54, 56, 62 n.68, 80, 91, 98, 131, 139, 150, 155–6, 159, 176, 211–25, 230, 265, 269, 275, 278
epidemics 8, 30–6, 40 n.81, 55, 59, 61–2, 69, 72, 75, 79, 95, 98, 100, 102, 140–1, 147, 153, 156, 174, 183, 188, 208, 221, 254–86, *see also* fever, plague, cholera, yellow fever

Evans, T. 100
exchange, concept of 10, 11, 12, 22, 186
experimental method 1, 2, 6, 27, 29, 41 n.82, 54, 57–8, 62, 66–7, 70, 91, 102, 112, 114, 134, 137, 146–71, 176, 215, 271

fatigue 102, 152, 200, 249, 259, *see also* non-naturals
fear 102, 115, 191, 20, 209, 221, 227, 229, 233, 234–6, 248, 253, 254, 265, 269, 270
Fellowes, Sir James 103, 273–5, 276, 277, 279
Fellowes, Sir Thomas 275
Ferguson, Adam 99
Fergusson, William 21, 185, 279
Fernando Po 212
Fernel, Jean 37
Ferriar, John 79
fevers 3, 5, 15, 19–20, 23, 27, 29–46, 57–63, 64–88, 92, 95, 99, 101–2, 105–8, 112–13, 121–8, 130–3, 136–7, 139–44, 146–7, 149–57, 161, 163, 165–6, 172, 175–7, 179–202, 207–8, 214, 216 n.23, 218, 221–3, 228, 230, 234–5, 242, 247, 249–50, 254–85, 288–9, *see also* epidemics, typhus, yellow fever
Ffrith, Dr 271
filararis, *see* elephantiasis
Fitzherbert, William 133, 144
Flemyng, Malcolm 62
flux, *see* dysentery
Fontanges, Dr 188
Fordyce, William 157
Fothergill, John 52–5, 57–8, 63, 131, 215, 216 n.23, 223
Fourcroy, A. F. 267
Fox, The 76
France 2, 3 n.13, 13, 15, 37, 39, 91, 109, 135, 137, 159, 172, 176, 188, 190, 195, 197, 202, 208, 220, 231, 235, 248, 256, 265–6, 280, 282, *see also* Paris medicine
Fryer, John 39–40, 44

Galenic medicine 28, 29, 31–2, 34, 51 n.21, 52 n.23, 59, 121, 272, *see also* humoral system
Galvani, Luigi 70
Gambia, the 208
gaols, *see* jails
Garthshore, Maxwell 268
gases, *see* air, chemistry
Gaudeloupe 109
Ganges, river 91, *see also* Hughly
Geach, Francis 162–3
Geddes, William 197
Geneva 263
George III, king 17, 215
George IV, king 261
Gentleman's Magazine, The 53
Ghazipore 177
Gibney, William 216–17, 220, 225
Gibraltar 13, 15, 19, 238, 268, 275–7, 279
Gillespie, Leonard 154, 187, 245, 290
Glasgow 57, 69, 71, 85, 152, 169, 186, 226, 261
Gloucestershire 140–1, 211–26
Goa 33–5, 38, 122, 123, 137–8
gonorrhoea, *see* venereal disease
Goodeve-Henry Hurry 92, 95–8, 100–1, 198
Gray, Dr 278
Great Britain 1–16, 22, 24, 27–8, 48, 53, 57–8, 61–6, 69–74, 77–9, 89, 91, 97–8, 100, 102, 107, 113, 115, 119, 127–8, 130, 137, 139–42, 145–6, 148–50, 156–9, 161, 166–9, 171–3, 178, 183, 185–6, 190–1, 195–6, 198, 201–3, 207–26, 227–9, 231, 233, 235–585, 287–91
Great Windmill Street Anatomy School 90, 169
Greece 190
Grenada 14, 111, 133, 263
Gujarat 138

Hales, Stephen 60
Halle 135, 137
Haller, Albrecht von 62

Halley, Edmund 44, 60, 74
Hamilton, Robert 156, 288
Hammick, Stephen 162–4
Harness, Dr 278
Harris, James, 1st Earl of Malmesbury, 157, 260
Harrowgate 225
Harvey, William 121
Havana 15, 274, 282
Heat 29–30, 33, 35–8, 40, 43–5, 48, 56–7, 60 n.63, 61–2, 64, 72, 76, 85–6, 92–3, 97–8, 106–7, 110, 112, 114, 122–3, 125, 128, 132, 140–1, 147, 161, 213–14, 215 n.20, 218, 221, 223, 230, 257, 272, 274, 276, *see also* climate, humidity, seasons, tropics
hepatitis 3, 5, 36, 92–3, 101–2, 114, 147, 149, 156–7, 192, 194–5, 214, 216, 221, 229–30, 289, *see also* bile, liver
Herbert, Sir Thomas 37–8
Hillary, William 54–8, 62–3, 70–1, 74–5, 83, 113, 126, 128
Hindus 123, 199 n.154, 231
Hippocratic medicine 4, 30–3, 37–41, 44–6, 48–52, 56, 59–60, 63, 74–5, 81, 113–14, 122, 141, 173, 272
Hobbes, Thomas 39
Holderness, Lord 261
Holland 13, 31–2, 42, *see also* Dutch East Indies, Leiden University, wars
Homer 246
Hooke, Robert 44
hospitals 1–5, 8–9, 11, 18–23, 27, 31, 35 n.45, 37, 42, 52, 53, 54, 57–8, 61, 64–6, 68–9, 72, 77–81, 83–4, 88–90, 97, 100–1, 104–5, 112–13, 119, 122–3, 133–4, 136, 142, 144, 146–8, 150, 152–3, 156, 162–9, 171, 173, 184–5, 187, 189, 193, 198, 202, 224, 256, 263, 267, 274–69, 283, 287–9
  Antigua 21, 218
  Batavia 35 n.45, 37
  Bombay 21–2, 158, 168
  Calcutta 21–3, 100–1, 174, 176, 183, 198–9
  Cheltenham 218
  Demerara 104
  Goa 122–3
  Haslar 18–19, 72, 79, 131, 240, 257, 278
  Isle of Wight 88
  Jamaica 19, 80, 84, 112, 1834
  Liverpool 165
  London 6, 42, 53–4, 57, 61 n.68, 80–1, 91, 105, 133, 165–6, 211, 214, 261
  Madras 21–2, 134, 146–8, 153
  Martinique 171
  Minorca 52
  Newcastle upon Tyne 77, 127, 156 n.51, 247
  Plymouth 18–19, 162–3
  St Domingue 182, 270
  Tangiers 19
  Tranquebar 136
  Trinidad 21
  Windward Islands 279
  Worcester 216
  Yarmouth 278
Houghton, The 176
Howard, John 262 n.35, 266
Howe, Admiral Lord 240
Huck, Dr 68–9, 252
Hugenots 138
Hughly, river 90, 92, 183
Hulme, Nathaniel 240
humidity 49, 69, 72, 87, 132–3, 229–30, *see also* damp, heat
humoral system 1, 30, 33, 37, 39, 44, 47, 52, 62, 68, 96, 98, 108, 122, 139, 141, 146–7, 172, 196, 198, 213–14, 241, *see also* bile, blood,Galenic medicine
humours, *see* humoral system
Hunter, John 83, 94, 112, 257
Hunter, William 261
Huntley, Harry 208, 212
Huxham, John 59–60, 124–5, 128, 132, 256 n.7
hydropathy, *see* Bath, Cheltenham, spas
hygiene 14, 17–18, 20, 66
hypochondriacism 227–9, 231, 233–4, *see also* nervous diseases

iatrochemistry, *see* antimonial drugs, chemistry, mercurial drugs, nitric acid
iatromechanism, *see* mechanical medicine
Iceland 70
impressment 237–8, 240, 242–4, 250–2, 259
improvement 76–7, 250, *see also* agriculture, cultivation
India 4–9, 13, 15–16, 21–3, 27, 29, 33–5, 38–40, 42, 50, 70, 74–7, 83, 89–103, 122–4, 126–7, 132, 134–41, 144, 146–53, 156–61, 165, 167–9, 173–9, 189–203, 207–8, 212–13, 215, 217–18, 220–1, 225–8, 234, 236, 254, 281, 287–9, *see also* East India Company
India Journal of Medical Science 97
Indians 93, 94, 97, 98–100, 101, 102
Indian Ocean 12
Indian practitioners of medicine 22, 96, 97, 101, 123, 124, 134, 136, 147–8, *see also* Ayurveda, Unani Tibb
Indian soldiers 9, 15, 94, 176
Industrialization 61, 209, 236, 237, 240, 245–7, 249, 252–3
inflammation 121, 123, 126–8, 134, 146, 149, 156–7, 176, 187, 189, 190, 193, 195–7, 199–200, 213, 219, 223, 230, 257, 268
Ingham, Dr 78
Ingram, Dale 266
invalids 88, 115, 131, 205–26, 227–36, 254, 257
Ireland 6 n.19, 16, 42, 52, 81 n.84, 90, 91, 185

Jackson, Robert 20, 105–9, 154, 179–88, 190, 192–3, 195, 214, 220, 245, 262, 269–70, 278
Jacobins 163, 176, 178, *see also* radicalism, revolutions
Jade, Prof 137
jails 65–6, 78, 256, 288
Jamaica 13, 14, 19–20, 23 n.107, 41–4, 46, 55, 72, 80, 83–4, 87, 94, 103, 112, 122, 126, 128, 133, 153, 155, 166, 176, 179–80, 183, 187, 270, 272, 278
James, Robert 142–3
  fever powders 142–5, 184, 221
Jameson, Thomas 215–20
jaundice, *see* hepatitis
Java 35–7, 76, 176, *see also* Batavia
Jefferson, Thomas 94 n.17
Jenner, Edward 165
Jodrell, Sir Paul 133, 150
Johnson, James 89–96, 99, 105, 110, 114, 191–5, 201, 203, 227–36, 237, 245, 248, 249, 254, 264, 283
Johnston, Dr 265
Joint Stock Farming Society 250
Jones, William, Sir 159
Jurin, James 59–60, 63

Kames, Lord 94 n.17
Kelso 74, 238
Kent, duke of 222, 275
Kier, James 69
Kingston 84
Knox, Robert 94
Koenig, J. G. 135

Laennec, R. T. H. 2
Lancet, The 194
Lavoisier, Anton 240
Lawrence, J. 196
leeches, *see* bloodletting
Leiden, University of 31, 35 n.45, 37, 42, 54, 124, 126
Lempriere, William 86–8
Lettsom, John Coakley 52 n.23, 131
Levant Company 57, 281
Levant, the 57–8, 137, 254, 262, 281, *see also* Middle East
Lind, James (1716–94) 17, 71–5, 79, 126–7, 131–2, 140–1, 144, 153 n.34, 156–7, 241, 256–7, 264
Lind, James (1736–1812) 69–71, 75–6, 86
Linnaeus (Karl von Linné) 135
Lisbon 150

Lister, S. W. 100
liver, the 92, 93, 101–2, 107, 110, 122–3, 127–8, 146–51, 156–7, 160–1, 165, 190, 192–3, 195, 198–9, 211–12, 218–19, 223, 227–30, 233, 245, *see also* bile, hepatitis, humoral system
Liverpool 165, 186, 238
Liverpool, Lord 178, 265
Locke, John 31
London 2, 6, 28, 42, 47, 50, 53–5, 57–8, 61–2, 65–6, 70, 74, 80–1, 90–3, 95, 100 n.51, 105, 107, 127, 139, 148, 150, 155, 156 n.53, 162, 165–6, 169, 211, 215, 217, 230, 233, 235, 261, 262 n.35, 265, 268, 277–8, 281
  Medical Society 195, 217 n.30 *see also* Royal College of Physicians and Surgeons of, Royal Society of
Lucretius 49
Lunar Society, the 69, 71, 163
luxury, *see* consumerism
Lyssons, Daniel 140–1, 156, 288

M'Cabe, James 107–8, 184–6, 220–2, 224, 234
Mabit, A. 188
MacBride, David 67, 69
Maclean, Allen 177
Maclean, Charles 1, 3, 8, 80, 105, 173–9, 184, 203, 281–4, 289
Madeira 46, 90, 161, 231
Madras 21–2, 69, 76, 90, 93, 96, 138, 146–9, 182–3, 262, 267–8
  Medical Board 95, 134, 196–7
  Medical College 97
  Medical and Physical Society 96
Madrid 281
Malabar coast 136, 147
malingering 244
Malvern, Great 216
Manchester 79
  duke of 260
  Literary and Philosophical Society 263
Manuchi, Dr 135
Marcet, Dr 166
Margate 233
marginality, concept of 11, 113, 196, 234
Martin, James Ranald 91, 201
masculinity 115, 209, 230, 236, 237–53
Mason, Abraham 129
Masulipatam 22
materia medica, *see* medicines
mathematics 47–8, 52 n.22, 69, 81, 124
Maxwell, Francis 152, 207
McGrigor, Sir James 94, 155, 168–70, 179, 185, 220, 222, 226, 249, 259–61, 264, 276, 278–80, 284
Mead, Richard 48, 81
mechanical medicine 27, 31–2, 46, 47–8, 49, 56, 59, 86, 113, 121, 124–5, 128
Medical Museum, The 156
Medical Repository, The 263, 271
medicines 4, 8, 10–12, 22, 34–5, 46, 58, 67, 92, 119, 121–4, 126–7, 130–45, 146–73, 175, 178, 180, 185, 187, 189, 192–3, 196–7, 201, 203, 211–14, 218, 222, 227, 233, 288–90
Medico-Chirurgical Review/Journal, The 90–1, 108, 191, 194, 234, 283
Mediterranean, the 12, 13, 27, 40, 50, 52, 57, 58, 103, 104, 221, 254, 256, 266, 273, 276–7, 279–80, 283–4
Melrose 238
mercurial drugs 92, 126, 134, 140, 146–58, 160–2, 165–8, 172, 175–6, 178, 180–1, 183–4, 187–9, 192–8, 201–3, 211–14, 219–21
meteorology 27, 30, 36, 40, 44–5, 51, 54–6, 58–60, 63, 70, 75, 96, 98, 228, 266, 274
metropole, concept of 10–11, 81, 145, 171, 290–1
miasma 38, 44, 64, 67, 76–7, 93, 98–100, 108, 141, 197, 259, 262–3, 268, 271–2, 274, 276, 282–3
microscopes 70
Middle East, the 50, *see also* Levant, Egypt
military, *see* Army
Millar, John 143
Milman, Francis 84, 119

Minorca 51–3, 57, 70, 81
missionaries 135–7
Mitter, Bysenaut 177
M'Lean, Hector 20–1, 104–5, 106–9, 176, 182–3, 262, 267–8
Modena 60
moisture, *see* damp
Monro, Donald 17
morbid anatomy, *see* pathological anatomy
morbidity rates 15, 18, 23, 30, 35–6, 207–9, 238
Morehead, Charles 97, 287
Morison, James 196, 213
monsoons 39, 40
morality 53, 55, 98, 102, 109, 112, 115, 266 n.51
mordechi 34
mortality rates 13, 15–17, 23, 35–6, 80, 84, 112, 207–9, 238, 268
Mortimer, W. 197, 212
Morton, Richard 121, 132, 143
Moseley, Benjamin 19–20, 80–5, 128, 133–4, 176, 193, 257–8
Mughals, the 34, 124, 138
Mulgrave, Baron 81 n.84
Munro, Alexander 21, 52
Murchison, Kenneth 76
Muslims 123, 154, 176, 199

Napoleon I 178, 190
Native Medical Institution 97
natural history 7, 8, 12, 25–120, 47–63, 64–88, 113–14, 135–7, 255, 263, 285
natural philosophy 6, 28–9, 31, 37, 42, 44, 47, 60, 66, 69–71, 77, 136, 176, 215, 240, 267
Navy, *see* Royal Navy
Neale, Adam 222–5
nervous system 62, 84 n.100, 85–8, 93, 95–6, 98, 101–2, 106–8, 110, 113–15, 140, 157, 172, 175, 180–1, 186, 188–99, 202, 227, 268
nervous diseases 85, 115–16, 209, 213–14, 220, 225, 228, 233–6, 240–53
networks 7, 11–12, 51–61, 63, 71–2, 254, 290–1
Nevis 46
Newcastle upon Tyne 77–9, 127, 156, 288
  Literary and Philosophical Society 77, 240, 247
Newfoundland 20
Newtonianism 7, 47–8, 59, 81, 86, *see also* mechanical medicine
New York 263–4
Nicaragua 84
Niger, river 212
Nitric acid 138–71, 197, 202–14, 220, 290
Non-naturals 34, 38, 49
Norfolk 156–7
Northumberland, The 176
nosography 29, 30, 37, 65, 68, 75, 81, 114
Nova Scotia 90, 100 n.51

O'Halloran, Thomas 279–82
Oliver, William 47, 139
Oonore 80
opium 173, 175, 189, 192–3, 196–7, 201–2, 203 n.167
ophthalmia 8, 254
orientalism 97, 150, 196 n.133
Orme, Robert 99
O'Shaughnessy, William 96–7
Ovington, John 138–9
Oxford, University of 5–6, 41, 61 n.68, 69, 140, 264

Padua 60
Paracelsian medicine 128, 142, 146, *see also* chemistry
Paris medicine 1–4, 9, 65, 80, 89, 91–3, 96, 112 n.119, 190, 203, 213, 289
Parliament 29, 41–2, 284
particulate theories 30–1, 40, 46–7, 86, 128
Pasley, Gilbert 69, 147–8, 150–1
pathology 2, 11, 37, 89–115, 119, 121, 169, 184–5, 189, 196, 257

pathological anatomy 4–6, 9, 23, 27, 35, 37, 50, 52, 64–5, 68, 75, 84, 89–115, 168–9, 172, 185, 190–1, 230, 288–90
patronage 72, 151, 169, 171, 260, 264, 275, 280 n.120, 291
Pearson, John 166–8
Peel, Sir Robert 285
Pelling, Margaret 98
Penang 189
periphery, concept of 10–11, 17, 290–1
Persia 38–9, 138
perspiration 47, 49, 62, 93–4, 139, 141, 144, 193, 228–9, 231
Pettelier, P. J. 197
Philadelphia 53, 57, 94 n.17, 155, 183, 254, 258, 262–3, 267
Philosophical Transactions of the Royal Society of London 54, 63, 66, 70
physicians 5–6, 13–14, 20, 27–8, 47–8, 50–5, 57–63, 66–8, 70–2, 77–81, 87, 90–1, 93, 95, 98, 102–3, 105, 109, 114, 119, 121–6, 128, 130, 132–3, 135–6, 138–40, 142–3, 145, 148–50, 152–4, 156–7, 160, 162, 164–8, 173, 178, 185–90, 192, 195, 200–1, 211–12, 214–16, 220–3, 225–8, 231, 234, 255–7, 260–2, 264–5, 268–70, 272–5, 277–8, 287–90, *see also* Royal Colleges of
physiology 62, 86–7, 89–115, 119, 121, 172, 187–92, 195–6, 198, 202, 213–14, 217 n.30, 236
Pinckard, George 14, 104, 110, 179, 183 n.62, 187, 262
Piso, Willem 48, 50 n.16
Pitcairn, William 58
Pitcairne, Archibald 124
Pitt, William (the younger) 252, 260, 265, 278
plague 30, 36, 40, 44, 50, 56–8, 85, 94, 102, 123, 129, 138, 146, 155, 166, 174, 208, 254–6, 260–2, 264–6, 271, 273, 276, 281, 284
plantations 5, 8–9, 13–14, 21, 48, 50, 119, 154, 263
pleurisy 153
Pneumatic Institute 163, 165, 167, *see also* Beddoes, Thomas, chemistry, Davy, Humphry, nitric acid
Pope, Henry 192
Port au Prince 182, 188
Port Royal 19, 42
Portsmouth 265–6
Portuguese settlements 34–5, 38, 122–3, 138, *see also* Daman, Diu, Goa
Powell, Charles 107
Priestley, Joseph 59, 66–7, 71, 159, 240
Prince of Wales, the 261
Pringle, Sir John 58 n.48, 61, 65–9, 74, 77, 126, 131, 142, 149 n.14, 156, 159, 191, 198, 240–1, 257 n.9, 258, 262 n.35
Privy Council, the 277–9
Protestantism 6 n.18, 135, 137, 234, *see also* Dissent *and individual denominations*
providence 39, 42–3, 46, 76, 93
Purhcas, Samuel 41
purgation 121–2, 127–8, 130–1, 133, 140, 143–4, 146, 149–51, 154–5, 157, 211, 213–16, 218–20
putrefaction 32, 36–7, 39, 44, 50, 52, 56, 58, 62, 64–72, 74–7, 80, 83–98, 107–8, 125, 127–8, 130–1, 146, 149, 153, 161, 172, 185, 198, 203, 241, 256–7, 262, 266, 271–2
Pym, William 105–6, 273, 275–9, 284

Quakers 42, 52 n.22, 53–5
quarantine 9, 105, 174, 178, 255–6, 260–7, 270–1, 273–8, 280–5, 290
Quier, John 154
quinine 197, 200–1

Race 45–6, 49, 83, 87, 89–115, 198–9, 202–3, 208–9, 249, 287, *see also* constitutions, degeneration
rainfall 76–7, 126, 131, *see also* monsoon, climates, seasons
Ramazzini, Bernadino 40, 60, 81
Ramsbottom, Dr 166

Rangoon 90
reform 1–6, 28, 30–1, 52–4, 57–8, 62 n.68, 71, 80–1, 91, 105, 136, 139, 150, 178, 234, 260, 264, 269–70, 272–3, 275–81, 290, *see also* Dissent, radicalism
regimen 38, 44, 74, 121, 139, 149, 162, 196, 219, 222, 230, *see also* diet
regiments, *see* Army
Register, The 225
Renaissance, the 30
Renny, Robert 14, 187 n.83
Republic of Letters 11
Restoration, the 42, *see also* Charles II
revolutions
  American 158, 208
  French 65, 70, 163, 208, 255, 260
Richerand, Dr 190
Richmond, duke of 260–1
Rider, Jacob 177
Ripon 54
Robertson, James 186–7
Robertson, Robert 134, 262
Rodney, Lord 157, 201
Romanticism 7, 88, 114, 208, 233 n.25, 240
Roman Catholics 43, 130, 135 n.34, 178, 266
Ross, Patrick 22
Rouppe, Lois L. 83
Roxburgh, William 135–7
Roxburghshire 74, 238
Royal College of Physicians of Edinburgh 70–1, 228, 268
Royal College of Physicians of London 2, 5–6, 28, 30–2, 52–4, 57–8, 62 n.68, 71, 80–1, 91, 105, 136, 139, 150, 178, 234, 260, 264, 269–70, 272–3, 275–8, 290
Royal College of Surgeons of London 54
Royal Medical Society of Edinburgh 216 n.25
Royal Ordnance 164
Royal Navy 1, 3, 5, 6 n.19, 14, 16–19, 21, 31, 35, 50–1, 54, 60, 64–7, 69, 71–2, 78–80, 81 n.84, 85, 90–2, 94, 103, 105, 112–13, 119–20, 150, 154, 156–7, 160, 162–4, 171–3, 184–7, 190–1, 202, 216, 227, 234, 237–3, 259, 261, 264–5, 269, 271, 283–5
Royal Society of London 10, 39–41, 44–5, 47, 54, 59–60, 63, 66–7, 70–1, 95, 113, 139, 150, 160, 162, 171, 240, 250, 263
Royal William, The 238
Rudling, John 22
Rusnock, Andrea 59
Russell, Alexander 57–8, 131, 262
Russell, Patrick 134, 262
Russell, William 101
Rush, Benjamin 155, 183, 203, 262–3, 267–8, 271, 273, 282
Ryan, Dr 214

Salisbury 62
salts 126, 143, 192, 211, 215–16, 221, 223–4, *see also* chemistry, spas
Samalkot 135–6
San Juan 84
Sanskrit 123–4
Saunders, William 93, 157, 211, 288
Savannah 153
Schwartz, Christian 134
science 69–70, 96–8, 105, 119, 134–5, 137, 158–9, 164, 171, 238, 250, 263, 280, 291, *see also* chemistry, experimental method, mechanical medicine, natural philosophy
Scotland 6, 11, 42, 53, 58 n.51, 62, 74, 85–6, 250, 261, *see also* Aberdeen University, Edinburgh, Glasgow, St Andrews
Scott, Helenus 158–71, 202, 214, 220, 290
scurvy 44, 66–7, 69, 71, 84 n.100, 131, 175, 238, 240–1, 243
seasoning 46, 49, 57, 64, 108–9, 112, 207, 268
seasons 33–4, 38–9, 45–6, 51, 55–7, 61, 76, 122–3, 126, 131, 200, 219, 221, 224–5, 246, 273, 276

Senegal 126
sensibility 114–15, 183, 188, 230, 233, 251, *see also* nervous system
sepoys, *see* Indian soldiers
Seville 188
sexes 32, 43, 72, 83, 209, 219
sexual intercourse 38, 43, 87
Shelley, Mary 70
Shelley, Percy Bysshe 70
Short, Dr 215
sickness *see* morbidity rates
Siddha 147
Sierra Leone 282–3
Silvester, Dr 148
Sinclair, Catherine 225
Sinclair, Sir John 249–50
Skillicorn, Nash 214
Slare, Frederick 139
slavery 5, 9–10, 111, 208, 237–8, 248–9, 251–2, 254, 271, *see also* Africa, Caribbean, West Indies
  slaves 5, 9, 13–14, 49–50, 55, 58 n.49, 110, 154, 160, 192, 199, 211, 214, 218, 219, 228, 230, 233, *see also* Africans, constitutions, race
Sloane, Sir Hans 46, 48, 51
smallpox 14, 44, 55–6, 77, 165, 178
Smith, John 178
Smith, Richard 208
Society of Collegiate Physicians 58
Society of Naval Surgeons 51
Southampton 266
Spain 13, 34 n.34, 37, 43, 103–4, 188, 190, 273–6, 279–82
Spit Head, mutiny at 251
St Andrews University 77
St Christophers 46, 109
St Domingue 15, 103, 109, 153–4, 180–2, 186, 207, 262, 265, 267–70, 273, 275
St Vincent 271
Stanhope-Smith, Samuel 94, 112
Stepan, Nancy 111
stimulants 173, 175–6, 184, 193, 196, 214, 233, *see also* medicines, tonics
Stock Exchange, the 234, 248
stomach, the 102, 104, 106–7, 126, 130, 139, 141, 144, 154, 160, 192, 199, 211, 214, 218–19, 228, 230, 233
Strasbourg 137
Strotter, Edward 47–8, 124
Stuart, J. 144
Stubbe, Henry 41, 63, 122
sublime, the 87–8
sugar 43, 48, 50, 231
surgeons 2, 5, 8, 13–14, 18, 22–3, 27–8, 31, 34 n.34, 35–7, 42, 50–1, 52 n.22, 53–4, 60, 64–5, 68–71, 74–6, 79–81, 84, 86–7, 89–91, 95–5, 100–1, 103–5, 107, 113, 121–3, 126–7, 132–3, 135, 137–8, 142, 144–8, 150–7, 162–6, 169, 171, 174, 176, 179, 182–6, 189, 191, 195–6, 198, 203, 207, 212, 216–17, 220, 224–7, 234, 238, 240–1, 243–5, 247, 254–7, 260–3, 266–9, 271, 273–5, 278–9, 283, 287–90
Swietenia febrifuga 136–7
Switzerland 171, 235, 263
Sydenham, Thomas 4, 28–33, 40, 47–50, 52, 59–60, 63, 68, 75, 81, 114, 124, 127, 130, 142, 181, 272
symptoms 30, 36–7, 65, 67, 75, 78, 85, 90, 106–7, 110–11, 122, 131, 141, 143, 153–4, 161, 165–6, 169, 172, 180–1, 182, 186, 192–3, 197–200, 229–30, 257, 267, 272
sympathetic action 93–4, 115, 227–8, 231
syphilis, *see* venereal disease

Tait, Dr 278
Tanjore Pill 112, 134–5, 137
Tangiers 19
Tavernier, J.-B. 138
Telegraph, The 177
Tewkesbury 216
therapeutics 2–5, 8, 12–14, 23, 27, 32, 34, 51, 54–8, 62 n.68, 65, 67–8, 71–2, 79, 88, 95, 99, 101, 104, 107, 108, 110, 114, 117–29, 130–45, 146–71, 172–203, 211–26, 227–36, 240, 257, 288–90, *see also* medicines

Thompson, E. P. 42
Thompson, Frederick 18
Thompson, Henry 215, 224
Thomson, James 110–1
Thomson, John 169
Thurston, John 109
Times, The 283
Tipu Sultan 80, 176
Tissot, S. A. A. D. 237
Tobago 186
tonics 88, 121, 192, 194, 197, 212, 227, 233
Tories 48, 59, 61, 234, 260
Torrid Zone, the 56, 63, 287, *see also* tropics, climates, heat
Towne, Richard 48–50, 83, 125, 128
Towns, Thomas 45
trade, *see* commerce
Trapham, Thomas
 (the elder) 42
 (the younger) 41–44, 50, 63, 83, 122, 214
Tranquebar 135–7
Transactions of the Medical and Physical Society of Bombay 287
treatment, *see* therapeutics
trials 2, 3, 58, 88, 119, 130, 133–7, 152, 156, 161–9, 171, 176, 181, 186, 189–90, 197, 203
Trinidad 21
Tropics, the 3–5, 8–10, 13–16, 19, 23, 27, 29, 33–4, 37–8, 41, 43–4, 46–64, 67, 69, 72, 74–5, 77, 84, 86, 88–9, 91–3, 98, 99 n.44, 105, 107–8, 110, 112, 114–15, 119, 122, 125–6, 128, 130–4, 136, 138, 140, 142, 144–5, 146, 148, 150–1, 154–7, 171–2, 178, 180, 184–6, 190–1, 192, 201–3, 207–9, 211–14, 218–24, 227–31, 233, 235–7, 240, 247, 249, 253, 256–9, 264, 266, 268, 287–91
Trotter, Thomas 157, 164, 237–53, 290
Turing, Robert 21
Turner, John 101
Twining, William 100–1, 108, 110
typhus 66, 241, 242–3, *see also* epidemics, fevers, contagion
Tytler, John 135

urbanization 61, 65, 77, 209, 227, 235
Unitarians 66, 74–7
Unani Tibb 97, 139, 147
Urquhart, Thomas 251–2
USA, *see* America, North

Vage, T. 167–8
valetudinarians, *see* invalids
Valiant, The 91
Van Helmont, J. B. 129, 142
Van Linschoten, Jan Huyghen 123
Van Swieten, Gerhard 143
vascular system 48–9, 99, 112, 181, see also blood, circulation, physiology
vegetables 196, 199 n.154, 213, 220, 231, *see also* diet
vegetation 64, 68, 98, 180, 259, 279, *see also* miasma
Vera Cruz 274
Vernon, Admiral Edward 19
venereal disease 43, 58, 71, 146, 147, 149, 162–71
venesection, *see* bloodletting
Vengeance, HMS 238
ventilation 18, 69, 78, 217, 230, 242, 262, 283
Venus, transit of 70
Vienna 2, 65, 68, 143
Virginia 45, 94 n.94, 122 n.7
Vizagapatam 134
vomits, *see* emetics
Von Humboldt, Alexander 114

Wade, Charles 150
Wade, John P. 150–1, 175–6
Wahrman, Dror 208
Wakefield 166
Wakley, Thomas 194
Walcheren 80, 88 n.115, 91, 185, 230
Warner, John Harley 203
Warren, Henry 50, 56, 125–6

wars 3, 7, 10, 12, 16–19, 27, 42, 64, 66, 68, 74, 81, 84, 135, 137, 143, 159, 237, 238, 246, 251–2, 254–5, 289–91
American (1812) 238, 251
American Independence 13, 15, 18, 20, 81 n.84, 84, 128, 157–8, 179, 238, 257
Anglo-Dutch 13
Austrian Succession 13, 16, 66, 81
English Civil 42
French Revolutionary 13, 15, 80, 88, 91, 103, 115, 159, 185, 230, 237–8, 240–3, 244, 251, 258, 260 n.23, 265, 269, 284, 290
Napoleonic 7–8, 90, 103, 115, 169 n.111, 220, 222, 224, 237, 244, 248, 265–6, 269, 274, 283 n.132, 284, 290
Seven Years 13, 16–17, 64, 68, 74, 256–7
Spanish Succession 13
Washington, George 158
Watson, Alexander 191
Watt, Dr James 191
Watt, James Jr. 69–70, 163–4
weather, *see* meteorology, seasons
Wellesley, Arthur, Duke of Wellington 168, 260, 264
Wellesley, R. C 176–8
West Indies 1, 3–5, 7, 12–16, 19–21, 23, 27, 33, 40–6, 48–9, 51, 54–5, 58 n.48., 63–5, 68, 71–2, 81, 83–7, 88 n.115, 103–12, 113–15, 119, 122, 126–9, 131–2, 134, 141, 143–4, 153–5, 157, 165, 171–3, 175–6, 179–84, 189, 191, 193–4, 201, 203, 207, 212–14, 217–18, 221, 238, 240, 248, 254–85, 287–91
Whytt, Robert 62, 140
Wight, Isle of 87–8
Wilkes, John 58
William IV, king 91, 178
William Pitt, HMS 174 n.41, 176
Williamson, Captain 192
Willis, Thomas 29 n.4, 32, 47, 122
Wilson, James 21
Wilson, John 147–8
Windsor 70, 75, 157
Wise, T. A. 196 n.132
women 72, 83, 108, 221, 230, 242, 247, *see also* sexes
Wright, William 133, 153, 264, 268–70
Wujastyk, Dominick 123–4
Wurzer, Professor 168
Wyndham, Charles 195

Yates, William 14–6, 179
yaws 14, 43
yellow fever 15, 27, 44, 56, 58 n.48, 68–9, 87, 103–9, 111, 126, 128, 129 n.48, 133, 143–4, 153–5, 165, 180, 183–8, 207–8, 221, 254–85, *see also* contagion, epidemics, fevers
York, duke of 81, 222 n.52; 264
Yorkshire 53–5

Zealand 80, *see also* Walcheren